THE QUALITY OF LIFE
OF CANCER PATIENTS

Monograph Series of the European
Organization for Research and Treatment of Cancer
Volume 17

MONOGRAPH SERIES OF THE
EUROPEAN ORGANIZATION FOR RESEARCH
AND TREATMENT OF CANCER

The Monograph Series of the EORTC deals with selected topics related to cancer treatment. Volumes are usually, but not necessarily, based on the proceedings of an EORTC symposium. The responsibility of the Editorial Advisory Board is to approve the subject of each monograph; the Board does not review individual manuscripts.

The Quality of Life of Cancer Patients

Monograph Series of the
European Organization for Research and
Treatment of Cancer
Volume 17

Chief Editors

Neil K. Aaronson, Ph.D.
The Netherlands Cancer Institute
Plesmanlaan 121
1066 CX Amsterdam, The
Netherlands

Joern H. Beckmann, Ph.D.
Department of Clinical Psychology
Odense University Hospital
Kloevervaenget 18
DK–5000 Odense C, Denmark

Associate Editors

Jan L. Bernheim, M.D., Ph.D.,
F.A.C.P.
Institut Médical Edith Cavell
32 Edith Cavell Street
1180 Brussels, Belgium

Robert Zittoun, M.D.
Department of Hematology
Hotel—Dieu de Paris
1, Place du Parvis Notre Dame
75181 Paris Cedex 04, France

Raven Press   New York

Raven Press, 1185 Avenue of the Americas, New York, New York 10036

Made in the United States of America

The material contained in this volume was submitted as previously unpublished material, except in the instances in which credit has been given to the source from which some of the illustrative material was derived.

Great care has been taken to maintain the accuracy of the information contained in the volume. However, Raven Press cannot be held responsible for errors or for any consequences arising from the use of the information contained herein.

Materials appearing in this book prepared by individuals as part of their official duties as U.S. Government employees are not covered by the above-mentioned copyright.

Library of Congress Cataloging-in-Publication Data

Quality of life of the cancer patient.

(Monograph series of the European Organization for Research on Treatment of Cancer; v. 17)
First publication of the EORTC Study Group on Quality of Life.
Includes index.
1. Cancer—Psychological aspects. 2. Cancer—Social aspects. 3. Quality of life. I. Aaronson, Neil K. II. Beckmann, J. III. EORTC Study Group on Quality of Life. IV. Series. [DNLM: 1. Attitude to Health. 2. Neoplasms—psychology. 3. Quality of Life. W1 M0559U v.17 / 0Z 200 Q116]
RC262.Q35 1987   616.99'406   86–31538
ISBN 0–88167–272–6

9 8 7 6 5 4 3 2 1

Preface

The EORTC monograph series has, to date, been devoted primarily to the documentation of advances in the medical treatment of cancer and to discussions of the interdisciplinary scientific and methodological problems in cancer research. While the psychosocial impact of cancer and its treatment has been touched on in earlier EORTC publications, it is both timely and appropriate to dedicate a volume in this series to an in-depth exploration of the conceptual, methodological, and substantive issues in quality of life research in cancer.

The quality of life of patients has always played a role, albeit often an implicit one, in the therapeutic objectives in oncology. While the evaluation of cancer treatments is focused primarily on biological outcomes (e.g., tumor response and disease-free and overall survival), judgments regarding therapeutic success also require consideration of the functional, psychological, and social burden associated with both conventional and experimental treatments. Yet, it is only in recent years that serious efforts have been mounted to provide a scientific structure for quality of life research in oncology. The development of such a structure, with both theoretical and methodological underpinnings, is essential if psychosocial research is to find a legitimate home in the oncology community.

Scientific advancement in the field of psychosocial oncology requires collaboration among many disciplines. Medical ethicists and social philosophers must grapple with the definition of quality of life and the role of individual, community, and cultural values in such a definition. Physicians, psychologists, social workers, and others involved in the care of cancer patients are needed to direct our discussions toward those specific domains of quality of life that are most relevant to the evaluation of cancer therapies. Finally, psychometricians, statisticians, and other research methodologists provide the technical expertise necessary to assure that both quantitative and qualitative research findings can weather the storms of scientific scrutiny.

The EORTC Study Group on Quality of Life was created in 1980 in response to an expressed need for collaborative efforts between physicians and behavioral scientists working in the cancer field in Europe. It is organized around a number of subgroups, each of which focuses on a particular aspect of research and clinical practice. Thus, there are subgroups concerned with conceptual issues in quality of life research, assessment of quality of life in adult cancer patients, psychotherapeutic interventions and psychosocial support, quality of life issues in childhood cancer, and terminal care. By means of annual conferences and informal contacts, the study group provides a forum for the exchange of ideas among European researchers interested in undertaking cross-cultural, cooperative research in psychosocial oncology. Of equal importance is its role as advisor to the clinical research groups of the EORTC with regard to the integration of quality of life issues in the objectives and evaluation of clinical trials.

This monograph represents the first major external publication of the EORTC Study Group on Quality of Life. To a great extent, the organization of the volume reflects the structure of the study group itself. Thus, there are major sections devoted to (1) conceptual views on quality of life; (2) methodological and measurement issues in quality of life research; (3) quality of life in pediatric oncology; (4) quality of life in adult oncology; and (5) quality of life of the terminally ill patient. A final section covers additional selected topics, including the role of patient self-help groups in oncology, the use of nonconventional therapies among cancer populations, and the doctor-patient relationship in oncology.

The contributors to this monograph also reflect the diversity of professional backgrounds, philosophical orientations, and research approaches found within the study group membership. Broadly speaking, two major paradigms are represented. First, there are those whose approach to the study of quality of life in cancer is holistic, inductive, and naturalistic. Those working within this tradition strive to provide, through the use of qualitative research approaches, an in-depth, detailed description of the world of the cancer patient. Second, there are those who follow the natural science paradigm of hypothetico-deductive methodology. Here, the emphasis is on quantitative measurement, experimental design, and formal statistical analysis.

Coexistence of these two scientific paradigms within the study group, combined with the mix of nationalities and cultures, has led to confrontation, debate, and dispute. While the clash of perspectives has sometimes been intense, it has also proved to be lively, fruitful, and creative. The principal lesson derived from these exchanges has been that neither scientific paradigm is intrinsically better than the other. Thus, in this volume we have attempted to give voice to both perspectives in the belief that they represent viable alternatives from which we can draw in formulating relevant research questions and in choosing research methodologies appropriate to answering those questions. At the same time, we have allowed ample room for expression of the many controversies that still surround the young science of psychosocial oncology.

NEIL K. AARONSON
JOERN H. BECKMAN
JAN L. BERNHEIM
ROBERT ZITTOUN

Acknowledgments

The editors would like to express their sincere appreciation to Birgitte Edlefsen for her skillful administrative assistance in the preparation of this monograph. The editorship of Dr. Neil K. Aaronson was supported by an EORTC research fellowship granted by the Koningin Wilhelmina Fonds, (The Netherlands Cancer Foundation).

Contents

Contributors

Neil K. Aaronson, Ph.D.
The Netherlands Cancer Institute
Plesmanlaan 121
1066 CX Amsterdam, The Netherlands

Willem Bakker, M.D., Ph.D.
Department of Pulmonology
University Hospital
Rijnsburgerweg 10
2333 AA Leiden, The Netherlands

Hans J. F. Baltrusch, M.D.
International Psychooncology Project
Bergstrasse 10
2900 Oldenburg
Federal Republic of Germany

Joern H. Beckmann, Ph.D.
Department of Clinical Psychology
Odense University Hospital
Kloevervaenget 18
DK–5000 Odense C, Denmark

**Jan L. Bernheim, M.D., Ph.D.,
F.A.C.P.**
Institut Médical Edith Cavell
32 Edith Cavell Street
1180 Brussels, Belgium

Sidney Bindemann, Ph.D.
Department of Clinical Oncology
Gartnavel General Hospital
University of Glasgow
1053 Western Road
GB–6B Glasgow G12 OYN
Scotland

H. W. van den Borne, Ph.D.
IVA, Institute for Social Research
University of Tilburg
Hogeschoollan 225
5000 LE Tilburg, The Netherlands

Gerjanne Bos, M.A.
Department of Obstetrics and Gynecology
University Hospital
Rijnsburgerweg 10
2333 AA Leiden, The Netherlands

Diana D. Bransfield, Ph.D.
Division of Cancer Prevention and Control
National Cancer Institute
Blair Building, Rm. 4A01
Bethesda, Maryland 20205

Pim Brouwers, Ph.D.
National Institutes of Health
Clinical Center—Room 4C110
Bethesda, Maryland 20892

Peter F. Bruning, M.D., Ph.D.
The Netherlands Cancer Institute
Plesmanlaan 121
1066 CX Amsterdam, The Netherlands

M. E. L. van der Burg, M.D.
Rotterdam Radiotherapy Institute
Groene Hilledijk 297
P.O. Box 5201
3008 AE Rotterdam, The Netherlands

Jeanette M. V. Burgers, M.D., Ph.D.
The Netherlands Cancer Institute
Plesmanlaan 121
1066 CX Amsterdam, The Netherlands

**Kenneth C. Calman, M.D., Ph.D.,
F.R.C.P., F.R.C.S.**
Dean of Postgraduate Medicine
University of Glasgow
Glasgow G12 8QQ, Scotland

Frits S. A. M. van Dam, Ph.D.
The Netherlands Cancer Institute
Plesmanlaan 121
1066 CX Amsterdam, The Netherlands

Gert Ditlev, M.A.
Institute of Philosophy
Odense University
5000 Odense C, Denmark

Peter M. Fayers
Medical Research Council
Tuberculosis and Chest Disease Unit
Brompton Hospital
Fulham Road
London SW3 6HP, England

Loma Feigenberg, M.D.
Karolinska Sjukhuset
Box 60500
10401 Stockholm, Sweden

Jacqueline Fournier
Centre Hospitalier Regional de Besancon
25030 Besancon Cedex, France

Johanna C. J. M. de Haes, M.S.
Institute of Social Medicine
University of Leiden
Wassenaarseweg 62
2333 AL Leiden, The Netherlands

Els Hamersma, M.S.
The Netherlands Cancer Institute
Plesmanlaan 121
1066 CX Amsterdam, The Netherlands

Gerrit J. F. P. Hanewald, M.S.
Department of Clinical Psychology
University of Amsterdam
Weesperplein 8
1018 XA Amsterdam, The Netherlands

Augustinus A. M. Hart, M.S.
The Netherlands Cancer Institute
Plesmanlaan 121
1066 CX Amsterdam, The Netherlands

Rudolphus J. J. Hermus, Ph.D.
The Institute Civo-Toxicology and Nutrition
TNO
P.O. Box 306
3700 AJ Ziest, The Netherlands

Richard Hillier, M.D.
Countess Mountbatten House
Southampton University Hospitals
Botley Road, West End
Southampton SO3 3JB, England

Sjouke J. Huisman, M.S.
The Netherlands Cancer Institute
Plesmanlaan 121
1066 CX Amsterdam, The Netherlands

David R. Jones, Ph.D.
Clinical Epidemiology and Social Medicine
St. Georges Hospital Medical School
Cranmer Terrace
London SW17 ORE, England

Robert P. Kamphuis, Ph.D.
Department of Pediatrics
University Hospital
Rijnsburgerweg 10
2333 AA Leiden, The Netherlands

Anne Kirkpatrick, M.A.
EORTC Data Center
Boulevard de Waterloo 125
1000 Brussels, Belgium

Everdina H. Klein Poelhuis, M.A.
The Netherlands Cancer Institute
Plesmanlaan 121
1066 CX Amsterdam, The Netherlands

Ferdinand C. E. van Knippenberg, M.S.
Department of Medical Psychology
Medical Faculty
Erasmus University
P.O. Box 1738
3000 DR Rotterdam, The Netherlands

Bob F. Last, M.A.
Children's Oncology Center
Emma Children's Hospital
Spinozastraat 51
1018 HJ Amsterdam, The Netherlands

Ghislain Ledure, M.D.
University Hospital St. Pierre
298 Rue Haute
1000 Brussels, Belgium

Jillian R. Mann, M.D.
Birmingham Children's Hospital
Ladywood Middleway
Birmingham B16 8ET, England

Eric Monpetit, M.D.
Centre Hospitalier Regional de Besancon
25030 Besancon Cedex, France

Tina Morris
Faith Courtauld Unit
The Rayne Institute
123 Coldharbour Lane
London SE5 9NU, England

J. P. Neijt, Ph.D.
Department of Internal Medicine
University Hospital
Catharijnesingel 101
3511 GU Utrecht, The Netherlands

Terrence J. Priestman, M.D., F.R.C.P.,
F.R.C.R.
Department of Radiotherapy
Queen Elizabeth Hospital
Birmingham B15 2TH, England

Jean F. A. Pruyn, Ph.D.
IVA, Institute for Social Research
University of Tilburg
Hogeschoollan 225
5000 LE Tilburg, The Netherlands

J. W. Raatgever, M.S.
Institute of Biostatistics
Erasmus University
P.O. Box 1738
3000 DR Rotterdam, The Netherlands

Darius Razavi, M.D.
Institut Jules Bordet
Tumor Center
University of Brussels
Rue Heger-Bordet 1
1000 Brussels, Belgium

Norman Sartorius, M.D., Ph.D.,
D.P.M., F.R.C. Psych.
Director, Division of Mental Health
The World Health Organization
1211 Geneva 27, Switzerland

Simon Schraub, M.D.
Centre Hospitalier Regional de Besancon
Boulevard Fleming
25030 Besancon Cedex, France

Jean Simons
Department of Social Work
The Hospital for Sick Children
Great Ormond Street
London WC1N 3JH, England

Michel Souris, M.D.
University Hospital St. Pierre
298 Rue Haute
1000 Brussels, Belgium

Anita L. Stewart, Ph.D.
The Rand Corporation
1700 Main Street
Santa Monica, California 90406

Anne M. H. van Veldhuizen, M.A.
Children's Oncology Centre
Emma Children's Hospital
Spinozastraat 51
1018 HJ Amsterdam, The Netherlands

E. Millard Waltz, Ph.D.
International Psychooncology Project
Bergstrasse 10
2900 Oldeburg
Federal Republic of Germany

John R. Yarnold, M.D.
Institute of Cancer Research
The Royal Marsden Hospital
Downs Road, Sutton
Surrey SM2 5PT, England

Nico van Zandwijk, M.D., Ph.D.
The Netherlands Cancer Institute
Plesmanlaan 121
1066 CX Amsterdam, The Netherlands

Robert Zittoun, M.D.
Department of Hematology
Hotel-Dieu de Paris
1, Place du Parvis Notre Dame
75181 Paris Cedex 04, France

The Quality of Life of Cancer Patients,
edited by N. K. Aaronson and J. Beckmann,
Raven Press, New York © 1987.

Definitions and Dimensions of Quality of Life

Kenneth C. Calman

Department of Oncology, University of Glasgow, Glasgow G12 9LY, Scotland

As an idea or a concept, the term "quality of life" is widespread, yet it is surprising how infrequently it is defined, as pointed out by Van Dam et al. (20). In a personal review of more than 250 references mentioning quality of life in the title, only a very small number gave any kind of definition as to what was meant by the phrase. This fact was also recognized by Aristotle (2) when he said:

> . . . when it comes to saying in what happiness consists, opinions differ, and the account given by the generality of mankind is not at all like that of the wise. The former take it to be something obvious and familiar, like pleasure or money or eminence, and there are various other views, and often the same person actually changes his opinion. When he falls ill he says that it is his health, and when he is hard up he says that it is money.

Clearly, quality of life means different things to different people, reflecting their own particular point of view. This chapter looks at some of the definitions that have been used and reviews some of the dimensions of quality of life. On some occasions the concepts have been paraphrased to make the ideas, often presented in book form, more succinct.

DEFINITIONS

The following definitions have been culled from the literature, and it is hoped that they reflect the breadth, depth, and diversity of the subject. The earliest comes again from Aristotle's "Ethics" (2):

> What is happiness? If we consider what the function of man is, we find that happiness is a virtuous activity of the soul. . . . Is happiness something that can be learnt, or acquired by habituation, or cultivated in some other way, or does it come to us by some form of divine dispensation, or even by chance? . . . Happiness demands not only complete goodness but a complete life. In the course of life we encounter many reverses and all kinds of vicissitudes . . . nobody calls a man happy who suffered fortunes like this and met a miserable end.

It highlights the importance of the complete life, as does the description by Oliver Wendell Holmes (10):

> The longer I live the more I am satisfied of two things. First that the truest lives are those that are cut rose-diamond fashion, with many facets. Second that society is always trying in some way or another to grind us down to a single flat surface.

Here the importance of how we view an individual is emphasized.

The World Health Organization's (22) definition of health as being "a state of complete physical, mental and social well being and not merely the absence of disease" makes the point of the wholeness of life and the relevance of the social component. This subject is also taken up by Burt et al. (3):

> An individual's evaluation of his or her quality of life derives from the level of consumption of socially valued goods and services relative to social norms. The extent to which an individual feels he has the power to determine his individual well-being within society.

Kaplan et al. (12) made a similar point:

> Levels of well-being are the weight, social preferences or measures of relative importance that members of society associate with each of the function levels and symptom/problem complexes.

Other definitions, given below, relate more to "happiness" and "satisfaction" as being the important feature, and several acknowledge that there is a spiritual dimension and an area of personal growth.

> The secrets of well-being include having meaning and direction of life, having experienced problems and overcome them, using failure constructively, having already attained several long term goals, being pleased with personal growth and development, being in love, having friends, being cheerful, having no major fears, being neither thick skinned nor too sensitive to criticism [18].

> Obtaining the necessary conditions for happiness [14].

> Happy are those who hear the word of God and obey it [Gospel according to St. Luke].

> Perhaps [quality of life] lies in creative fulfillment. It must surely relate to freedom and maintenance of the dignity of each of us to choose his own path through life and develop it fully [9].

> Global satisfaction in several life domains. The attributes of specific domains related to satisfaction [1,5].

> Living the authentic self, living in harmony with nature, living at peace with God, living in the fulfillment of our children, living at ease in our mind, living in our own biological heritage [16].

> Quality of life involves value judgments that are highly subjective and associated with profound satisfaction from the activities of daily life [7].

A further definition emphasizes the breadth of the term quality of life.

> Measures of "socio-personal" or "quality of life" should include physical, social and emotional function, attitudes to illness, personal features of patients' daily life, including family interactions and the cost of illness [19].

The final group of definitions takes a slightly different point of view and sees quality of life as something related to the individuals' own perception and how they view the gap between what can be accomplished or achieved and what cannot.

> Perceived health status is an important adjunct to quality of life [11].

> . . . comparing the importance of specific aspects of life with their actual presence [13,17].

> The prevalence of psychiatric disorders is less related to the objective way of life than to whether people do or do not live according to their wishes. Confirming Otto's work who regarded the discrepancy between the desires and the actual life situation as stressful factors . . . [w]e should not aim at imposing our values on the population at large but rather should try to help individuals to determine and fulfill their desires in actual life. The perceived fulfillment of their desires had the highest association with their health and well-being [13].

> Quality of life is measured by the degree to which an individual succeeds in accomplishing his desires, despite the constraints put upon him by a hostile or indifferent nature, God or social order [8].

> Happiness occurs when self space and life space come closer [6].

It is hoped that these quotations reveal the range of ideas involved in any discussion of quality of life. Despite their diversity there is some unanimity. The concept relates to individuals, covers many aspects of life, and in several of the definitions points to the level of fulfillment and the perceived and actual quality of life. This theme is taken up later when a further definition is proposed. Because of the spectrum of life areas that could be involved, the next section is concerned with the dimensions of quality of life.

DIMENSIONS OF QUALITY OF LIFE

This section deals with the varying dimensions of quality of life, particularly as they might apply to cancer patients. Consideration of these dimensions provides a framework for applying the quality of life concept within the context of clinically relevant psychosocial research.

Dimensions Related to Physical Problems

Physical Dimension

The presence or absence of physical symptoms, e.g., pain, nausea, and immobility, may have a major effect on quality of life. To some observers this factor is the most obvious one that influences life and well-being, but it is clearly not the only one. Equating quality of life with the absence of symptoms is too simplistic.

Toxicity Dimension

For some groups of patients and their relatives, the toxicity dimension can be the aspect of life that is most distressing. Coping with the side effects of radiotherapy, chemotherapy, or surgery can have a major impact on life style. Many of the questionnaires used to investigate such patients concentrate on this aspect of life.

Body Image and Mobility Dimension

Because of the effect of both treatment and the disease, the body image may be altered. This change has been documented best in patients with mastectomy and colostomy. The decreased mobility and the loss of the ability to carry out simple tasks such as washing, shaving, or using the toilet has a devastating effect on some people. These aspects must be considered in any study of quality of life.

Dimensions Related to Psychological, Social, and Spiritual Factors

Psychological Dimension

The psychological dimension overlaps some of the dimensions already discussed. It is particularly concerned with the ability of the individual to cope with problems, physical and psychological, and to deal with times of anxiety and depression. A great deal has been written about mind and cancer in relation to modifying the course of the disease and altering the quality of life. Many of the techniques used to improve quality of life are directed at changing the psychological response of the individual.

Interpersonal Dimension

At any stage in the process of cancer management interpersonal relationships are critical and may be one of the most important factors in maintaining the quality of life. These relationships extend not only to the immediate family but to friends and medical and nursing staff. Sexual relationships may be very important, as is the presence of a loving environment. Crises of any sort strain such relationships, particularly if physical illness or a reduction of libido associated with treatment also occurs. This period is a time when relationships can break up and pent up problems surface. The "ripple" effect of illness must be recognized.

Happiness Dimension

The happiness dimension is often the way in which a "good" quality of life is recognized. Words such as satisfaction, fulfillment, and *joi de vivre* are used in this context. They are very subjective words, and the associated feelings are often short-lived. Pleasure is usually associated with the individual himself, though it can be associated with giving pleasure to others. A broader way of looking at this area is to use the term well-being.

Spiritual Dimension

A very personal yet important aspect of life that can be easily overlooked is the spiritual dimension. It is a difficult, and some would say embarrassing, subject to discuss with patients. Yet it may be the most important source of strength in the individual's life, the central philosophy, and the mainstay of support. The spiritual dimension can be in many forms and implies a strong personal belief system. It is sometimes interpreted as "living with nature" or "that peace which passes all understanding." Spiritual aspects of life do not necessarily imply belief in God.

Financial Dimension

The cost of treatment, travel, and loss of earnings due to illness can have a profound effect on the quality of life. Special foods and extra heating and lighting can eat into savings. There may be concern for the long-term financial security of the family and the home.

Wider Dimensions

Individual Dimension

Most of the definitions agree that quality of life is an individual matter and is specific to the patient. What matters to one person may not matter to another, and it is inappropriate for an observer—medical, nursing, or nonprofessional—to judge the quality of that individual's life. Personal factors that are important include ambitions and priorities, work, hobbies, and accomplishments. These factors may be a very important aspect of the patient's life and may be underrated by those concerned with cancer care.

Cultural Dimension

The cultural dimension can be relevant to patients and their families who do not fit the cultural norm. Cultural values of quality of life may vary from group to group, and it is a mistake to assume that one particular culture has it right.

Culture in this sense is meant to cover not only ethnic differences but differences between groups of the same nationality and variations in socioeconomic status. In this respect the values of any counterculture must be looked at in the same way.

Political Dimension

Because of the differences in earnings, housing, food intake, and amenities between different groups, there is a clear political dimension to quality of life. Why should some groups, races, and countries have less or more than others? Such differences form the basis of much conflict in society, with the imposition of one group's values on others. This chapter does not discuss this subject further, though it is clearly of importance. The political philosophy of a country or a government determines for some individuals a major part of their quality of life, employment, salary, housing, and health and social services. At least one country has written "life, liberty and the pursuit of happiness" into its constitution.

Philosophical Dimension

The philosopher for many hundreds of years has been trying to define happiness and to unify thinking on the subject. The two major schools of philosophical thought look at happiness in different ways, and these ways are reflected in the differences in attitude among doctors. The first of these schools is utilitarianism. The three elements of utilitarianism are hedonism (pleasure and happiness), consequentialism (the value of an action is determined by its consequences), and maximization (the greatest happiness to the greatest number). This school contrasts with deontological theories, which are concerned with rights and duties. Of the several principles underlining this approach, some are of direct relevance to the determination of quality of life. For example, it is important not to cause pain or inflict harm and to promote happiness. Promises should be kept, and the truth should be told. There are special relationships to be kept, particularly among family and friends. The duty to others is greater than that to ourselves. These two views of life find echoes in the way individual doctors, nurses, and patients see the relative importance of some aspects of quality of life. Discussions on the philosophical aspects of life lead to thoughts on the meaning of life and its purpose. This area, however, is beyond the scope of this chapter.

Time Dimension

The time dimension covers a wide range of life factors and concerns the whole patient, bringing together some, but perhaps not all, of the components of quality of life. However, to see this process in a dynamic way, one further dimension must be added—that of time. Time changes many things, and so it is with the quality of life. As individuals grow older, their hopes and aspirations change. They expect more, or sometimes less, from life. Events, problems, and success, which were at one time very important, change with time and achieve some kind of perspective. This change may be seen particularly with the advent of illness, when priorities are suddenly altered, relationships changed, and an alteration in life span considered. The time dimension also implies that for every individual, well or ill, there are natural ups and downs from day to day, week to week, and year to year. It is for this reason, therefore, that it is necessary (though not always desirable) to consider quality of life at a particular period of time, rather than to assume that the quality of life expected, and achieved, at the start of illness is necessarily the same at the end of the illness or during treatment.

What is critical, therefore, is that the phrase quality of life must cover many aspects of life, be related to the individual's own perception of life, and may change with time. How, then, can we define quality of life?

DEFINITION OF QUALITY OF LIFE

The many attempts to define quality of life have been detailed in previous sections, together with the dimensions of the concept. Few attempts have been made to develop a definition that would both assist in its understanding and be of practical value to the patient. The following definition is not claimed to be original, but it tries to synthesize some of the concepts and ideas already described. It focuses on three major issues. The first is that quality of life can be related only to individuals. The second is that the concept must be broad and cover all areas of life. The third is to suggest ways by which the quality of life might be improved and emphasizes the importance of personal growth and development. It is also considered important that such a definition be critically examined and tested.

Potential for Growth

The quality of life can be described and measured only in individual terms, and it depends on past experiences and future hopes, dreams, and ambitions. Quality of life must include all areas of life and experience, and take into account the impact of illness and treatment. A good quality of life can be said to be present when the hopes and expectations of an individual are matched and fulfilled by experience. The opposite is also true. A poor quality of life occurs when the hopes and expectations do not meet with the experience. Quality of life changes with time and under normal circumstances can vary considerably. The priorities and goals of an individual must be realistic and therefore are expected to change with time and be modified by age and experience. To improve the quality of life, therefore, it is necessary to try to narrow the gap between hopes and dreams and what actually happens. The aim therefore is to try to help the person to reach his or her set goals and to grow and develop. A good quality of life is usually expressed in terms of satisfaction, contentment, happiness, fulfillment, and the ability to cope.

From this definition of quality of life certain implications follow.

1. It can only be described by the individual.
2. It must take into account many aspects of life.
3. It must be related to individual aims and goals.
4. Improvement is related to the ability to identify and achieve these goals.
5. Illness and treatment may modify these goals.
6. The goals must, in general, be realistic, though the individual may well wish to retain for himself or herself the hope of achieving special goals.
7. Action is required to narrow the gap, either by meeting goals or by reducing expectations. This action may be by the patient via personal growth and development or with the help of others.
8. The gap between expectations and reality may be the driving force for some individuals.

Quality of life therefore measures the difference, at a particular period of time, between the hopes and expectations of the individual and the individual's present experience. It is concerned with the difference between perceived goals and actual goals. It is an assessment of the potential for growth. This concept has been developed further (4).

The concept, as developed here, is essentially a task analysis or goal-oriented approach and as such fits into such current concepts as the nursing process (15) and problem-oriented medical records (21). It represents a pragmatic approach to the quality of life, which might allow improvements to be made in the individual.

According to the definition proposed and the implications that follow, four stages of action are required to modify the quality of life:

1. Assessment and definition of the problems and priorities of the individual.
2. Planning of care with full patient involvement. This step requires full discussion with the patient and family and requires insight by the patient with the dynamics of the situation.
3. Implementation of the action plan, by either the patient or the caring team. This goal may be accomplished by improving physical symptoms, altering the psychological status, or reducing the expectation of the individual while still retaining hope.
4. Evaluation of the results of intervention and reassessment of the problem. This part is an essential component of the definition.

Such a cyclical process should allow the dimensions of quality of life to be fully considered and provide further refinement of the definition of quality of life.

REFERENCES

1. Andrews, F. M., and Withey, S. B. (1976): *Social Indicators of Well-being in America: The Development and Measurement of Perceptual Indicators*. Plenum, London.
2. Aristotle (1976): *Ethics*. Penguin Books. Harmondsworth, England.
3. Burt, R. S., Wiley, J. A., Minor, M. J., and Murray, J. R. (1978): Structure of well-being: Form content, and stability over time. *Soc. Methods Res.*, 6:365–407.
4. Calman, K. C. (1984): The quality of life in cancer patients—an hypothesis. *J. Med. Ethics*, 10:124–127.
5. Campbell, A., Converse, P. E., and Rodgers, W. L. (1976): *The Quality of American Life*. Russell Sage Foundation, New York.
6. De Bono, E. (1979): *The Happiness Purpose*. Penguin Books, Harmondsworth, England.
7. Dubos, R. (1976): The state of health and the quality of life. *West. J. Med.*, 125:8.
8. Gerson, E. M. (1976): On the quality of life. *Am. Soc. Rev.*, 41:793–806.
9. Gillingham, F. J. (1982): The quality of life. *Aust. N.Z. J. Surg.*, 52:453–460.
10. Holmes, O. W. (1860): *The Professor at the Breakfast Table*. Routledge & Son, London.
11. Hunt, S. M., McKenna, S. P., McEwen, J., Backett, E. M., Williams, J., and Papp, E. (1980): A quantitative approach to perceived health status: A validation study. *J. Epidemiol. Community Health*, 34:281–286.
12. Kaplan, R. M., Bush, J. W., and Berry, C. C. (1979): Health index status: Category rating versus magnitude estimation for measuring levels of well-being. *Med. Care*, 17:501–525.
13. Krupinski, J. (1980): Health and the quality of life. *Soc. Sci. Med.*, 14a:203–211.
14. McCall, S. (1975): Quality of life. *Soc. Indicators Res.*, 2:229–248.
15. McFarlane, J., and Castledine, G. (1982): *A Guide to the Practice of Nursing Using the Nursing Process*. C. V. Mosby, London.
16. Meares, A. D. (1976): *Let's Be Human: New Recreation for the Old*, pp. 209–220. Fontana Books, London.
17. Otto, R. (1976): Patterns of stress, symptoms awareness and medical help seeking among men and women in selected occupations. Ph.D. thesis, Melbourne. Quoted in Krupinski (13).
18. Sheehy, G. (1982): *Pathfinders*. Bantam, Toronto.
19. Spitzer, W. O., Dobson, A. J., Hall, J., Chesterman, E., Levi, J., Shepherd, R., Battista, R. N., and Catchlove, B. R. (1981): Measuring the quality of life of cancer patients: A concise QL-index for use by physicians. *J. Chronic Dis.*, 34:585–597.
20. Van Dam, F. S. A. M., Somers, R., and Van Beek-Couzijn, A. L. (1981): Quality of life some theoretical issues. *J. Clin. Pharmacol.*, 21:166S–168S.
21. Weed, L. L. (1969): *Medical Records, Medical Education and Patient Care*. Case Western Reserve University Press, Cleveland.
22. World Health Organization *Constitution*. WHO, Geneva.

The Quality of Life of Cancer Patients,
edited by N. K. Aaronson and J. Beckmann,
Raven Press, New York © 1987.

Measurement of Quality of Life: An Imperative for Experimental Cancer Medicine

Jan L. Bernheim

Edith Cavell Institute, 1180 Brussels, Belgium; and UCB Pharmaceutical Sector, 1420 Braine-l'Alleud, Belgium

> Death I understand very well, it is suffering I cannot understand.
>
> Isaac B. Singer

> So, among the experiments that may be tried on man, those that can harm are forbidden, those that are innocent are permissible, and those that may do good are obligatory.
>
> Claude Bernard

From the vantage point of the medical oncologist, the juxtaposition of the above thoughts poses a major challenge. Experimental cancer treatment is seldom innocent but is, rather, potentially harmful when, as is often the case, it is unsuccessful. This chapter expands on some dilemmas facing us in our double task of giving every patient optimal care and seeing to it that the experience gained in treating each patient benefits others in the future.

When two or more equally valuable (or equally unsatisfactory) treatment modalities are available—one of them standard treatment and the other an experimental procedure—the medical oncologist (like other physicians) has no choice. He has the ethical obligation to choose the one that contributes to the body of biomedical knowledge that serves to prevent or alleviate similar suffering in the future. Admittedly, the physician's primary responsibility is toward the patient, but clinical research is a secondary concern and a transcendental responsibility that can never be neglected.

The problem therefore is to make sure that the medical oncologist's double task does not create a frustrating antagonism between loyalties to the patient and those to medical science, but allows these two goals to be cross-fertilizing. The ideal way for the oncologist to combine the two tasks is to treat patients in the framework of carefully planned clinical trials that unassailably meet ethical standards (2–4,16,17,23,24). Only few cancer patients are treated according to a study protocol, even in countries with a reputation for excellent clinical research. For example, in the United Kingdom in 1979 only 4% of cancer patients were so treated (19).

Several factors contribute to this rather deplorable state of affairs.

1. Investigational treatments tend to be more complicated and expensive. The present economic crisis is also reflected in lower research budgets.

2. Clinical research treatment is time-consuming and usually carries no other than intellectual rewards. Indeed, insofar as economic constraints mandate "productivity," research activities tend to be officially discouraged.

3. Many physicians are also restricted by lack of training in clinical research.

4. Serious doubts exist among the public and physicians about the net benefit of experimental treatment to the individual patient. This is because, in a diffuse way, experimental treatment for advanced cancer is associated with poor results for the patients, not only in duration of survival but in terms of quality of life. Some sectors of the now universal "quality of life" and "patients' rights" movements tend to discredit clinical experimentation in cancer as contradictory to their ideals. They take the view that "society has more to lose from erosion of its ethics by unwarranted human experimentation than by delaying of investigation that could technically be done today" (10). This pessimism is shared by the many physicians who, though theoretically willing to contribute to research, choose rather to be on the safe side by applying only standard treatment. Thus the legitimate concern to preserve ethical standards in clinical investigation (4) has tended to override Claude Bernard's exhortation to perform the investigations that are ethically obligatory (16).

The central and badly defined issue raised by the latter position is that of "quality of life." My contention is that introducing the parameter "quality of life" into clinical research practice is a useful proposition in its own right and goes some length toward solving the above stated medical ethics problem.

Two series of medical-ethical considerations seem to make consideration of this proposition imperative. The first series concerns reflections on the ethical consequences of developments in the biosociological background of health care in general and medical oncology in particular. The second stems from the present-day efficacy of the medical-oncological area.

BIOETHICAL AND SOCIOLOGICAL IMPERATIVES FOR THE MEASUREMENT OF QUALITY OF LIFE

It is a matter beyond debate that medical efforts primordially aim at preserving life. In quantitative terms, the prime dimension of life is time; hence it is necessary to maximize the number of lived person-years for the patients under one's care. Each physician functions under this mandate from the community. This statement, however, must be supplemented by the concept of *quality* of life as an important amendment.

Physicians operate under the basic assumption that every form of life is meaningful and worth preserving. Even when they may have personal doubts about the desirability of the prolongation of certain severely handicapped lives, their opinion counts for little and the wishes of the patient must dictate their action. Arguably, even this last rule may not always hold. Insofar as in many religious perspectives life is not a property but an endowment, even the patient may not be authorized to stop fighting for its preservation. In practice, however, most agree that from some degree of irreversible suffering and infirmity onward, mere survival ceases to be a positive value and, if the result of treatment, is to be considered an unwanted effect. Both religious (14) and judicial (7) authorities have allowed physicians to act in some cases according to their judgment of what is in the best interest of their patients. In some cases this action implies withholding life, prolonging treatment, and giving priority to the patient's comfort at the expense of lengthening of survival. In the hierarchy of medical priorities, the preservation of life still comes first, but quality of life often runs a strong second. Because they often bear the responsibility to choose which management strategy is in the patient's best interest, physicians must be informed about the impact of the options on quality of life.

It is generally acknowledged that public health and social progress have accounted for a much larger part in the increase of life expectancy during the last century and a half than therapeutic medicine. Moreover, it is sobering to realize that much of therapeutic medicine is not curative but palliative. Before the advent of therapeutic medicine and the access to it of the masses, the total amount of per capita physical suffering was probably less than it is now, as ailments that today are palliable at the cost of major medical treatment, painful therapy, and lengthy infirmity were previously rapidly fatal. This state of affairs is unlikely to change in the foreseeable future, as it is enforced by both ethical standards and unalienable technical acquisitions. However, it does impose on the medical research community the task to find means to improve quality of life. In order to do so in a scientific way, we are faced with the necessity to measure this quality of life.

If, in the future, resources for health care were to be allocated on the basis of obtained person-years, emergency medicine and pediatrics would compete for the top areas of the priority list, and psychiatry, dermatology, geriatrics, neurology, and solid-tumor medical oncology would inevitably be near the bottom. For example, in 1 year of practice, a pediatrician is apt to preserve more person-years than a solid-tumor medical oncologist can hope to do in a lifetime. In fact, if preservation of life were the only goal of medicine, and its success rate were the yardstick by which medical efficacy should be judged, considerable sectors of present-day medicine would make little sense. This whole idea is intolerable because the basic assumption underlying it is wrong: Answering every call for assistance, alleviating suffering, and promoting the quality of life has become almost as important as preserving life.

Because it has become clear that simultaneous economic growth and development of all health care areas is materially impossible, cost-benefit analysis and accounting are going to determine health care policy (20). Abhorrent as the principle of financial accountability of the health care professions to the community may be, no amount of ethical incantation is going to avert systematic cost-benefit analysis.

If the medical and consumer partners in the social contract do not come up with acceptable techniques to quantitate the variable quality of life, the economy-oriented partners will unavoidably tend to disregard it.

Growing segments of public opinion perceive many aspects of standard modern health care as contradictory to their new conceptions of quality of life. This trend often takes the form of alternative modes of treatment that are at variance with classic medicine in that they are largely uncontrolled by scientific evaluation. (18). Inevitably, some of these activities are of widely inferior quality and give rise to financial exploitation. Health care authorities are in the uneasy situation of having to find compromises between protection of public health and of civil liberties. Under the paradigm that health care is a service to the community and mandated by it, there is bound to be a permanent interaction between what medicine as a technology has to offer and what the public as consumers want to receive. We cannot escape the conclusion that, especially in the field of cancer medicine, the message conveyed to us by the proliferation of alternative modes of management is that we have been paying too little heed to the evaluation of the quality of life of our patients.

QUALITY OF LIFE AND THE PRESENT EFFICACY OF MEDICAL ONCOLOGICAL TREATMENT

To discern in what way the medical oncologist confronts the dual task of optimal care and clinical investigation, a summary overview of the state of the art is necessary (6,12,13). At the present time, clinical oncology is among the most rapidly expanding clinical areas, in terms of both the human and financial resources it drains and the amount of research devoted to it. In view of the enormity of the problem it is poised to alleviate, this expansion appears well justified. Because over the last 30 years the rate of expansion of radiotherapy and oncological surgery has by and large followed the pace set by most other clinical areas, the recent growth of clinical oncology is essentially due to the addition of medical oncology, mainly chemotherapy. Indeed, chemotherapeutic results have been impressive in leukemias, lymphomas, germinal tissue carcinomas, embryonic and childhood tumors, and small-cell anaplastic bronchial carcinoma, and highly encouraging in mammary carcinoma and osteosarcoma (13). Most of these treatments are aggressive and pose a heavy burden on the patient. There is, however, no doubt that they save lives or significantly prolong them, so their net benefit to the patients is beyond reasonable debate. For this category of diseases, the medical oncologist's goal is to find more successful treatments, with the understanding that success can reside in either better survival rates or better tolerance of the therapy—preferably both. To ascertain the latter type of improvement, evaluation of the effects of new treatments on the quality of life are necessary.

On the other hand, the fact must be faced that for most advanced solid malignancies, e.g., non-small-cell bronchial, head and neck, gastrointestinal, and genitourinary tract carcinomas, gliomas, and melanoma, no decisively active chemotherapeutic regimens have been found. On the whole, the "standard" or experimental chemotherapeutic treatment of these conditions remains subject to grave doubts in terms of *net benefit* to patients (1). It must be stressed that these doubts also apply to those chemotherapeutic regimens that have yielded up to 50% objective response rates and significantly longer survival in responders than in nonresponders. Two main reasons explain this state of affairs.

First, too few therapeutic trials were controlled, and among those that were very few have included an "only supportive treatment" arm. For example, for lack of such a control it cannot be excluded that chemotherapy inducing a partial or complete response in 20 to 50% of metastatic melanoma patients could actually shorten the survival of nonresponders, thereby statistically canceling out whatever benefit has been gained by responders (8).

Second, if one is to try to evaluate the net benefit to patients, the variable of the *quality of survival* is inescapable. Taking the example of intensive radiotherapy and chemotherapy for metastatic or recurrent epidermoid bronchogenic carcinoma, the question must be asked if the benefits of treatment outweigh debilitating nausea, vomiting, hair loss, and frequent traumatic removal from the home environment (1).

Because for most metastatic solid tumors results of treatment in terms of net benefit to patients are highly unsatisfactory, the prime task of the chemotherapist is to find new drugs, new administration schedules, or new combinations of drugs that would prove effective in at least lengthening the survival of patients. This step has to be done using the technique of clinical trial experimentation (5). In phase I trials one determines the mode of administration of a new agent by giving progressively increasing doses and trying out different administration schedules (15). In phase II trials a drug or drug combination for which a safe mode of administration has been found in a phase I trial is so given to a series of patients in order to explore its side effects and its activity on disease. If the response rate is vastly better than that with conventional treatment, one may dispense with phase III trials. If not, a phase III trial serves to establish the value of the new treatment by comparing it with the best available treatment(s).

The ethics of phase II and III trials are beyond the scope of this chapter and have been thoroughly discussed elsewhere (21). Suffice it to say that the clinical usefulness of comparative (randomized) trials would be greatly enhanced if results were also expressed in terms of quality of life. The major ethical problem involving quality of life resides in phase I trials. In these studies, for obvious reasons, only drugs are given that, after *in vitro* and animal experimentation, offer a reasonable chance to prove effective in man. However, improvement of the clinical condition and regression of tumor masses are not the expected endpoints of phase I trials. In fact, patients treated according to such protocols are usually those in whom all standard treatment has failed, for whom no effective standard treatment is available, or who have unmeasurable disease, e.g., diffuse organ infiltration, atelectasis, and pleural or peritoneal carcinomatosis.

In effect, objective improvement of the clinical condition, although theoretically possible, rarely occurs during phase I trials, whereas side effects and the inconveniences of being subjected to an experimental protocol (frequent tests, hospitalization) are the rule rather than the exception. However, such trials are carried out by oncologists under the following assumptions.

1. The frequent interactions between patient and chemotherapist-investigator, which are necessary for the safety and the information yield of phase I and phase II protocols, also provide maximal opportunity for treatment of disease-related and intercurrent complaints.

2. There is a rational, albeit minimal chance that the patient will obtain an objective improvement.

3. Even when, as in most cases, it does not eventuate, the patient psychologically benefits from actively participating in a rational struggle and from the caring, empathy, enthusiasm, and interest the therapist-investigator provides.

In summary, the main therapeutic result of most experimental treatment of solid tumors may be akin to the placebo effect. This working assumption is plausible but unproved. For lack of an instrument to measure quality of life, no randomized study exists on the respective quality of survival of patients who are treated in phase I (or phase II) protocols and those who receive only supportive or standard low efficacy treatment. The question therefore is the proper selection of patients for these trials. Experience and a successful and intense relationship between physician and patient may help in the choice of which course to take. However, experience is mainly the result of trial and error, and errors in this matter are well-nigh intolerable. As for the "successful and intense relationship between physician and patient," when for whatever reason it is not achieved, the necessity of making the right decisions is no less stringent. Clearly, more precise guidelines are desirable.

At first sight, informed consent appears to wholly dispose of the problem: Only "volunteer" patients pass this hurdle into clinical trials. This chapter is not the place to discuss informed consent in depth. In brief, however, it implies the possibility for the patient to choose from among the various therapeutic options the one that looks the most promising to him—and so seems to shift the responsibility for engaging in experimental treatment from the physician to the patient (9,11). However, informed consent does not solve the medical ethical problems of experimental treatment for two main reasons.

First, the burden of information remains on the physician. In order to inform the patient usefully of the consequences of the therapeutic options, it would be helpful if better than intuitive data on the quality of life were available. Second, obtaining informed consent may be inhumane and become a callous substitute for medical ignorance of what the psychological consequences of the treatment options are likely to be. There are obvious ethical restrictions on its usage, as exemplified by the statement of the Medical Research Council (MRC) of Great Britain on responsibility in investigations on human subjects. On the duty to inform patients, the MRC stated: "Occasionally, however, to do so is contraindicated. For example to awaken patients with a possible fatal illness to the existence of

such doubts about effective treatment may not always be in their best interest''
(21). Furthermore, for complex and respectable cultural reasons, full patient information on diagnosis and prognosis of fatal diseases is yet the exception rather than the rule in many countries that nevertheless adhere to basically the same ethical standards as the United States. As a corollary, the informed consent procedure as understood in the United States is rather exceptional. In these countries, the entire responsibility for therapeutic choices rests squarely on the physician. Even more than in the informed consent situation, experimental data on quality of survival would help to make a more fully informed decision.

Quality of life studies in cancer should include psychosocial data on the patients. For example, a psychological personality profile might allow positive correlations between certain personality traits and a better quality of life under different management strategies to emerge. Such results might serve as elements of information for patients confronted with an informed consent procedure and would provide valuable guidelines for the responsible physician in the management of individual patients, when in other circumstances the responsibility for therapeutic decisions rests mainly with the physician.

PERSPECTIVES

From a utilitarian perspective, some form of assessment of the quality of life or quality of survival of treated cancer patients would meet a number of socioeconomic and ethical requirements. Oncologists in fact spend much time pondering and discussing what might be the fate of their individual patients depending on the chosen management strategy; quality of life has always been the next preoccupation after lengthening of survival. This awareness was also expressed by a World Health Organization report on standardization of results of cancer treatment as recommendations relating to subjective response and quality of life (22):

> An accurate assessment of subjective response is not possible as the methodology does not exist. In reporting results of treatment, performance status of patients should be recorded by an approved scale during, as well as before, treatment, and subsequently at regular intervals and assessed as a measure of the quality of life. The patient's weight should also be regularly recorded and reported, together with some measure of toxicity or side-effect from treatment. All collaborating groups concerned with evaluating treatment should attempt to develop reproducible scales which might further measure the quality of life.

Accurately quantitating the quality of life is obviously a futile proposition and at first sight a contradiction in terms. However, reasonable approximates should be satisfactory.

ACKNOWLEDGMENTS

This work was supported in part by grant 2822225500 of the Belgian National Lottery via the Nationaal Fonds voor Wetenschappelijk Onderzoek, and by a grant from the Franqui-Foundation. The secretarial work of Ms. M. De Bruyne and A. Vanhaelewijck is gratefully acknowledged.

REFERENCES

1. Aisner, J., and Hansen, H. H. (1981): Commentary: Current status of chemotherapy for non-small cell lung cancer. *Cancer Treat. Rep.,* 65:979–986.
2. American Medical Association (1973): Human experimentation: Statement of the American Medical Association. *Conn. Med.,* 37:365–366.
3. Barber, B. (1976): The ethics of experimentation with human subjects. *Sci. Am.,* 234:25–31.
4. Beecher, H. K. (1966): Ethics and clinical research. *N. Engl. J. Med.,* 274:1354–1360.
5. Buyse, M., Staquet, M., and Sylvester, R., eds. (1983): *Cancer Clinical Trials: Methods and Practice.* Oxford University Press, Oxford.
6. Cortes-Funes, H., and Rozencweig, M., eds. (1982): *New Approaches in Cancer Therapy.* Raven Press, New York.
7. Curran, W. J. (1978): The Saikewics decision. *N. Engl. J. Med.,* 298:499–500.
8. De Wasch, G., Bernheim, J., and Kenis, Y. (1978): Combination chemotherapy with three marginally effective agents, CCNU, vincristine and bleomycin in the treatment of stage III melanoma. *Cancer Treat. Rep.,* 60:1273–1276.
9. Epstein, L. C., and Lasagna, L. (1969): Obtaining informed consent: Form or substance. *Arch. Intern. Med.,* 123:682–688.
10. Jonas, H. (1974): Philosophical reflections on experimenting with human subjects. In: *Philosophical Essays: From Ancient Creed to Technical Man,* edited by H. Jonas. Prentice-Hall, Englewood Cliffs, New Jersey.
11. Medical Research Council (1964): Responsibility in investigations on human subjects: Statement by the Medical Research Council. *Br. Med. J.,* 2:178–180.
12. Milsted, R. A. V., Tattersall, M. H. N., Fox, R. M., and Woods, R. L. (1980): Cancer chemotherapy: What have we achieved? *Lancet,* 1:1343–1346.
13. Pinedo, H., ed. (1983): *Cancer Chemotherapy 1083. The EORTC Cancer Chemotherapy Annual 4.* Excerpta Medica, Amsterdam.
14. Pius XII (1957): The Pope speaks, prolongation of life. *Observatore Romano,* 4:393–398.
15. Rozencweig, M., Dodion, P., Nicaise, C., Piccart, M., and Kenis, Y. (1982): Approach to phase I trials in cancer patients. In: *New Approaches in Cancer Therapy,* pp. 1–13, edited by H. Cortes-Funes and Rozencweig. Raven Press, New York.
16. Shimkin, M. B. (1979): Scientific investigations on man: A medical research worker's viewpoint. In: *Biomedical Ethics and the Law,* pp. 229–238, edited by J. M. Humber and R. F. Alineder. Plenum Press, New York.
17. Strauss, M. B. (1973): Ethics of experimental therapeutics. *N. Engl. J. Med.,* 288:1183–1184.
18. Subcommittee on Orthodox Therapies, American Society of Clinical Oncology (1983): Ineffective cancer therapy: A guide for the layperson. *J. Clin. Oncol.,* 1:154–163.
19. Tate, H. C., Rawlinson, J. B., and Freedman, L. S. (1979): Randomised comparative studies in the treatment of cancer in the United Kingdom: Room for improvement? *Lancet,* 2:623.
20. Williams, A. (1974): The cost benefit approach. *Br. Med. Bull.,* 30:252–256.
21. Wing, J. K. (1975): The ethics of clinical trials. *J. Med. Ethics,* 1:174–175.
22. World Health Organization (1977): *Meeting on Standardisation of Reporting Results of Cancer Treatment: WHO Report CAN/77.1,* Geneva.
23. World Medical Association (1962): Draft code of ethics on human experimentation. *Br. Med. J.,* 2:1119.
24. World Medical Association (1977): Declaration of Helsinki: Recommendations guiding medical doctors in biomedical research involving human subjects. In: *Ethics in Medicine: Historical Perspectives and Contemporary Concerns,* pp. 328–329, edited by S. J. Reiser, A. J. Dyck, and W. J. Curran. MIT Press, Cambridge.

The Quality of Life of Cancer Patients,
edited by N. K. Aaronson and J. Beckmann,
Raven Press, New York © 1987.

Cross-Cultural Comparisons of Data About Quality of Life: A Sample of Issues

Norman Sartorius

Division of Mental Health, World Health Organization, 1211 Geneva 27, Switzerland

The development of methods for measuring quality of life of people affected by a disease is a difficult but important effort. This is so for at least three reasons. First, it reminds all concerned that health care is essentially a human transaction where comfort, pain, satisfaction, fear, and other emotions are the targets and codeterminants of all action. Second, the lack of adequate methods for such measurement prevents the scientific evaluation of the impact that a disease or treatment given for it have on quality of life. This lack in turn is an obstacle to efforts aiming at improving quality of life. Third, methodological progress in the measurement of quality of life in people suffering from a disease may help in the production of methods needed to monitor effects of economic, technological, and social innovations and changes on the quality of life.

Quality of life is a vague term used for a variety of purposes and in a variety of situations. It is used as a political statement, as a philosophical proposition, as an advertising slogan, in research, and in training. For the purposes of this chapter it is expressed in terms of distance between a person's position and his goals.

A person's goal can be defined by the individual himself, a group of peers (e.g., the community), and society. The congruence between these groups of goals varies from person to person, community to community, and society to society. Furthermore, immediate and long-term goals are not necessarily the same; nor do long-term goals necessarily have a commanding influence on short-term goals.

Even within the same universe of discourse there may be conflicting goals: Moving toward one may mean moving away from another. Herein lies the difference between the concepts of quality of life and satisfaction. Satisfaction refers to the achievement of a goal (or to the sense of approaching it); quality of life is a derivation of the levels of achievement of the various goals a person may have. Quality of life may therefore be high, even if some of the goals are not achieved and if there are serious difficulties the individual may face. Satisfaction may also refer to the achievement of a goal that may have been set for a person by others but which does not significantly affect his or her quality of life.

The distance between a person and his goals can be assessed by the individual himself, his peers, a third party, and an assessor designated by a scientific, political, or other authority (Table 1). The estimates of distance may vary depending on who makes the assessment.

It is easy and probably interesting to argue which goals are the most important ones when assessing the quality of life of patients affected by cancer and which method should be used to measure the distance between a person and his goals. Some swear that it is the distance between the person's position and the goals set by society, measured by an objective assessor, that truly describes the quality of life, the way of life of people. A societal goal, for example, may be that each person as a member of the society who is of a certain age should be employed, and that whether he or she is employed should and can be assessed by a person designated for this statistical exercise—an authority. Regardless of whether the individual in question likes working, whether the job is of any interest to him/her, and whether he/she is in any way productive in the performance of this job is often not entered into this statement.

Others argue that quality of life presents the individual's own assessment of the distance between his position and the goals he himself has set. The goals he has may only in part be congruent with the goals which society or a group of peers are setting for him. This fact, however, within certain broad limits, is of no relevance for the measurement. This group of thinkers thus argues that it may be more important—the quality of life would be better—for a person who does not like to work to have no obligation to do so. Similarly, they argue that a person who has an impairment that prevents him from functioning at a high level may decide that he has achieved his goals or that his distance from them is small, even though he can perform only in a simple job. He would therefore refuse to take part in a rehabilitation program and would not only be entitled to do so but could and should be counted as a person who has a satisfactory quality of life.

The pitfalls of these two extreme positions are obvious, and yet both are defended with fervor and many apparently powerful arguments. For purposes of this discussion, it is proposed to take an intermediate position, with some leaning toward the left-hand side of Table 1; that is, for measurements of quality of life in patients it is the individual's feeling about his distance from his goals that should have a preference or greater weight than the judgment of his peers of how well or how

TABLE 1. *Assessment of distance to goals*

Distance to goal measured by	Goals set by		
	Individual	Peers	Society
Individual			
Peers			
Assessor designated by an authority			

badly he fares, and both of these groups of judgments are preferred to the judgments of an assessor. Also, greater weight is given to goals set by the individual so long as they are within the broad framework set by vital needs of communities and societies.

With this definition in mind the following assumptions must be fulfilled to allow the measurement of quality of life in an individual suffering from a serious disease such as cancer.

1. The individual can set and define his own goals in clear enough terms to allow an estimation of how close or distant he is from them.

2. The individual can express his estimation in terms that are understandable to others. Following this rule is only partly possible in children, for example, who can express their satisfaction or dissatisfaction only in a gross and global way.

3. There is enough stability in the goals to allow measurement and to allow comparisons over brief periods of time, e.g., months.

4. Cancer—or any other serious disease—affects the quality of life. The relation between the disease and the quality of life is under this assumption curvilinear; that is, in very early stages of the disease there is no relation between the two; similarly, in very far progressed forms of disease the relation is difficult to establish because the very manifestations of life are enormously reduced.

5. The measurement of quality of life is subject to no other difficulties than those inherent in all measurement of emotions; that is, emotions are difficult to assess while felt and difficult to remember once they pass (1).

Each of these assumptions is wide open to cultural invalidation. In some cultural settings it is apparently impossible to imagine that an individual could set his own goals. Goals are always collective goals. They are shared with other members of the community, cast, or social group. This rationale makes it easier to understand or to verbalize the goals of patients, provided of course that the rule that everyone has the goals of the collective self also holds when disease and pain are present.

The capacity to grasp and verbalize distance from goals or from events in one's memory also varies among cultures as much as concepts of time and distance are known to vary. Time can be conceptualized in a linear fashion, with chronologically ordered events strung on the axis of time, like pearls on a necklace. Other cultures tend to understand time differently, in a punctual, summative fashion in which events in time superimpose themselves on each other, like leaves of a book. Still other settings report that time is grasped as a spiral of progression in which the events are ordered but their understanding depends on the position from which they are regarded.

To discover (therefore) if any one of the above assumptions is true in another culture, it is necessary to reach out of the realm of question-and-answer situations and to explore the very meaning of the words used in the communication. It is possible that this exploration can be done only by investigators from the culture in which the patient lives. At the same time, however, the techniques for the exploration of the conceptual universe of a culture can probably be borrowed from anthropologists, social psychologists, and epistemologists in the same or a different culture and used in a valid way. Long and detailed discussion between investigators and social scientists can help to make them aware of the peculiarities of their own culture and concepts that sounded so easy and self-evident (2).

IMPACT OF DISEASE

The impact of diseases on individuals in different cultures is poorly explored. It is known that almost all people feel pain, for example. However, the number of questions about the impact of disease on the individual's psychology, for which we have no answer, is much larger than the number of questions for which answers are available. It is unknown, for example, if the presence of a disease affects equally, in all cultures, the capacity of individuals to talk about themselves as they were or as they would like to be.

It is also unclear if there are differences between people in their comprehension of bodily changes. The answer to this question depends to a large extent on whether people believe in a mind–body dichotomy. In some African countries, for example, it is easy to make a patient accept that a purely bodily symptom has a psychological origin. On the other hand, even the suggestion of such a link raises strong objections by many patients in Europe who, when told that it is impossible to find a change in an organ where they feel pain, turn away offended. The perception of disease varies greatly among people in different cultures and so does the way in which its causal pathways are understood.

CROSS-CULTURAL CONSIDERATIONS

The fact that the assumptions which underlie the measurement of quality of life may be invalid in another culture is no reason to give up the objective of comparing data obtained in different cultures. The significant advances in our knowledge about cross-cultural psychology and psychiatry make it possible to devise methods in a way that ensures the comparability of data collected from people of different cultures. Several major cross-cultural studies have confirmed this. They have also demonstrated the important gains in knowledge that can be obtained from cross-cultural studies of disease and its manifestations (3,4). These studies and others underline the importance of the following four principles:

1. No instrument for the assessment of psychological states is culture-free. In each instance the validity, objectivity, and other metric characteristics of the instrument must be assessed in the culture of application. The assessment must be done under the conditions of field use: Hindi-speaking patients hospitalized in Sweden are not the group to be assessed with an instrument that would be used

in India. The equivalence of a question (and of an answer!) in two different cultures is a *sine qua non* rather than a (literary) similarity of form in which it is asked or answered.

2. The comparability of an item of information obtained in studies carried out in two or more cultures is limited in time. Cultures sometimes change slowly and almost imperceptibly, but they change. The rate of change is not necessarily the same in different cultures or across time within the same culture. Old data are interesting, useful, fascinating, telling, but they are usually not comparable with data collected years later.

3. Achieving equivalence of instruments and comparability of data takes time and patience. Undoubtedly one of the most useful ways to learn about a culture or about the way in which an instrument can be used in such a culture is to talk with investigators from the other culture about all things, big and small, including diseases, ways of talking about them, and ways of dealing with them.

4. It is easier to communicate summary assessment from one culture to another than to translate detailed parts of an overall assessment. Global judgments are usually based on items included in the assessment or on other, invisible items that are often perceived without a conscious effort. The investigator is different from an adding machine in that he not only takes into account all numbers but also their variations and possible corrections. This statement does not mean that global judgments should replace a careful record of items about which information was obtained: It means simply that in general a global judgment by an experienced investigator who standardized the scope of his enquiry might be the best piece of information to use in comparisons across cultures.

Finally, it is important to say a word about the value of knowledge that can be obtained from cross-cultural investigations. Today it is in no way necessary to travel a thousand miles to come into a foreign culture; many towns in Europe, for example, are composed of groups of people from different countries or stemming from different sociocultural settings. Even within rural areas of the same country, cultural differences abound. The old are often as profoundly uprooted in time and distance from the young in their own country as from members of another culture.

Members of a different social class may have ways of thinking, traditions, styles of behavior that are much more distant from their doctors' culture than are the ways of thinking and behavior of doctors living in a country that had once a very different culture. Knowledge therefore about different cultures and skills in the ways of cross-cultural investigation can be helpful even without being involved in internal or transcontinental investigations; it can be used in daily work, practice, and research.

Such knowledge about cultures and an involvement and effort to understand them, however, has another more important function. It makes us remember the larger family of man and the obligation to learn how to help others, regardless of their looks and addresses, their races, size, and language. It also brings to mind the many ways in which it is possible to go wrong and right in being with others of the same culture or of another.

REFERENCES

1. European Organization for Research on Treatment of Cancer (1983): Proceedings of the 4th Workshop of the EORTC Study Group on Quality of Life, Birmingham, England, 4–5 February 1983. Odense University Hospital, Odense, Denmark.
2. Kisker, K. P., et al., eds. (1979): *Cross-Cultural Psychiatry (Psychiatrie der Gegenwart)*, 2nd ed., pp. 711–737. Springer-Verlag, Berlin.
3. World Health Organization (1974): *International Pilot Study of Schizophrenia*, Vol. 1. WHO Offset Publ. No. 2, ISBN 92 4 170002 5. WHO, Geneva.
4. World Health Organization (1979): *Schizophrenia: An International Follow-Up Study*. Wiley, Geneva.

The Quality of Life of Cancer Patients,
edited by N. K. Aaronson and J. Beckmann,
Raven Press, New York © 1987.

Theoretical Framework for Developing Measures of Quality of Life and Morale

Hans J. F. Baltrusch and E. Millard Waltz

*International Psychooncology Project, D-2900 Oldenburg,
Federal Republic of Germany*

The development of instruments for adequately measuring quality of life (QOL) of cancer patients and for discriminating between individuals with high and low QOL is facilitated if we have a theoretical framework of major adaptive tasks and processes triggered by neoplastic diseases. QOL appears to be closely connected to the ability of the individual to cope with the stress of illness. The outcome of various adaptive processes may therefore be posited as useful empirical indicators of QOL. The theoretical framework suggested in this chapter is an integration of two research traditions. One consists in clinical observations and epidemiological research on how individuals adjust to cancer and other types of serious illness (3,11,23,35; R. Lichtman, J. Wood, and S. Taylor, *unpublished observations*). This body of behavioral literature provides a rich descriptive base for focusing on salient aspects of adaptation and relating them to QOL. The second research tradition is the work of community psychologists who have probed into the nature and determinants of QOL (5,7,44). Good health, marital and job satisfaction, and an adequate social network in the larger community appear to be important correlates of QOL in the general population. The somatic and psychosocial sequelae of illness may alter the life space of the cancer patient so that positive determinants of QOL are substantially decreased and negative ones increased. In this framework, self-esteem and depression are viewed as psychological mediators between health-related and socioenvironmental variables on the one hand and the individual's level of QOL (3,25,44).

DEFINITION OF THE CONCEPT OF QUALITY OF LIFE

Quality of life is a fairly malleable concept and one which has received a great deal of attention from behavioral scientists (5,7,8). Due to progress in the field of neuroimmunomodulation, the salience of this psychosocial factor will most undoubtedly increase as we learn more about how positive and negative emotions influence neuroendocrine processes and the initiation and course of malignant tumors. When people think about QOL, they frequently have two things in mind. On the one side, they are referring to dysphoric feeling states triggered by adverse life situations, daily hassles with other people, and chronic problems-in-living. Problems related to their health or family and work situations are important sources of negative emotions linked to a low sense of well-being. On the other side, they are thinking about the positive aspects of their lives and the daily uplifts provided by interaction with their social environment. These include the gratification of socioemotional needs in the family and larger community, such as those for intimacy, affection, and social recognition. Work and leisure activities are a source of personal achievement and daily uplifts, likewise associated with positive feeling states. QOL, in a very general sense, may therefore be defined as the balance between euphoric and dysphoric feeling states. Adaptation to a life with cancer or the maintenance of a reasonable level of QOL may be viewed relative to the reduction of dysphoric emotions and the creation of a life situation with adequate sources of personal gratification and daily uplifts.

Zautra (44) proposed a two-factor model of QOL, linking positive and negative environmental influences with same-domain feeling states. This model is suggested here as useful for conceptualizing QOL in the wake of serious illness due to its focus on changes in different groups of health-related variables. It allows an integration of our knowledge about coping processes and subjective well-being. Generally speaking, physical illness and impairment lead to a reduction in positive sources of QOL and to a notable increase in anxiety, uncertainty about the future, and other dysphoric feeling states. According to the two-factor model, this alteration in the life situation of the tumor patient is synonymous with a decrease in QOL.

Cohen (13) coined the term *psychosocial morbidity* to describe the negative influences triggered by cancer. She viewed malignancy as a "massive assault on the physical and psychological integrity" of the person.

The neoplastic diseases, perhaps more so than other types of serious illness, should be considered as a threat to physical existence; they are associated in the minds of most people with fears of dying, damage to one's body, and loss of independence. Psychosocial morbidity is defined as the distress arising in various stages of the patient career, beginning with the discovery and diagnosis of malignancy (1,12,13). Surgery, irradiation, or chemotherapy may each hold its own special terrors, and the pretreatment period is usually one of high emotional upset (17,19,26,31). In addition, functional impairment or disfigurement from the cancer, treatment, or both is a severe threat to the individual's sense of bodily integrity (28). A self-image of being healthy and able and having a normal, attractive body is central to most people's views of themselves and probably to their sense of environmental control. Neoplasia and its physical sequelae pose a threat to one's previous self-concept and frequently necessitate changes in self-image (27,30).

Physical disfigurement may also lead to self-stigmatization, social withdrawal, and adverse changes in interpersonal relationships (15,42). Many marriages are severely strained by the sexual and emotional problems related to cancer and its treatment (30). This question has been most thoroughly investigated among mastectomy patients (20,30; R. Lichtman et al., *unpublished observations*), although as Mantell (21) has noted, it probably also applies to persons with cancer at other sites. Problems in other major social roles, e.g., the work role, can likewise have a wide-reaching impact on the total life space of the individual (16). Forced retirement in the wake of malignant disease can entail a loss of opportunities for personal achievement and social recognition, as well as social isolation and withdrawal into the nuclear family. The loss of the work role may be a salient symbolic and object loss for those individuals who received a great deal of personal gratification from their jobs. Charmaz (10) has therefore described chronic illness as a severe restriction of the life space of the individual leading to a loss of the self. In the two-factor model of QOL, the social sequelae of illness reduce positive sources of QOL and simultaneously entail social isolation and other negative feeling states.

Summarizing research on the social and psychological consequences of serious illness, cancer may be viewed as a threat to bodily integrity and comfort, as well as to the individual's self-concept, belief systems, social and occupational functioning, values, commitments, and emotional equilibrium (11,13). The dysphoric emotions associated with the losses and threats of cancer have been used to define psychosocial morbidity. These factors include anxiety, depressed mood, anger, social isolation, and feelings of helplessness and low self-worth. At the same time, illness may considerably restrict the opportunities for daily uplifts and gratifying social interaction with other people. The physical and psychosocial aftermath of cancer and its treatment can tip the balance between negative and positive affective states to the negative side with a marked decrease in QOL(33).

CONCEPTUAL FRAMEWORK OF ADAPTATION AND QOL

There is a growing body of behavioral research suggesting that cancer patients adjust to their altered life situation in very different manners (23; R. Lichtman et al., *unpublished observations*). Many patients are able to restructure their lives in such a way as to maintain or regain a reasonable level of happiness and life satisfaction. Others, as Charmaz (10) described them, lead a very restricted life with little opportunity for uplifting and gratifying social interaction with other people. Moos and Tzu (24) have described coping behavior and adaptive tasks related to the maintenance of QOL in the wake of physical illness. These tasks encompass the following.

1. Stress management and the maintenance of emotional equilibrium
2. Preservation of positive-self-images and a sense of mastery
3. Maintenance of adequate interpersonal relationships

The QOL of individuals who have survived neoplastic illness depends on the same factors that influence happiness in healthy individuals. In addition, they must cope effectively with the psychosocial stress and distress caused by their illness.

A conceptual framework for investigating QOL among cancer patients should encompass major adaptive processes influencing adjustment and well-being. Clinical studies with small samples and exploratory research using qualitative methods have provided a descriptive basis for developing such a conceptual framework. Patient concerns and problems (2,13,37,38) have been identified and adaptive processes delineated. The following sections focus on coping processes related to stress management, self-concept, and maintenance of interpersonal relationships. These areas may be considered salient aspects of adjustment affecting happiness and well-being.

At the operational level, QOL can be measured using general appraisals of happiness and life satisfaction developed for national surveys on QOL (5,8). One such general measure of affective aspects of QOL is Bradburn's positive and negative affect subscales (7). Variables tapping the outcome of various adaptive processes linked to well-being are also suggested. These should correspond to the World Health Organization (WHO) conceptualization of physical, psychological, and social well-being. Profiles of process variables, e.g., somatic concerns, psychological distress, body image, self-esteem, social and occupational functioning, and degree of social isolation or loneliness, appear useful for providing a differentiated picture of adjustment. These outcome measures may be viewed as correlates of QOL in the wake of serious illness (3).

COPING WITH PSYCHOLOGICAL DISTRESS

Cancer has been described as entailing various types of symbolic and object losses: (a) at the somatic level: amputation of limbs, physical mutilation, and the forfeit of previous good health and functional capacity; (b) at the social level: the forfeit of prized roles and activities or disability in these areas; (c) at the psychological level: losses related to the individual's pre-illness construction of reality and psychological future.

Cognitive and emotional adaptation requires the individual to mourn these symbolic and object losses and to restructure his ways of looking at himself and his world. Any major life change requires effort and can be distressing, as previously adequate patterns of thinking must be given up and new, more effective ones developed (35). This is especially true of life with malignant disease. Cancer as a series of loss events can lead to depressed mood, demoralization, and even clinical depression (13,14,19,20,22–24,31,41).

The fears and anxiety engendered by malignancy include the threat to life itself, as well as extreme uncertainty about the future. The threat of serious illness to the person and his assumptive world is a source of psychological distress. QOL entails adjustment processes associated with the management of dysphoric emotions and the maintenance of psychological equilibrium. Several studies have shown that the outcome of cognitive and affective adaptation is substantially influenced by the social support of significant others, above all by the emotional and confiding support of the spouse (32; R. Lichtman et al., *unpublished observations*).

Social Support from the Family

Successful coping with the emotional impact of cancer is probably facilitated if the family fulfills certain functions related to cognitive and emotional adaptation that have been subsumed under the concept of *social support*. At the cognitive level the family influences how the individual perceives and interprets the stressful life situation confronting him. In a coherent, stable, and supportive family environment, adverse life events are appraised as less threatening and more controllable. Second, the family group provides a refuge into which the patient can withdraw when necessary for "tanking-up" psychologically and getting a new perspective on things. Third, cognitive processes of adaptation can be shared through confiding and reality reassurances. These supports play a pivotal role in aiding the person who is restructuring his assumptive world.

At the emotional level of adjustment, supportive families meet the increased needs of the patient for love, social approval, succorance, security, and a sense of belongingness. Symbolic and object losses can be mourned together and sufficient grief work performed. Sustained by a sense of reliable reliance with significant others, the threat of illness to physical and psychological integrity is less emotionally menacing. Hence dysphoric emotions are moderated. Anxiety and other types of psychological distress are reduced owing to the mere presence of trusted others and through supportive interaction. This type of emotional support should buffer the impact of the stress of illness and enable the individual to go out and master his problems.

MAINTENANCE OF A POSITIVE SELF-CONCEPT

The physical and social sequelae of neoplastic disease have been discussed as impinging on the person's attitudes toward himself and his self-appraisal of environmental control. A number of theoretical dimensions of the self-concept may be speculated to reflect the impact of illness and the coping success of the individual during the recovery process. Particularly salient in respect to cancer patients are aesthetic and functional body images. The disfigurement and physical mutilation associated with surgery and irradiation may adversely affect body images, but this effect can be buffered by the social support of significant others, as several studies seem to suggest (15,18,21,27,30,31,40; R. Lichtman et al., *unpublished observations*).

Other dimensions of the self include self-esteem and self-confidence, two aspects of self-appraisal that are frequently related but conceptually distinct. The latter has been termed self-efficacy, internal locus of control, sense of mastery, and efficacy-based self-esteem (43). Self-esteem is the judgment the person holds about his own self-worth. It is linked to self-respect and therefore distinguishable from self-confidence or sense of environmental control. Cancer may severely influence the individual's views about his degree of self-worth owing to changes in appearance and functional capacity. The loss of prized social roles may further lead to an erosion of self-esteem if role-related achievements were an important source of personal enhancement, supporting positive views of the self. Sexual problems and forced retirement may provide a substantial blow to self-worth. The same is true of social withdrawal and the loss of everyday opportunities for ego-bolstering interpersonal interaction in the larger community. Charmaz (10) has succinctly described the impact of these consequences of chronic illness on self-evaluations.

A further aspect of the self-concept encompasses feelings of self-confidence, personal efficacy, and environmental control. This type of self-judgment relates to the ideas the person holds about his own ability to influence the factors that importantly affect his life. There is a considerable conceptual overlap among such terms as self-confidence, personal efficacy, and internal locus of control. The theme common to all these concepts is that of feeling oneself to be an active and competent agent. It is the anticipation of successfully mastering challenges and overcoming obstacles, as Rosenberg (29) has formulated it. Whereas self-esteem refers to self-acceptance and feelings of self-worth, the former concept refers to the belief that the individual can make things happen in accord with inner wishes (43).

Malignancy is a particularly virulent type of threat to such self-images. It is very difficult to maintain a sense of mastery and personal control when the person is confronted with cancer and its impact on his total life space. The high degree of uncertainty in the biomedical sciences about factors involved in the etiology and course of neoplastic diseases favors the emergence of feelings of powerlessness and helplessness. The patient experiences a lack of medical and individual control over his fate. The constant threat of recurrence and possible death intensifies such feelings of loss of control. The illness per se, its medical treatment, and many of the social consequences already discussed seem highly inimical to the maintenance of feelings of self-agency. Self-confidence may also be impinged on by changes in body image and self-esteem described earlier in this section. Many patients are able to cope with the threat of cancer to their pre-illness self-concept. One factor facilitating the maintenance of positive attitudes toward one's body and self-worth is the marital situation of the patient (15,35,42; R. Lichtman et al., *unpublished observations*).

Marital Situation and Self-Concept

Social support from the spouse has generally been found to be an important personal resource when coping with the adverse effects of illness on the self-concept (described earlier). Experiencing that one means very much to a significant other and that one is valued for one's own intrinsic worth is an important provision of a close interpersonal relationship. Mastectomy patients, for example, need clear signals from the spouse that they are loved, valued, and sexually attractive (R.

Lichtman et al., *unpublished observations*). This mechanism might be termed love-based self-esteem. An emotionally close conjugal bond may be viewed as buffering feelings of self-respect and self-worth from the negative impact of cancer.

A second type of social support is a sense of reliable alliance or the feeling of being able to rely on one's spouse in case of need. This provision of interpersonal relationships may be seen as strengthening self-confidence and, through it, self-esteem. This mechanism might be termed efficacy-based self-esteem.

The types of social support described above probably influence QOL directly as well as indirectly, as mediated by their favorable influence on the self-concept. In contrast, a marital situation characterized by conflict or by a lack of emotional intimacy probably severely encumbers the maintenance of a positive self-concept. Chronic role strains or unresolved problems-in-living in the marital sphere have been shown to lead to an erosion of self-esteem and feelings of personal efficacy (25). Persons who had such a marriage prior to illness appraise themselves more negatively at the time of diagnosis and are more vulnerable to the assault of cancer on their self-judgments. This topic is discussed in more detail in the next section.

MAINTENANCE OF ADEQUATE INTERPERSONAL RELATIONS

The maintenance of adequate interpersonal ties in the wake of illness is a major coping task of cancer patients. Social support as a provision of adequate interpersonal relationships has already been discussed in regard to cognitive and emotional adjustment. In this section, the direct effect of such relations on QOL is the main focus. A great deal of research on QOL has investigated the types of social networks people have and the quality of their ties to various network members. Zautra (44) summarized the findings from this research as follows. "National surveys . . . leave little doubt that when people talk about the quality of their lives (or the lack of it) they often have social resources on their minds." The term social resources here refers to the positive and negative aspects of interpersonal relationships. In a two-factor model of QOL, Zautra posited the daily uplifts and needs gratification arising from positive social interaction with other persons to be reflected primarily in the positive feeling domain. Social isolation and interpersonal conflict, in contrast, are mirrored primarily in the negative affect domain. Cancer can adversely affect the balance between positive and negative feeling states and therefore lead to a drop in QOL due to a wide-reaching impact it may have on the social relations of patients (42).

Malignancy frequently has repercussions on the social ties of the individual in the family, in his network of friends and relatives, and in the larger community. These repercussions may lead to a feeling of being emotionally and socially isolated (42). A breakdown in communication between the cancer patient and his social environment and the inability to speak candidly about health-related concerns are problems reported by many individuals. Self-stigmatization and social withdrawal may aggravate this tendency toward the emotional isolation of many patients. Self-stigmatization is especially strong when the patient believes his cancer to be highly visible. The feeling of no longer having an attractive, normal physique may cut the individual off from his social environment. This withdrawal is due to the expectance of negative reactions from others. The loss of previous social roles and their interpersonal networks may intensify such tendencies toward withdrawal from the larger community. When the social network at the workplace was a major site for socializing and experiencing social recognition, forced retirement may lead to strong feelings of loneliness, boredom, and marginality. All of these repercussions of cancer on interpersonal ties impinge on QOL.

An important determinant of QOL noted by Zautra (44) is the gratifying social interaction with others that results from everyday participation in family, occupational, and community activities. These factors include ties to various groups of people in their social network, both weak and strong interpersonal ties. Strong ties encompass those with the spouse and other family members as well as close friends and relatives. Weak social ties are those with work colleagues, acquaintances, and similar persons. A lack of strong human bonds is associated with what Weiss (34) has defined as emotional isolation, or "pining for someone to be close to." QOL depends on the gratification of emotional needs for love and affection, as well as for intimacy opportunities. A lack of weaker ties in the larger community is related to social isolation or "pining for social activity." Socializing, a sense of belongingness and group affiliation, and the social recognition provided by others are human needs linking the interpersonal environment and QOL. The provisions of strong and weak ties also influence the ability of the cancer patient to cope with his illness. They can aid in the maintenance of favorable body images and self-esteem. Characteristics of the social environment should therefore be viewed as affecting psychological well-being directly and indirectly. Indirectly, the social resources of the patient can support or aggravate psychosocial recovery. Directly, they are a major determinant of QOL, as most national surveys have shown (3,5,7,8,44).

PRACTICAL IMPLICATIONS

The development of short, easy-to-use measures of QOL is currently a pressing need for those engaged in clinical and research work in cancer. It was argued that we could most effectively select appropriate measures if we understand how individuals adjust to a life with cancer and the relation between adaptation and QOL. The questionnaires and interview schedules we use should discriminate between patient groups who are doing well according to various criteria and those who are developing into "social and psychological invalids." Various adaptive tasks suggested in the psychooncology literature may be used to operationalize psychosocial adjustment and QOL.

An attempt was made at adaptation of a model developed in QOL research to the specific situation of life after cancer. The two-factor model utilized by Bradburn,

Zautra, and other community psychologists for explaining QOL distinguishes between positive and negative aspects of everyday experiences and their reflection in two separate affective domains. The social environment, a potential source of both social support and social stress, is a particularly salient component of this model. Generally speaking, a diagnosis of cancer impinges on QOL by increasing negative emotions and by severely constricting opportunities for positive experiences. The physical, social, and psychological sequelae of cancer may therefore be viewed as having an impact on both the positive and negative affective domains. The activities of the patient to cope effectively with his or her new life situation are thus aimed at a reduction of dysphoric emotions and the creation of a life with adequate sources of personal gratification and daily uplifts. The two-factor model allows us to focus on various aspects of life after cancer and their corresponding impact on QOL as the balance between positive and negative emotions.

Quality of life can be quantified using single-item measures or scales, such as that of Bradburn (7), which have been used with success in representative national surveys. It was further suggested that other measures be used which monitor the coping effectiveness of the individual relative to a number of important adaptive tasks. Scales measuring anxiety, depression, and dysphoric mood states in the wake of illness are negatively associated with QOL. The same is true of empirical measures of the level of somatic concerns and health-related problems. The maintenance of positive views about the self and adequate interpersonal relations with significant others were emphasized as major aspects of QOL. Scales are available for measuring body image, self-esteem, self-confidence, and other dimensions of the self-concept. These empirical measures may be viewed as tapping the success of the patient in coping with cancer and in maintaining supportive social ties. Because of the salience of social adaptation relative to QOL, it is necessary to develop measures for assessing the degree of social integration of the patient in the family, at the work place, and in the larger community. Satisfaction with major social roles and interpersonal ties has been found in national surveys to be determinants of QOL. The same is true of cancer patients. Scales measuring loneliness or emotional isolation may be most appropriate for tapping social adjustment.

REFERENCES

1. Ahmed, P., ed. (1981): *Living and Dying with Cancer, Coping with Medical Issues.* Elsevier, New York.
2. American Cancer Society (1979): *Report on the Social, Economic, and Psychological Needs of Cancer Patients.* American Cancer Society, San Francisco.
3. Badura, B., and Waltz, M. (1984): Social support and the quality of life following myocardial infarction. *Soc. Indicators Res.,* 14:295–311.
4. Baltrusch, H. J., and Waltz, M. (1985): Cancer from a biobehavioural and social epidemiologic perspective. *Soc. Sci. Med.,* 20:789–794.
5. Beiser, M. (1974): Components and correlates of mental well-being. *J. Health Soc. Behav.,* 15:320–327.
6. Bloom, J. (1978): *Psychological Aspects of Breast Cancer.* Publ. No. NO1-CN55313 (DHEW). National Cancer Institute, Washington, D.C.
7. Bradburn, N. (1969): *The Structure of Well-Being.* Aldin, Chicago.

8. Campbell, A., Converse, P., and Rogers, W. (1976): *The Quality of American Life.* Sage, New York.
9. Cantor, R. (1980): Self-esteem, sexuality and cancer-related stress. *Front. Radiat. Ther. Oncol.,* 14:51–54.
10. Charmaz, K. (1983): Loss of self: A fundamental form of suffering in the chronically ill. *Sociol. Health Illness,* 5:168–195.
11. Cohen, F., and Lazarus, R. (1980): Coping with the stress of illness. In: *Health Psychology,* edited by G. Stone, F. Cohen, and N. Adler. Jossey-Bass, San Francisco.
12. Cohen, J., Cullen, J., and Martin, R. (1982): *Psychosocial Aspects of Cancer.* Raven Press, New York.
13. Cohen, M. (1982): Psychosocial morbidity in cancer: A clinical perspective. In: *Psychosocial Aspects of Cancer,* edited by J. Cohen, J. Cullen, and R. Martin. Raven Press, New York.
14. Craig, T. J., and Abeloff, M. D. (1974): Psychiatric symptomatology among hospitalized cancer patients. *Am. J. Psychiatry,* 131:1323–1327.
15. Dyk, R., and Sutherland, A. (1956): Adaptation of the spouse and other family members to the colostomy patient. *Cancer,* 9:123–138.
16. Feldmann, F. (1982): Work and cancer health histories. In: *Psychosocial Aspects of Cancer,* edited by J. Cohen, J. Cullen, and R. Martin. Raven Press, New York.
17. Gyllenskold, K. (1978): Psychological reactions of breast cancer patients to radiotherapy. In: *Breast Cancer,* edited by P. C. Brand and P. A. van Keep. University Park Press, Baltimore.
18. Jamison, K. R., Wellisch, D. K., and Pasnau, R. O. (1978): Psychosocial aspects of mastectomy: The woman's perspective. *Am. J. Psychiatry,* 135:432–436.
19. Leigh, H., Ungerer, J., and Percarpio, B. (1980): Denial and helplessness in cancer patients undergoing radiation therapy. *Cancer,* 45:3086–3089.
20. Lewis, F., and Bloom, J. (1979): Psychosocial adjustment to breast cancer: A selected review of the literature. *Int. J. Psychiatry Med.,* 9:1–10.
21. Mantell, J. (1982): Sexuality and cancer. In: *Psychosocial Aspects of Cancer,* edited by J. Cohen, J. Cullen, and R. Martin. Raven Press, New York.
22. McCorkle, R., and Quint-Benoliel, J. (1983): Symptom distress, current concerns, and mood disturbance after diagnosis of life-threatening disease. *Soc. Sci. Med.,* 17:431–438.
23. Mendelsohn, G. (1979): The psychological consequences of cancer: A study of adaptation to somatic illness. *Cah. Anthropol.,* 2:53–92.
24. Moos, R. H., and Tzu, V. (1977): The crisis of physical illness: An overview. In: *Coping with Physical Illness,* edited by R. H. Moos. Plenum Press, New York.
25. Pearlin, L. I., Lieberman, M. A., Menaghan, E. G., and Mullan, J. I. (1981): The stress process. *J. Health Soc. Behav.,* 22:337–356.
26. Peck, A. (1972): Emotional reactions to radiation treatment. *AJR,* 114:591–599.
27. Polivy, J. (1977): Psychological effects of mastectomy on a woman's feminine self-concept. *J. Nerv. Ment. Dis.,* 164:77–87.
28. Ray, C. (1978): Adjustment to mastectomy: The psychological impact of disfigurement. In: *Breast Cancer: Psychosocial Aspects of Early Detection and Treatment,* edited by P. C. Brand and P. A. van Keep. University Park Press, Baltimore.
29. Rosenberg, M. (1979): *Conceiving the Self.* Basic Books, New York.
30. Schain, W. (1980): Sexual functioning, self-esteem, and cancer care. *Front. Radiat. Ther. Oncol.,* 14:12–19.
31. Silberfarb, P. M., Philibert, D., and Levine, P. M. (1978): Psychosocial aspects of neoplastic disease: Affective and cognitive effects of chemotherapy in cancer patients. *Am. J. Psychiatry,* 137:597–601.
32. Spiegel, D., Bloom, J., and Gottheil, E. (1983): Family environment as a predictor of adjustment to metastatic breast cancer. *J. Psychosoc. Oncol.,* 1:33–44.
33. Spitzer, W. (1981): Measuring the quality of life of cancer patients. *J. Chronic Dis.,* 34:585–597.
34. Weis, R. (1975): *Marital Separation.* Basic Books, New York.
35. Weisman, A. (1979): *Coping with Cancer.* McGraw-Hill, New York.
36. Weisman, A., and Sobel, H. (1974): Coping with cancer through self-instruction: A hypothesis. *J. Hum. Stress,* 5:3–8.
37. Weisman, A. D., Worden, J. W., and Sobel, H. (1980): Psychosocial screening and intervention with cancer patients. Research Report. National Cancer Institute, Bethesda.

38. Wellisch, D., Landsverk, J., Guidera, K., Pasnau, R., and Fawzy, F. (1983): Evaluation of psychosocial problems of the home-bound cancer patient. *Psychosom. Med.,* 45:11–21.
39. Wells, L. E., and Marwell, G. (1976): *Self-Esteem: Its Conceptualization and Measurement.* Sage, Beverly Hills.
40. Wirsching, M., Druner, H., Hehl, F., Herrmann, C., and Köhler, K. (1977): Psychosoziale Rehabilitation von Anuspraeterträgern. *Med. Psychol.,* 3:119–128.
41. Worden, J. W., and Weisman, A. D. (1977): The fallacy of post-mastectomy depression. *Am. J. Med. Sci.,* 273:169–175.
42. Wortman, C., and Dunkel-Schetter, C. (1979): Interpersonal relationships and cancer: A theoretical analysis. *J. Soc. Issues,* 35:120–155.
43. Wylie, R. (1974, 1978): *The Self-Concept.* Vols. I and II, revised ed. University of Nebraska Press, Lincoln.
44. Zautra, A. (1983): Social resources and the quality of life. *Am. J. Community Psychol.,* 11:275–289.

The Quality of Life of Cancer Patients,
edited by N. K. Aaronson and J. Beckmann,
Raven Press, New York © 1987.

Quality of Life and Empirical Research

Joern Beckmann and *Gert Ditlev

*Department of Clinical Psychology, Fyns Amts Sygehusvaesen, and *Institute of Philosophy,
Odense University, DK-5000 Odense C, Denmark*

> Whoever engages in research without having first stated
> his problem is like a person who does not know where he
> is going or whether or not he has found what he wants.
> Aristotle, *Metaphysics*, Book Beta

This chapter explores some of the theoretical problems involved in the quality
of life project.

EMPIRICAL RESEARCH

It seems that most quality of life research is dominated by empirical research,
called the empirical-quantitative approach. This approach gives rise to six questions—questions that are not raised to oppose the empirical-quantitative approach
but, rather, to attempt to clarify problems basic to the research situation of empirical
science.

1. Which factors are involved in the seeming unwillingness to use a theoretical
approach? This aversion is seldom discussed openly. It may be explained by either
a lack of knowledge of other procedures or an attitude that the choice is too
obvious to discuss.

2. What are the reasons for the rejection of a theoretical approach? This type
of research may be considered too abstract or unrealistic when compared with
empirical-quantitative analysis, which is perceived as concrete and reality-oriented.
The theoretical approach may be perceived as inexact and unscientific, in contrast
to the seeming precision of the empirical-quantitative approach.

3. Is empirical-quantitative analysis the only form of empirical research applicable
to quality of life studies? An alternative model can, in fact, be developed (model
2) and is presented here in contrast with the empirical-quantitative approach (model
1).

Parameter	Model 1: empirical-quantitative	Model 2: empirical-qualitative
Method	Monologue	Dialogue
Approach	General	Individual
Basis	Natural science	Humanism
Results	Semiinvestigative	Interpretive
Procedure	Subject to object	Subject to subject

4. Is the empirical-quantitative approach without theoretical considerations? What scientifically justifies the use of this approach? Scientific study is composed of research models, reasoning, and reflections. It cannot be empirically, quantitatively proven that the empirical-quantitative approach is the only form of scientific thinking.

5. Is it possible to empirically assess quality of life without the existence of a quality of life theory? The empirical-quantitative approach selects research categories according to two criteria or theories. First, categories are selected on the basis of one definite theory of science: The categories shall be operational or empirically unambiguous. Second, and this is the central point in our argumentation, research categories are also selected on the basis of a theory of quality of life. The theory of science can declare only which terms are operational or "scientific." It cannot say anything about which terms are *relevant* to the subject of quality of life, and it cannot declare when *all* the relevant terms have been brought forward. Each empirical-quantitative analysis thus necessarily presupposes a theory of quality of life.

6. What progress, if any, is made by the use of the empirical approach to quality of life? "Progress" means an advance in defining the research categories utilized (a norm of exactness or in increasing or decreasing their number).

The extension or restriction of the number of research categories in the empirical approach paradoxically does not occur through a systematic empirical method because it is not the facts that create the categories but the categories that create the facts. This form of progress is therefore arbitrary and has a purely theoretical basis. As a result, one theory of quality of life is arbitrarily exchanged for another without the benefit of critical discussion. Quality of life research demands that the empirical-quantitative and the empirical-qualitative methods be integrated and combined with theoretical considerations.

PARADIGMS OF QUALITY OF LIFE

The current quality of life debate has been confined to discussions of the merits of the natural science versus the humanistic approaches. These discussions have resulted in an exchange of preconceived, untenable viewpoints.

Both approaches define quality of life as "happiness" but define "happiness" in different ways. The natural science approach utilizes the concept of hedonism, through the categories of pleasure–displeasure. In the biological-mechanical paradigm the human being is viewed as "nature" or an isolated, mechanical being. The humanistic paradigm utilizes the concept of eudaemonism to define "happiness" through the categories of self-realization, inner peace, and harmony. The human being is seen as "culture," or a conscious social being.

The disagreement between the eudaemonists and the hedonists over the definition of happiness has become, in part, a discussion of the two paradigms. The argument here is that the problem is theoretically unsolvable. The result has been that many researchers have given up the debate regarding the definition of happiness and begun to measure quality of life without having previously defined it.

A NEW PARADIGM

It is possible to present a new paradigm that incorporates the concept of choice into the definition of happiness. A concrete, universal definition of happiness is impossible, as this concept varies from person to person. According to our new paradigm, the highest possible degree of personal freedom is necessary for an individual to choose and realize his goals for happiness.

In the natural science paradigm, "illness" is defined as disharmony with the biological-physical necessity. Within the humanistic paradigm it equals a collapse of meaning. Within our new paradigm, "illness" is defined as a restraint on or reduction of freedom.

The task of treatment in the natural science paradigm is to reestablish the harmony of necessity, and in the humanistic paradigm it is to reestablish meaning. The new paradigm defines it as the maximizing of freedom.

QUALITY OF LIFE AND THERAPEUTIC METHODS

The new concept of quality of life is not only a criterion for decision and choice but also an important part of a therapeutic method. Crisis situations become the new starting point for this paradigm.

Cancer, in contrast to many other diseases, creates two crises that are interrelated. The double crisis theory presents an opportunity to evaluate not only the crisis of integration but also the crisis caused by a diagnosis of cancer. Usually, however, only the crisis of the integration of the cancer experience is described.

The fundamental crisis occurs when everyday life collapses as the loss of the outside world is contemplated. The person is no longer an "anonymous being" but, instead, becomes an "I" who must deal with fright, both *for* and *of* himself. The inevitability of life is shaken, and the individual must depend on his own resources. The ego is shattered, and the individual is confronted with his basic lack of self. The security and confidence of being an anonymous being are revealed as illusory. The "I," rather than the surroundings, assumes control in a fundamental crisis.

The second part of the crisis of cancer revolves around integration of the illness into goal-oriented attitudes and behavior. If this crisis is treated in isolation, serious problems can arise. The patient, at this point, is reconstructing himself. The integration therefore is not of new into old but of new into new. The patient must also deal with the fact that he must try to solve his fundamental crisis alone, although it may be basically unsolvable. In addition, the process of solving the crisis of integration may block the solution of the fundamental crisis. Hospitalization further contributes to the individual's loss of self, conditioning him to patterns and values that belong to the institution, rather than to himself.

In summary, our paradigm demonstrates that quality of life is not only a criterion necessary for choosing a treatment strategy but also a concept that in and of itself becomes a therapeutic method. This method can be utilized in the complex crisis situations that result from an individual's withdrawal from a given value system that is no longer functional. The individual must construct a new system, using only himself as both a basis for and a test of validity. These new values are not "anonymous being" values but "I" values and therefore push the individual further into crisis. This crisis can force him to uphold and defend his decisions and values—and be strengthened by them.

The Quality of Life of Cancer Patients,
edited by N. K. Aaronson and J. Beckmann,
Raven Press, New York © 1987.

Measuring and Analyzing Quality of Life in Cancer Clinical Trials: A Review*

David R. Jones, *Peter M. Fayers, and **Jean Simons

*Clinical Epidemiology & Social Medicine, St. Georges Hospital Medical School, Cranmer Terrace, London SW17 ORE; *MRC Tuberculosis and Chest Diseases Unit, Brompton Hospital, London SW3 6HP; and **Hospital for Sick Children, London WC1N 3JH, England*

Many treatments for cancer are extremely unpleasant and often highly toxic, and too frequently they result in little if any prolongation of survival. Consequently many physicians are becoming increasingly interested in assessing the quality of life of patients on different treatments; a treatment that yields only minimal improvement in survival may be rejected because of its adverse side effects. Despite this fact, most current clinical trials evaluate only length of survival or the response of the tumor to treatment and simply describe the more obvious side effects such as adverse reactions and reduced blood counts.

Developing interest in quality of life is reflected in the increasing number of references that mention this phrase in the title: We found more than 200 such papers published during the period 1978 to 1980. The European Organization for Research on Treatment of Cancer (EORTC) has responded to this rise in interest by setting up a Study Group on Quality of Life (16). In a review of publications of cancer trials, Bardelli and Saracci (3) reported that over the period 1956 to 1976 fewer than 5% of trials measured quality of life as distinct from toxicity; of those that did, most used either the Karnofsky scale (30), Zubrod (66) method, or similar scales to assess functional status. Furthermore, most attempts to evaluate psychosocial, as distinct from physical, side effects of therapy have been confined to patients with breast cancer (4,12,47,51,52) and often to those treated by mastectomy (13,37,41,54,57).

Although clinical trials of drug treatments intended to give relief from pain (36) and from psychiatric symptoms such as depression (34) and insomnia (45) provide useful starting points for the development of methods of assessing quality of life, the principal objective of these treatments is to alleviate the symptoms that were the primary reason for presentation and hence often relatively clearly defined. The term "quality of life" and various synonyms are widely used throughout

---

* This chapter is a revised and extended version of the paper published in *Statistics in Medicine*, 2:429–446, 1983.

the social, psychological, and medical sciences, but definitions are elusive. Although most people have an intuitive understanding of quality of life, it is extremely difficult to define, and an adequate index of "quality" is probably impossible to construct. Rather than attempt a formal definition, we describe various indices and measurements that represent facets of the generally accepted concept of quality of life.

This chapter reviews methods of assessing quality of life with particular emphasis on techniques appropriate to clinical trials of cancer therapies in which the treatment frequently consists in cytotoxic chemotherapy given over a period of many months, possibly in pulses every few weeks. Other reviews (17) are available to complement this chapter; in particular, van Dam et al. (60) gave a general review and Krauth (33) considered analysis and philosophical issues in detail.

MEASURING QUALITY OF LIFE

Many of the problems in measuring the quality of life are those of measuring subjective variables, perceptions, attitudes, and judgments, perhaps exacerbated by the need to obtain information at a time when the patient is likely to be especially under stress and particularly sensitive to questions relating to the illness or its treatment. Furthermore, the form of the question may need to be restricted because some patients are unaware of the nature of their illness.

The problem of making subjective measurements in surveys is well known and is reviewed in detail by Kalton and Schuman (29), but many aspects of the problem remain to be answered. Furthermore, complications arise when data are collected by means of a self-assessment questionnaire, as is often the case in clinical trials. The response obtained depends on the ability of the investigator to (a) conceptualize the issues which are to be investigated, and (b) communicate these concepts to the respondent; the ability of the respondent to (c) read and understand the questions, (d) recall the relevant information, and (e) formulate the answer; and the respondent's (f) perception of the social acceptability of the answers he/she is considering, and (g) willingness to devote effort to answering the questions.

The training and experience of the assessor and his or her relationship with the patient may be expected to affect the patient's compliance and the assessments of quality of life obtained. Even when self-assessment is not used there are problems: Many clinicians experience difficulties even in making reliable assessments using the relatively familiar Karnofsky scale (27,64). If the assessor is a close relative of the patient and is responsible for reporting on the patient's quality of life, problems may result from confounding of the patient's view and the views of the observer. The danger that the assessor confuses his or her anxieties about the patient's disease with anxieties expressed by the patient must be regarded as severe. There may even be inconsistencies in assessments of relatively objective aspects of quality of life, e.g., the frequency and severity of vomiting and of sleeplessness.

What Questions Should Be Asked about Quality of Life?

Which facets of quality of life to assess depend on the nature of the disease and the treatment; for example, mastectomy for breast cancer produces different psychosocial problems from cytotoxic chemotherapy for lung cancer. The relative importance attached to each of these facets varies from subject to subject, as does the willingness to accept increased discomfort for a potential increase in survival (39). In the context of clinical trials a detailed assessment of quality of life may not be required, and often resources are not sufficient to allow, say, an extensive interview with each patient; those facets that may be affected by the treatment policies are of primary importance. However, the possibility that other aspects of quality of life interact with those most directly associated with the disease and its treatment should not be ruled out. Thus, for example, financial worries might result from restricted ability to work following disease or therapy, and such worries may adversely affect the quality of life following treatment.

Several standard scales have been used in those cancer trials in which an attempt has been made to assess quality of life. The best known is the Karnofsky scale (30), which is shown in Table 1. It is intended to assess the patient's overall ability to perform certain physical activities, using an 11-point scale (within three broad categories). In a similar way Zubrod et al. (66) evaluated patients on a 5-

TABLE 1. *Karnofsky performance status scale*

Condition	Performance status (%)	Comments
A: Able to carry on normal activity and to work. No special care is needed.	100	Normal. No complaints. No evidence of disease.
	90	Able to carry on normal activity. Minor signs or symptoms of disease.
	80	Normal activity with effort. Some signs or symptoms of disease.
B: Unable to work. Able to live at home and care for most personal needs. A varying degree of assistance is needed.	70	Cares for self. Unable to carry on normal activity or to do active work.
	60	Requires occasional assistance but is able to care for most of his needs.
	50	Requires considerable assistance and frequent medical care.
C: Unable to care for self. Requires equivalent of institutional or hospital care. Disease may be progressing rapidly.	40	Disabled. Requires special care and assistance.
	30	Severely disabled. Hospitalization indicated, although death not imminent.
	20	Hospitalization necessary, very sick, active supportive treatment necessary.
	10	Moribund. Fatal processes progressing rapidly.
	0	Dead.

point scale, and Carlens et al. (9) and Burge et al. (8) used a 6-point scale. The World Health Organization (62) advocated the use of a scale similar to that of Zubrod.

Although considered to be relatively objective, the reliability and validity of these scales, as discussed below, are questionable. (A "reliable" measure is one that is able to detect systematic patterns; a "valid" measure has general, predictive value outside the context of the present study—see below). In particular, they rely heavily on an overall assessment of physical performance; indeed, the Karnofsky scale was introduced as a measure of nursing dependency. Such scales may correlate poorly with the patient's feelings and perceptions of quality of life (56).

Craig et al. (13) extended the standard approach by asking two questions about physical performance and four questions about psychosocial functioning of patients with breast cancer. Some of the questions are of a very general nature, and others are much more specific. A similar approach was used by Morris et al. (41) and Roberts et al. (54).

A mixture of general and specific questions is also seen in the influential study by Priestman and Baum (52) with a related study reported by Baum et al. (4). In the first study 10 questions were asked of each patient relating to the general feeling of well-being, mood, level of activity, degree of pain, nausea, appetite, ability to perform housework, social activities, and general level of anxiety, with the final very general question "Is treatment helping?" In the later study, which was also concerned with the quality of life of women receiving chemotherapy for advanced breast cancer, 25 questions were asked. Ten were concerned with symptoms and side effects, 5 related to anxiety and depression, 5 more concerned personal relationships, and the last 5 were about aspects of physical performance. A broadly similar approach is represented by the work of Padilla et al. (46) and Palmer et al. (47), in which questions were asked about physical condition, side effects, and ability to perform important activities, together with broad questions about quality of life. A similar approach is adopted in a questionnaire designed by the EORTC Quality of Life Study Group (16) that comprises 28 questions.

There were differences between the Karnofsky, Zubrod, and other scales used to assess performance, and not surprisingly the more detailed ad hoc questionnaires show even greater variation in the wording of questions and in the form of scale used for the assessment (see below). For example:

1. EORTC (16): "Were you feeling low spirited yesterday?" (yes, no) "Overall, did you feel ill yesterday?" (yes, no)

Padilla et al. (46): "How good is your quality of life?" (linear analogue scale) "Is your life satisfying?" (linear analogue scale)

Palmer et al. (47): "Did you feel off color?" (4-point scale) "How much did the course of treatment interfere with your life?" (4-point scale)

The interpretation of the results obtained should take into account the dependence of the response on the wording and form of the question (see below).

Although studies that report quality of life assessments usually assess toxicity as well, it is perhaps worth noting that with aggressive cytotoxic therapy the dosage may be deliberately increased until it is unacceptable or dangerous to go further. Conversely, if excessively high toxicity has been reported, the dosage of subsequent pulses may be reduced. It is important to record changes in therapy, as these changes and the reasons for them may modify the aspects of quality of life being reported.

When to Ask about Quality of Life

Ideally the data collected should describe quality of life of patients before, during, and after treatment, giving a continuous picture of any changes. More practically, however, reports may be sought on the quality of life during specified time periods or between clinic visits, the patient being asked to give an overall measure of quality of life over that time period. The choice of time scale on which to make these inquiries must depend on the natural history of the disease and the timing and pattern of treatment. If there is an expectation of life of many years, the quality of life is unlikely to be estimated more frequently than monthly or at each outpatient or clinic visit, as in most studies involving mastectomy for breast cancer. On the other hand, during an intensive period of treatment it may be important to have frequent measures of the quality of life, perhaps at intervals of 1 to 2 days. Priestman and Baum (52), in their breast cancer study, asked questions about the quality of life before treatment and 3 months later, as well as 3 days after each major pulse of treatment to assess toxicity.

There are several constraints on the frequency and timing of inquiries about quality of life. If investigations are too infrequent, transient effects, most likely during and after each treatment pulse, may be missed. On the other hand, inquiries that are too frequent may well be construed as an imposition on the patient, especially as it may be a time of particular stress because of the disease and its treatment. It has been suggested that patients might find frequent and detailed questioning tedious, irksome, and even depressing. However, in contradistinction to this, van Dam et al. (60), among others, has suggested that the inquiry may itself have some therapeutic or cathartic value. Patients may regard the inquiry as reflecting real interest in the quality of their life or as offering an opportunity to communicate their feelings to the physician. In either case, even the act of making an inquiry may modify the quality of life. Noncompliance has, however, been a severe problem in some of the studies in which a detailed attempt to assess quality of life has been made. For example, Baum et al. (4) reported that only 51 of 91 patients filled in assessments, and nearly a half of them did so only sporadically. Compliance is likely to depend on the way in which the assessment forms are explained to patients if self-assessment is required, the degree of encouragement given, and the frequency with which the completed forms are collected and inspected. Hence in a multicenter trial patient compliance may vary considerably from center to center.

Who Should Ask and Who Should Be Asked

Few clinical trials of cancer treatment have involved assessments by medical staff other than doctors (e.g., nurses or social workers), although it could be argued that concern with a patient's quality of life is more directly a responsibility of the social worker than of the clinician. Furthermore, an experienced and sympathetic nurse or social worker may be more able than a clinician to gain the patient's confidence and is more likely to hear any unfavorable comments on treatment; some patients may try to please their doctor and therefore may refrain from disclosing their feelings.

When quality of life is assessed it is usual to address the questions to the patient; however, some trials include assessments by a relative. For example, a study by Hinton (25) included and contrasted similar mood assessments made by the patient, the spouse, and a nurse. Few studies describe a baseline assessment, either for patients before treatment or for control subjects.

Method Effects: Dependence of Responses on the Form of the Question

"Method effects," i.e., the dependence of responses on the form and context of the questions, have received considerable attention from psychometricians. A summary of basic results is given in textbooks on questionnaire design, such as that of Sudman and Bradburn (59).

The questions fall into two major categories; they can either be *open* questions, to which the respondent is free to make any response, or *closed* (fixed choice or precoded) questions in which the respondent is supplied with a list of alternative responses or a fixed scale on which to mark a response. Open questions may be less likely to influence or restrict the possible responses but are clearly less easy to categorize and analyze than the responses to closed questions. Hence open questions are rarely used on their own, except that "any other comments" are often invited, though are less frequently analyzed. When closed questions are used, two decisions about their form have to be made. Should a continuous or a categorical scale be offered? Should a standard scale or an ad hoc scale specifically be constructed for the current trial be used? Many of the general recommendations for the design of forms for use in clinical trials made by Wright and Haybittle (63) also apply to the collection of information about the quality of life of patients in a clinical trial, whether the forms are to be completed by the patient or by someone else.

Measurement Scales

Continuous (Linear Analogue) Scales

Linear analogue scales are often used to assess subjective symptoms such as mood, and it has been suggested that these scales are easier to complete than categorical closed questions. For each variable or aspect of interest, a fixed-length line is presented to the respondent, the ends of the line being labeled with words describing the two extreme states of the variable if the scale is bipolar, or a neutral state and an extreme state if it is unipolar. The respondent is asked to mark a point on the line appropriate to the perceived value between the extremes indicated by the ends of the line. The distance of the point from one end (or possibly from the midpoint) of the scale is recorded. This method can be used for assessment by either the patient or an observer. It is clear that fine discrimination is provided in theory by this analogue method, in contrast to the discrete categories provided by categorical scales. However, when Remington et al. (53) compared the use of categorical scales and the linear analogue self-assessment scale in reporting the result of Wing's Present State Examination (PSE) (61) for classification of psychiatric patients, they found that the reliability and validity of the linear analogue self-assessment scale was not markedly superior to that of the categorical representation. (It should be borne in mind that the PSE was originally designed for use with a categorical scale.) In practice, ease of administration, coding, and analysis may be major factors militating in favor of categorical scales.

Bond and Lader (6) provided a brief historical review of the use of analogue scales in rating a variety of subjective feelings and gave some prominence to the work of Aitken (1) in developing such techniques in trials of acute effects of drug therapy. Early and influential examples from breast cancer trials were studies by Priestman and Baum (52), and Padilla et al. (46) provided a more recent example.

Categorical Scales

Although categorical scales have the advantages of being more familiar, requiring less instruction for their use, and being precoded for analyses, a number of problems arise when they are used.

1. It may be difficult to ensure that the categories are both appropriate and clearly placed in an ordinally correct position, especially if there is any suggestion that the scale being measured in a particular question has more than one dimension. For example, if pain is perceived as unidimensional, it should not be difficult to use phrases that rank the various categories of pain in an increasing order. However, if duration, intensity, character, and degree of localization of pain vary, it may not be possible to place the categories in an order that is widely accepted: The relative positions of a short bout of acute pain and a longer bout of less severe pain are not obvious.

2. The choice of the number of categories to be offered is clearly interrelated with the issues of the previous paragraph. Too many categories may lead to difficulties in distinguishing shades of meaning for adjacent categories, and too few are likely to leave the respondent with a choice in which no category closely matches

the answer the respondent wishes to give. Too many categories may also lead to unreliability in the sense that respondents do not consistently choose the same answer from the closely adjacent possibilities in the same circumstances (5,32,38).

In a small experiment using a well established method for assessing psychiatric symptomatology, i.e., the PSE (61), Remington et al. (53) compared the reliability of categorical scales with different numbers of categories. They concluded that, in this context, reliability does not alter materially with the number of categories, up to a value of 4. Lissitz and Green (35), however, suggested that a 5-point scale is the optimum, whereas, exceptionally, Ferguson (18) reported an increase in reliability with the number of categories. It seems likely that, for many assessments, a 4- or 5-point scale is appropriate.

3. The question arises whether to allow a middle alternative (e.g., in a 3-point scale) or not (e.g., a 4-point scale). Presser and Schuman (50) found that, although many respondents selected the neutral middle category if offered, these respondents came proportionately from the two extremes and so the balance between the extremes was not affected.

Standard Scales

The above problems could indicate a need to use a standard and well tested scale such as the Karnofsky, Zubrod, or Carlens scale. However, even the most frequently used scale of physical performance, the Karnofsky scale, was found by Hutchinson et al. (27) and Yates et al. (64) to have poor reliability.

The standard questionnaires for collecting information on psychosocial aspects of quality of life may have better reliability. In general, however, these questionnaires take some time to apply and require training and experience on the part of the interviewers. In the field of cancer several scales originally developed for use in psychiatric populations have been used, although their suitability for this purpose is untested. For example, the Psychosocial Adjustment to Illness Scale (15) was used in a study of patients with Hodgkin's disease (42); the Hamilton Rating Scale (23) for depression was used by Morris et al. (41) in a study of mastectomy for breast cancer, and the PSE (61) was used by Maguire et al. (37) in a study of breast cancer patients. Studies of cancer patients by Cooper et al. (12), Craig et al. (13), Gordon et al. (22), and Plumb and Holland (49) used other questionnaires. Standard scales have also been developed for the assessment of "health status" in a wider context. The Nottingham Health Profile (26) and perhaps Goldberg's General Health Questionnaire (21) may be applicable to the assessment of quality of life in cancer trials.

Interpretation of the Questions and Answers

There are a number of problems associated with the wording of questions and their answers. For example, most patients have their own interpretation of the meaning of such terms as "anxiety" and "depression," but it may not accord with the more specific meaning used by psychologists and varies from person to person. Psychologists generally consider a set of multi-item questions more reliable and valid than a single question about, say, mood.

Moreover, when categories labeled "normal" or "as usual" are employed, it may be unclear whether the patient is intended to infer additional phrases such as "normal for someone of my age," or "as usual before my illness," or "as usual before my treatment but since my illness." Duration of illness and the patient's memory may be relevant factors as well. Furthermore, some patients (and even some healthy subjects) may continually complain of being miserable or depressed. Pain thresholds and discomfort tolerances vary considerably; some patients are stoical and maintain they are "fine" despite clear evidence to the contrary. In particular, even the reported severity of relatively objective symptoms, e.g., the amount of vomiting, may bear little relation to the level of discomfort suffered by the patient. Furthermore, there may be only loose linkage between the objective conditions and a patient's perception of well-being. For example, in a question about nausea and vomiting, whereas nausea might appear to an observer to be less important than vomiting, to a patient it is often much "worse" than the vomiting, which may be of shorter duration.

For such reasons it is especially difficult to describe the quality of life in a single group of patients. It may be, however, that many of the problems are reduced if only the differences between two groups of well-matched patients are analyzed, the assumption being that any bias in the assessment is similar in each group.

ASSESSMENT OF METHODS

If a new method has been developed for measuring quality of life or if a question-naire has been transferred to a different environment, it is necessary to evaluate its *reliability* and *validity*. More obviously, it is also important for scales to be *sensitive* and able to detect meaningful changes in a patient's quality of life. The assessment of measurement methods was fully discussed by Zeller and Carmines (65).

Reliability of Quality of Life Data

Because there are no "true" or absolute measures of quality of life to act as a yardstick, the meaning of any assessment is open to some conjecture. In such circumstances it is important to evaluate the repeatability of the assessment when made at different times under similar circumstances, using the same questionnaire. Similarly, the repeatability should be evaluated using different assessors (patient/spouse/nurse/doctor) and perhaps in different places (home/hospital). Thus, for example, Priestman and Baum (52) compared assessments of quality of life made by their patients when alone with those made in the presence of a doctor a day earlier, whereas Padilla et al. (46) reported the results of comparing one assessment with another made by the same individual after a short interval. Failure to find good agreement between two such sets of data is likely to be worrying, although sometimes the assumption that the conditions in the first and second assessments are the same is not valid, particularly if the time interval between the two is substantial or if there is reason to expect that two assessors have a different perception of the variables assessed. This may be the case if the assessments of a clinician are compared with those of a patient—or even if a patient's assessment is compared with that of the spouse.

The methods of analysis used in reliability assessment are simple and familiar; plotting a scatter diagram of the test–retest scores is particularly valuable (52), and Cohen's tests (27) for the agreement of two or more judges form a natural method of analysis (11,53). Fleiss and Cohen (19) reviewed measures of agreement and recommended the use of weighted kappa as an intraclass correlation coefficient. Cichetti (10) proposed an alternative measure.

There is, unfortunately, a tendency to regard correlation coefficients between the test and retest scores as an adequate measure of the reliability of the sample. This approach is questionable as Altman and Bland (2) indicated in some detail in their paper on method comparison studies. They recommended various solutions, such as plotting the within-patient standard deviation against the mean. Padilla et al. (46) suggested using the proportion of retest scores that lie within a small distance of the corresponding original test score, e.g., the proportion of linear analogue retest scores lying within 10% of the original test score.

Validity of Quality of Life Data

Whereas reliability is concerned with the extent to which the measurements are consistent and repeatable, validity is concerned with the broader and more difficult question of how well the measurements actually assess the variables of interest. Unfortunately, no absolute values are available for a direct check of validity. There are two broad areas to be considered. The first, which is called *content validity,* is the extent to which the measurements included in the assessment appear to cover all of the issues of interest and appear to be applicable for such a purpose. Consensus approval before use is a practical approach to assessments of this kind of validity.

The second, *construct validity,* is a widely recognized issue although not one on which a clear-cut approach to evaluation can be found. The validation has to be indirect and carried out by attempting to ascertain if the relation between the variables measured is consistent with prior expectations on the basis of an underlying theory (or some less formal conceptualization) of the aspects of quality of life investigated. For example, Padilla et al. investigated the construct validity of their 14 questions by performing principal component analysis; three major factors were identified, and because these corresponded broadly with the three areas of content originally identified for investigation it was concluded that the questionnaire had sufficient construct validity. Naturally it is important to check that the responses to interrelated questions are plausible and consistent. Thus in general we would not expect answers to broad questions about the overall tolerability of treatment to indicate that the treatment was acceptable if several of the key questions about specific aspects of quality of life indicated that that quality is actually very poor. Similarly, if a patient's condition is deteriorating rapidly, with objective symptoms such as weight loss being apparent, it is likely that some of the other aspects of quality of life (e.g., anxiety) should reflect a change.

Morrow et al. (43) indicated an attempt to perform construct validity in their study of children with Hodgkin's disease; van Dam et al. (60) referred to further investigations at The Netherlands Cancer Institute and drew attention to the important point that questionnaires tapping psychosocial distress have usually been validated using patients with psychiatric problems; it is not clear to what extent the construct validity thus established applies to cancer patients.

Several mathematical methods have been suggested for examining construct validity. Morrow (42) gave an example of "multitrait-multimethod" analysis of a correlation matrix, and Zeller and Carmines (65) described various methods of analysis.

ANALYZING QUALITY OF LIFE DATA

In general, observations are made at intervals, not necessarily evenly spaced; if linear analogue methods have been used, the data may be regarded as continuous, although perhaps not from a normal distribution. However, categorical scales yield discrete data, often ordered, sometimes dichotomous. In studies in which questions are asked only once there are few special problems of describing or comparing groups of data, e.g., Palmer et al. (47); it is the repetition of measurements over time that leads to difficulties.

Analyses can be considered under two main headings: *description* of the data collected and *comparison* of patients in different groups (usually treatment groups).

Description of Quality of Life Data

The questions that may be posed for analysis of quality of life include: (a) How many and which patients suffer impaired quality? (b) For how long, how frequently, and when (relative to treatment) does this occur? (c) How severe is it? (Severity usually varies with time.) If the data are continuous, simple descriptions of groups of patients are provided by estimates of location and dispersion of the measurements and their changes over various time intervals. For example, Baum et al. (4) plotted patient-group means and standard errors of each variable at each time interval. They presented such a plot for depression. However, it is difficult to regard this plot as an absolute or informative measure: What is average depression over a group of patients? Baum et al. used these means and standard errors primarily to compare groups of patients, as discussed below, which is likely to be a more realistic use of the data.

For discrete data, statements such as "75% of the patients vomited more than once after their treatment pulse, but 30% of these vomited only for the first day" provide summaries of the patterns experienced. This type of report leads naturally to descriptions of the pattern of change of various components of quality of life in an individual patient over time. Similarly, it may be of interest to describe the changes experienced by groups of patients, especially during development of the disease and its treatment. In particular, the relations between the prevailing levels before, during, and after treatment are likely to be important.

Most of these analyses can be accomplished by simple statistical methods. The most important issues are to what extent the assumptions usually implied by use of such methods are valid and to what extent interesting and important features of the data are obscured by the summarizing measures. For example, can a patient who vomits twice in one day be equated to two patients who vomit once each or to one patient who vomits once on each of two successive days? Although descriptive methods are generally used, life-table analysis may also be applicable. Herson (24) gave an example of analysis of toxicity data.

The pattern of quality of life over time for individual patients is perhaps best presented graphically. An interesting example of this approach is given by Nou and Aberg (44) who presented Carlens vitagrams for each patient, showing a broad summary of quality of life on a scale not dissimilar to that of Karnofsky. They claimed to recognize and classify the patients into several distinct patterns of changing quality of life. Although this approach is an appealing descriptive tool, it is questionable if it is valid to compare over subgroups the proportions of patients classified, subjectively, into each type of vitagram; there is a danger of forcing patients artificially into preconceived patterns. However, such graphic techniques are clearly of importance as exploratory tools to suggest appropriate groupings and methods of analysis. For example, such a graph aids the decision about the period of time over which to report a mean level of quality of life after treatment.

More sophisticated methods than those indicated above can be used for the description of patterns over time for individual patients. The data collected on quality of life over a series of time intervals take the form of sets of interrelated time series of data, and formal time series modeling of these data sets and estimation of trends, autocorrelation, and so on is possible. There are, however, some difficulties. Often the data are categorical rather than continuous. Relatively few time series methods are directly applicable to such data, and it seems likely that transient nonperiodic behavior of the quality of life data is of special interest. The stationarity assumption is therefore in question and the effort involved in fitting time series models is probably not justified in practice. The data are also unlikely to have been collected with complete regularity, and there are likely to be missing observations, further complicating the practical application of time series models, although this problem may be less than in psychiatric trials.

It is likely to be even more difficult to model the interrelations between the time series corresponding to different aspects of quality of life, although, for example, it would be of interest to see whether anxiety increases as the level of pain increases or in a different way. A whole series of such interrelationships could in principle be explored by regression modeling of the sets of time series for individual patients. In the same way the dependence of anxiety on background variables describing the prognosis of the patient could be contemplated.

In summary, at the *individual patient* level little more than application of graphic display of patterns over time and ad hoc use of descriptive measures ("the level of pain was reported as acceptable or better for the period 6 weeks after treatment onward") is likely to be worthwhile. This approach was used by Gilbert et al. (20), who reported time interval averages of the Karnofsky rating and in particular whether the rating was "good" for a substantial period of follow-up.

All of the above problems are encountered again when descriptions of patterns of quality of life experienced in *groups of patients* as a whole are to be made. The definition of summary measures, such as definition of the time interval over which to average results, must generally be made after inspection of the data on individual patients. However, in some cases there is prior knowledge, enabling expected patterns to be defined. It is usually of interest to see how the patterns change during the period immediately after each pulse of treatment, although the definition of the duration of this period is of course important. For example, Schottenfield and Robbins (57) compared the proportions of women with breast cancer who were working before and after treatment, but both of these proportions, particularly the latter, depend strongly on the time at which the observations were made relative to the treatment.

Descriptions of patterns are in general straightforward; the proportion achieving prespecified levels of quality of life by a given time is typical of the measures used. When the data are continuous, as they are if obtained from linear analogue scales, it may be desirable to transform the data to achieve approximate normality before describing the quality of subgroups. Bond and Lader (6), Aitkin (1), and Baum et al. (4) referred to logarithmic transformation of data obtained from analogue scales to achieve approximate normality.

Comparative Data Analysis

In phase III cancer clinical trials outcome is usually measured in terms of survival (or time to regression or relapse of disease) and response to treatment. We are now advocating the addition of quality of life assessments and comparisons among treatment groups. The principal problems that arise are first that the quality of life variables are relatively "soft," with the consequence that a particular choice of measure may not be universally acceptable, and second that a multiplicity of measures must be used because of the multidimensional aspects of quality of life to be investigated. Apart from the obvious extra complexity, the lack of knowledge about the interrelations and the inferential difficulties resulting from the multiplicity of measures may be severe. However, in the comparative approach biases in and uncertainties of interpretation of particular components of the quality of life measurements may be effectively canceled between the two groups compared, so that although the absolute measure is in doubt the comparison between the two groups is more secure.

The initial approaches to comparative data analysis of this kind clearly parallel the methods proposed earlier for description of the patterns seen in a group of patients. They similarly parallel methods used for analysis of the more traditional outcome measures, such as survival or response to treatment. Thus a natural approach is to compare the proportions of the two treatment groups who report, for example, sleeplessness, nausea, or anxiety during a certain period or beginning a certain time after treatment (or even in anticipation of a further pulse of treatment). Simple statistical techniques such as t-tests, possibly after variance stabilizing transformation, may be used (4). Rosenman and Choi (55) applied survival-curve analysis to a Karnofsky scale by defining a grade of "less than 60" as the event of interest.

Analysis of Quality and Duration of Survival

In a cancer clinical trial, survival from treatment to some key endpoint such as death or relapse is very likely to be an important, and perhaps paramount, outcome measure. Separate analyses are thus likely to be made for quality of life and for survival. However, one theoretical solution is to combine duration and quality of survival in a single model for the purposes of the comparison.

An informal weighting of duration of survival against its quality is probably made by the clinician when weighing the pros and cons of the various courses of management for a particular case. A less effective treatment (in terms of survival) might be chosen because the side effects are also less severe. However, it is difficult to quantify and generalize such a decision process. Thus, for example, equating 1 day on which the respondent reported himself or herself free of pain to, say, 3 days on which there was severe pain (and so on for the other aspects of the quality of life) would permit the construction of a quality-weighted duration of survival for each patient. Standard survival analysis techniques could in principle be used to analyze and compare weighted survival times in the treatment groups.

The weight functions could come from several sources such as (a) guesses or prejudices of the medical staff involved in the trial or (b) questioning patients about the relative values they attach to different lengths of survival and different qualities of survival (58). McNeil et al. (39,40) and Pauker and Kassirer (48) have derived "utility" curves for individual patients and recommended that each patient's attitudes be examined in detail and by formal utility analysis techniques before the physician decides on a course of hazardous or unpleasant treatment. However, the patients are likely to be under considerable stress and might not make consistent decisions. Also, although the physician may have information about *group* survival probabilities, he is unlikely to be able or willing to predict the effect a treatment may have on an individual patient.

An alternative and more easily justified approach is to separate the quality and duration of survival variables and to regard the endpoints used in defining survival together with particular levels of some of the quality of life variables as multiple endpoints for simultaneous stochastic processes. The choice of the endpoint is again arbitrary. Data of this kind could be analyzed by several methods. Extensions of the simplest models are required for survival data, in which there is just one possible endpoint (usually death) for each patient. For example, the proportional hazards model (7,28) could be extended to allow several possible failure types or endpoints, e.g., death, the onset of severe depression, or the onset of chronic pain. As described by David and Moeschberger (14) and by Kalbfleisch and Prentice (28), estimates can be made of the distribution of the latent interval to each type of endpoint. Other useful extensions would be to multistage and multistate models (31). Such models are unlikely to be appropriate for analysis of the short-term transient effects of treatments such as cytotoxic chemotherapy but may be more suitable for evaluating trends in quality of life, e.g., after mastectomy.

TWO NEW METHODS FOR ASSESSING QUALITY OF LIFE

We now illustrate how the methods and problems described above have determined two questionnaires that are currently being used for quality of life assessments.

Diary Card

The diary card was developed by the Medical Research Council's (MRC) Tuberculosis and Chest Diseases Unit and the Clinical Oncology and Radiotherapeutics Unit. It is currently in use in several MRC cancer treatment studies.

Because cytotoxic treatment is given in pulses, with accompanying side effects that may be either immediate but transient (e.g., vomiting) or longer-lasting and perhaps less immediate in onset (e.g., alopecia), it was decided that daily answers to several questions would be desirable. This decision determined that: (a) self-assessment as outpatients was necessary; (b) linear analogue scales would be impractical as several questions per day per patient would need to be answered; (c) only a few simple questions could be asked. It was decided to use 5-point scales and to select obvious and relatively objective side effects (nausea and vomiting) as well as less objective questions on mood and general condition. A particular point to note is that, as already mentioned, categories such as "average" mood are ambiguous: perhaps "normal for me before my present illness" is preferable, but such distinctions are difficult to convey succinctly and clearly on a simple card or form.

The card illustrated in Fig. 1 is prefolded and compact. The word "cancer" does not appear on it because some patients may be unaware of the exact disease they suffer. For similar reasons, disease-specific symptoms such as "pain" were avoided. Ample space has been left for the patient to add extra information or comments.

A new card is provided at each clinic attendance, and the patient is assisted in completing the information for the first day of the period. Although most patients require only minimal explanation on how to complete the card, it is essential to explain *why* the information is required. Patient compliance in completing the card varies greatly from center to center; some centers report that their patients dislike and refuse to complete the cards, whereas in others patients meticulously complete them and add extra messages or comments directed to their physician. The cards can thus provide both potentially valuable information for the comparative trial and much useful detail about the patient's condition for the physician.

When the patients attend the clinic the physician also makes assessments of general condition and activity and asks about toxicity. The use of psychotropic and other drugs that might induce a symptom or mood-modifying behavior is noted, although it might be reasonably argued that such drugs are part of the overall policy of management and that it is only the outcome that is relevant. Other mood-modifying events, which are unfortunately almost impossible to measure, are the times when patients first learn that they have cancer or metastases, or when they realize that their disease is not responding to treatment.

Possible descriptions of the data are the following.

1. Approximately 73% of patients vomited at least once after their treatment pulse, but 48% of these vomited only during the first day.

2. While chemotherapy was being given, 5% of patient-days were accompanied by nausea without vomiting, and a further 7% of patient-days included vomiting.

3. After the first pulse of chemotherapy 30% of patients reported feeling "very miserable," but after the fifth pulse this figure was reduced to 20% of patients.

The validity and reliability of the data collected in these studies are being assessed and will be published elsewhere. We hope to examine if the card is sensitive enough to at least detect known changes in the patients' health, and, conversely, if major changes in the patients' reporting appear to relate to changes observed by the physician. We will be considering both the absolute levels reported on the cards and the changes since previous cards.

Examples of analyses being made include the following.

1. Comparison of patients' assessments with physicians' assessments

2. Relation of patients' assessment to more objective variables that might reflect overall health (e.g., weight loss and survival)

3. Assessment of the relative magnitude of short-term changes (e.g., between

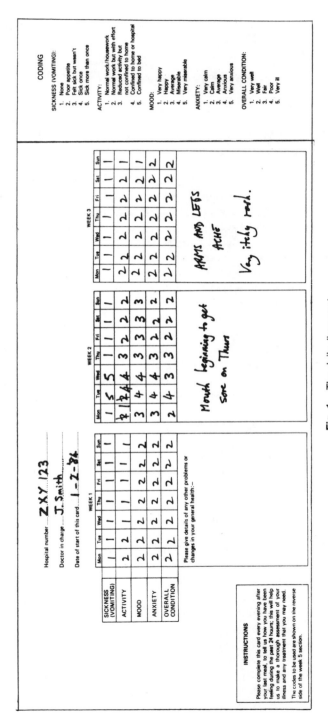

Fig. 1. The daily diary card.

pulses 1 and 2) in contrast to changes over a longer period (pulses 1 and 6), and if these changes relate to general deterioration or improvement of the patient

Self-Assessment Questionnaire

A second example is provided by a randomized multicenter controlled trial of two therapies for poor risk neuroblastoma (European Neuroblastoma Study Group). A parent of each child in the trial is asked to complete a "self-assessment" questionnaire each week during and for the first 4 months after treatment. Clinicians are asked to record briefly at each outpatient visit their impression of the child's quality of life. The two assessments will be compared. The questionnaire comprises mainly closed questions, but an open question invites any comments the parent wishes to make on the child's health, attitudes, and treatment during the week. The answers given to this question will be subjected to a content analysis. It is hoped that this will give useful guidance on the issues to be covered by questions of closed form in subsequent questionnaires as well as provide information of interest per se. The closed questions are in categorical form, the parent being asked to assess the degree to which the child's activity has been restricted by the illness, levels of pain, sickness, fever, appetite, hearing difficulty (a potential side effect of the trial therapy), sleeplessness, degree of worry about hair loss, and apprehension about the next hospital visit.

The parents are also asked to make an overall assessment of the child's happiness and enjoyment of life and to record *their* level of worry about their child's health and *their* perception of the acceptability of the treatment. Details of medications for pain, insomnia, and vomiting are requested.

The quality of life data collected in this way will not be analyzed and presented until recruitment to the trial and allocation to treatment has ceased. However, the reaction of parents of the first 20 children who used the assessment form at The Hospital for Sick Children, London is reported briefly. At this hospital the form is given to parents by their medical social worker, who explains its purpose and offers guidance on how to complete it. Completed forms are collected by the same person at subsequent hospital admissions or clinic visits. Introducing and supplying the form helps to initiate and consolidate the parent–social worker relationship; discussion of the form and of the parents' answers helps to identify and facilitate discussion of the medicosocial problems associated with the illness and its treatment. Collection of the form by someone other than the treating clinician encourages open reporting of problems with the treatment and care received. On the whole, the reaction of the parents to use of the form has been favorable, with only three of the 20 families discontinuing its use. Several parents commented that using the form was beneficial to them as it offered the opportunity to contribute to the treatment in some way.

Apart from minor problems with the layout of the assessment form, one major criticism emerges from its early use: Questions about the response of family members to the child's illness and treatment as well as cross-validating questions are too limited, as a consequence of keeping the form as short as possible.

CONCLUSIONS

There are difficulties inherent in almost all aspects of the definition, collection, and analysis of data about quality of life in patients undergoing treatment for cancer. Nonetheless, such data describe an important aspect of treatment and should not be ignored merely on the grounds of the practical and theoretical difficulties involved. It may be argued, however, that in view of the problems of data definition and collection too much sophistication in analysis would be misguided—that methods used for analysis should broadly match the quality of the data. With so many difficulties the only hope for progress is the careful step-by-step evaluation of each assumption made in the collection and analysis of the data. This approach is advocated by Kalton and Schuman (29) in the wider context of investigating the influence of survey methodology on the responses obtained. As a large program of detailed investigations is required, some standardization and coordination of methods and investigation seems desirable if progress is to be made quickly. It is hoped that this will result from an increased interest in these issues on the part of statisticians involved in clinical trials.

ACKNOWLEDGMENTS

The authors wish to thank members of the MRC Working Parties and of the European Neuroblastoma Study Group for their cooperation in studies involving assessment of quality of life, and *Statistics in Medicine* (John Wiley) for permission to adapt and extend our earlier paper (17). Laurence Freedman and Alison Pickett were closely involved in developing the diary card and contributed to many of the ideas presented in this chapter.

REFERENCES

1. Aitken, R. C. B. (1969): Measurement of feelings using visual analogue scales. *Proc. R. Soc. Med.*, 62:989–993.
2. Altman, D., and Bland, J. M. (1983): Measurement in medicine: The analysis of method comparison studies. *Statistician,* 32:307–318.
3. Bardelli, D., and Saracci, R. (1978): Measuring the quality of life in cancer clinical trials: A sample survey of published trials. *UICC Techn. Rep.*, 36:75–94.
4. Baum, M., Priestman, T., and Jones, E. M. (1979): A comparison of the quality of life in a controlled trial comparing endocrine with cytotoxic therapy for advanced breast cancer. In: *Breast Cancer: Experimental and Clinical Aspects,* edited by H. T. Mauridson and P. Palshof. Pergamon Press, London.
5. Bendig, A. W. (1954): Reliability and the number of rating scale categories. *J. Appl. Psychol.,* 38:38–40.
6. Bond, A., and Lader, M. (1974): Use of analog scales in rating subjective feelings. *Br. J. Med. Psychol.,* 47:211–218.
7. Breslow, N. E. (1975): Analysis of survival data under the proportional hazards model. *Int. Stat. Rev.,* 43:45–58.
8. Burge, P. S., Prankerd, T. A. J., Richards, J. D. M., Sare, M., Thompson, D. S., and Wright, P. (1975): Quality and quantity of survival in acute myeloid leukaemia. *Lancet,* 2:621–624.

9. Carlens, E., Dahlstrom, G., and Nou, E. (1970): Comparative measurements of quality of survival of lung cancer patients after diagnosis. *Scand. J. Respir. Dis.*, 51:268–275.
10. Cichetti, D. V. (1976): Assessing inter-rater reliability for rating scales: Resolving some basic issues. *Br. J. Psychiatry,* 129:452–456.
11. Cohen, J. (1960): A coefficient of agreement for nominal scales. *Educ. Psychol. Meas.*, 20:37–46.
12. Cooper, A. F., Meadle, C. S., Russel, A. R., and Smith, D. C. (1979): Psychiatric morbidity associated with adjuvant chemotherapy following mastectomy for breast cancer. *Br. J. Surg.*, 66:362.
13. Craig, T. J., Comstock, G. W., and Geiser, P. B. (1974): The quality of survival in breast cancer: A case-control comparison. *Cancer*, 33:1451–1457.
14. David, H. A., and Moeschberger, M. L. (1978): *The Theory of Competing Risks.* Griffin, London.
15. Derogatis, L. R. (1976): *Scoring and Procedures Manual for PAIS.* Clinical Psychometric Research, Baltimore.
16. EORTC (1981–1982): *Proceedings of the EORTC Quality of Life Workshops (May 1981, November 1981, June 1982).* EORTC, Brussels.
17. Fayers, P. M., and Jones, D. R. (1983): Measuring and analysing quality of life in cancer clinical trials: A review. *Stat. Med.*, 2:429–446.
18. Ferguson, L. W. (1941): A study of the Likert technique of attitude scale construction. *J. Soc. Psychol.*, 13:51–57.
19. Fleiss, J. L., and Cohen, J. (1973): The equivalence of weighted kappa and the intraclass correlation coefficient as measures of reliability. *Educ. Psychol. Meas.*, 33:613–619.
20. Gilbert, H. A., Kagan, A. R., Nussbaum, H., et al. (1977): Evaluation of radiation-therapy for bone metastases—pain relief and the quality of life. *AJR*, 129:1095–1096.
21. Goldberg, D. P. (1972) *The Detection of Psychiatric Illness by Questionnaire.* Oxford University Press, London.
22. Gordon, W. A., et al. (1980): Efficacy of psychosocial intervention with cancer patients. *J. Consult. Clin. Psychol.*, 48:743–759.
23. Hamilton, M. (1967): Development of a rating scale for primary depressive illness. *Br. J. Soc. Clin. Psychol.*, 6:278–296.
24. Herson, J. (1980): Evaluation of toxicity: Statistical considerations. *Cancer Treat. Rep.*, 64:463–468.
25. Hinton, J. (1979): Comparison of places and policies for terminal care. *Lancet*, 1:29–32.
26. Hunt, S. M., McKenna, S. P., McEwen, J., Williams, J., and Papp, E. (1981): The Nottingham Health Profile: Subjective health status and medical consultations. *Soc. Sci. Med.*, 15A:221–229.
27. Hutchinson, T. A., Boyd, N. F., and Feinstein, A. R. (1979): Scientific problems in clinical scales as demonstrated in the Karnofsky index of performance status. *J. Chronic Dis.*, 32:661–666.
28. Kalbfleisch, J. D., and Prentice, R. L. (1980): *The Statistical Analysis of Failure Time Data.* Wiley, New York.
29. Kalton, G., and Schuman, H. (1982): The effect of the question on survey responses. *J. R. Stat. Soc. (A)*, 145:42–73.
30. Karnofsky, D., and Burchenal, J. H. (1949): Clinical evaluation of chemotherapeutic agents in cancer. In: *Evaluation of Chemotherapeutic Agents*, edited by C. M. Macleod. Columbia University Press, New York.
31. Kay, R. (1982): The analysis of transition times in multistate stochastic processes using proportional hazard regression models. *Communications Stat.*, 11:1743–1756.
32. Komorita, S. S., and Graham, W. K. (1965): Number of scale points and the reliability of scales. *Educ. Psychol. Meas.*, 4:987–995.
33. Krauth, J. Objective measurements of the quality of life. In: *Proceedings of the Second Symposium on Clinical Trials in Early Breast Cancer.* Heidelberg.
34. Lader, M. (1981): The clinical assessment of depression. *Br. J. Clin. Pharmacol.*, 11:5–14.
35. Lissitz, R. W., and Green, S. B. (1975): Effect of the number of scale points on reliability: A Monte Carlo approach. *J. Appl. Psychol.*, 60:10–13.
36. Littlejohns, D. W., and Vere, D. W. (1981): The clinical assessment of analgesic drugs. *Br. J. Clin. Pharmacol.*, 11:319–332.
37. Maguire, P., Tait, A., Brooke, M., Thomas, C., and Sellwood, R. (1980): Effect of counselling on the psychiatric morbidity associated with mastectomy. *Br. Med. J.*, 281:1454–1455.
38. Matell, M. S., and Jacoby, J. (1971): Is there an optimal number of alternatives for Likert scale items? Study 1: Reliability and validity. *Educ. Psychol. Measurement*, 31:657–674.

39. McNeil, B. J., Weichselbaum, R., and Pauker, S. G. (1978): Fallacy of the 5-year survival in lung cancer. *N. Engl. J. Med.,* 299:1397–1401.
40. McNeil, B. J., Weichselbaum, R., and Pauker, S. G. (1981): Tradeoffs between quality and quantity of life in laryngeal cancer. *N. Engl. J. Med.,* 305:982–987.
41. Morris, T., Greer, H. S., and White, P. (1977): Psychological and social adjustment to mastectomy. *Cancer,* 40:2381–2387.
42. Morrow, G. R. (1980): Clinical trials in psychosocial medicine: Methodologic and statistical considerations, part iii. *Cancer Treat. Rep.,* 64:451–456.
43. Morrow, G. R., Chiarello, R. J., and Derogatis, L. R. (1978): A new scale for assessing patients' psychosocial adjustment to medical illness. *Psychol. Med.,* 8:605–610.
44. Nou, E., and Aberg, T. (1980): Quality of survival in patients with surgically treated bronchial carcinoma. *Thorax,* 35:255–263.
45. Oswald, I. (1981): Assessment of insomnia. *Br. Med. J.,* 283:874–875.
46. Padilla, G., Presant, C. A., Grant, M., Baer, C., and Metter, G. (1981): Assessment of quality of life in cancer patients. *Proc. Am. Assoc. Cancer Res.,* 22:397.
47. Palmer, B. V., Walsh, G. A., McKinna, J. A., and Greening, W. P. (1980): Adjuvant chemotherapy for breast cancer: Side effects and quality of life. *Br. Med. J.,* 281:1594–1597.
48. Pauker, S. G., and Kassirer, J. P. (1980): The threshold approach to clinical decision making. *N. Engl. J. Med.,* 302:1109–1117.
49. Plumb, M. M., and Holland, J. (1981): Comparative studies of psychological function in patients with advanced cancer. II. Interviewer-rated current and past psychological symptoms. *Psychosom. Med.,* 43:243–254.
50. Presser, S., and Schuman, H. (1980): The measurement of a middle position in attitude surveys. *Public Opinion Q.,* 44:70–85.
51. Priestman, T. J. (1984): Quality of life after cytotoxic chemotherapy: Discussion paper. *J. R. Soc. Med.,* 77:492–495.
52. Priestman, T. J., and Baum, M. (1976): Evaluation of quality of life in patients receiving treatment for advanced breast cancer. *Lancet,* 1:899–901.
53. Remington, M., Tyrer, P. J., Newsom-Smith, J., and Cichetti, D. V. (1979): Comparative reliability of categorical and analogue scales in the assessment of psychiatric symptomatology. *Psychol. Med.,* 9:765–770.
54. Roberts, M. M., Furnival, I. G., and Forrest, A. P. M. (1972): The morbidity of mastectomy. *Br. J. Surg.,* 59:301–302.
55. Rosenman, J., and Choi, N. C. (1982): Improved quality of life of patients with small-cell carcinoma of the lung by elective irradiation of the brain. *Int. J. Radiat. Oncol.,* 8:1041–1043.
56. Schmale, A. H. (1980): Clinical trials in psychosocial medicine: Methodologic and statistical considerations, part 1. *Cancer Treat. Rep.,* 64:441–443.
57. Schottenfeld, D., and Robbins, G. F. (1970): Quality of survival among patients who have had radical mastectomy. *Cancer,* 26:650–654.
58. Spiegelhalter, D. J., and Smith, A. F. M. (1980): Decision analysis and clinical decisions. European Symposium on Medical Statistics, Rome.
59. Sudman, S., and Bradburn, N. (1982): *Asking Questions.* Jossey Bass, San Francisco.
60. Van Dam, F. S. A. M., Linssen, A. C. G., and Couzijn, A. L. (1983): Evaluating quality of life: Behavioural measures in clinical cancer trials. In: *The Practice of Clinical Trials,* edited by M. Staquet, R. Sylvester, and M. Buyse. Oxford University Press, New York.
61. Wing, J. K., Cooper, J. E., and Sartorius, N. (1974): *Measurement and Classification of Psychiatric Symptoms.* Cambridge University Press, Cambridge.
62. World Health Organization (1979): *Handbook for Reporting Results of Cancer Treatment.* WHO Offset Publ. 48. WHO, Geneva.
63. Wright, P., and Haybittle, J. (1979): Design of forms for clinical trials. *Br. Med. J.,* 2:529–530, 590–592, 650–651.
64. Yates, J. W., Chalmer, B., and McKegney, P. (1980): Evaluation of patients with advanced cancer using the Karnofsky performance status. *Cancer,* 45:2220–2224.
65. Zeller, R. A., and Carmines, E. G. (1980): *Measurement in the Social Sciences.* Cambridge University Press, Cambridge.
66. Zubrod, C. G., Schneiderman, M., Frei, E., et al. (1960): Appraisal of methods for the study of chemotherapy of cancer in man: Comparative therapeutic trial of nitrogen mustard and triethylene thiophosphoramide. *J. Chronic Dis.,* 11:7–33.

The Quality of Life of Cancer Patients,
edited by N. K. Aaronson and J. Beckmann,
Raven Press, New York © 1987.

Multidimensional Approach to the Measurement of Quality of Life in Lung Cancer Clinical Trials

Neil K. Aaronson, *Willem Bakker, **Anita L. Stewart,
Frits S.A.M. van Dam, Nico van Zandwijk, †John R. Yarnold,
and ‡Anne Kirkpatrick

*The Netherlands Cancer Institute, 1066 CX Amsterdam, The Netherlands; *Department of Pulmonology, University Hospital, 2333 AA Leiden, The Netherlands; **The Rand Corporation, Santa Monica, California 90406; †Institute of Cancer Research, The Royal Marsden Hospital, Surrey SM2 5PT, England; and ‡EORTC Data Center, 1000 Brussels, Belgium*

Evaluation of clinical modalities for the treatment of cancer is focused on such biomedical outcomes as length of survival, retardation of the disease process, and control of major physical symptoms. Clinical decision-making is similarly guided by these biological endpoints, with relatively little systematic attention being paid to how varied treatments affect the quality of life of the patient. In recent years, however, increased interest has been voiced in determining the extent to which medical treatments impact on the physical, psychological, social, and economic life of the individual. Thus the scope of inquiry in cancer research has been gradually broadened to include variables that allow for some judgment regarding the tradeoff between biological and psychosocial endpoints of care.

A precise definition of "quality of life" is elusive, and a review of the relevant literature underscores its multidimensional nature. Included under this rubric are such factors as the control of physical symptoms, the toxicity or side effects of treatment, limitations in functional status, disruption of social roles and relationships, disease- or treatment-related psychological distress, pain, and sexual dysfunction. More positive aspects of the quality of life construct include satisfaction with medical care, feelings of well-being, and general life satisfaction.

Although interest in the quality of life of cancer patients has increased substantially, rhetoric in this area has far outpaced performance. For example, in a review of cancer clinical trials undertaken between 1956 and 1976, Bardelli and Saracci (7) found that fewer than 5% of published studies included outcomes that, in the

63

broadest sense, could be construed as measuring the effects of treatment on quality of life. Although a more recent review of the literature (20) has unearthed more than 200 papers that employ the term "quality of life" in the title, many such studies limit assessment to physician ratings of patients' physical performance status as measured by the Karnofsky scale (28), the ECOG/WHO scale (54), and similar clinical observation methods. Furthermore, as Fayers and Jones (20) pointed out, the range of cancer types and treatments that have been evaluated from a psychosocial perspective has been relatively narrow, with most effort evidenced in the assessment of the psychological consequences of breast cancer and mastectomy.

A particularly notable gap in the quality of life literature concerns the psychosocial aspects of the treatment of the most prevalent of cancer types—lung cancer. A limited number of studies of the postoperative adjustment of bronchial carcinoma patients have included clinical observation of performance status using the Carlens Vitagram method (16,36–39). Similarly, Bakker et al. (6) used the Karnofsky scale and changes in body weight to assess the impact of maintenance chemotherapy on the quality of life of 57 patients with small cell lung cancer. Silberfarb and his colleagues (44) employed the Profile of Mood States to assess depression and fatigue among small cell lung carcinoma patients receiving varied chemotherapy regimens.

The paucity of studies of the quality of life of lung cancer patients is quite disconcerting when one considers the slow progress that has been made in extending the period of survival of such patients and the increasingly toxic nature of many of the available treatment regimens. There appear to be at least two principal factors that account for this hesitancy to include psychosocial parameters in the assessment of treatment outcome. First, physicians have little training or experience in evaluating systematically nonmedical outcomes of patient care. Although quality of life issues are often implicitly factored into clinical decision-making, such judgments concerning the qualitative aspects of care may reflect the personal values, philosophical orientations, and subjective assessments of the physician, rather than those of the patient.

Second, and perhaps more importantly, the physician interested in assessing the psychosocial impact of both routine medical care and experimental treatments is confronted with a confusing array of measurement tools. At one end of the spectrum are extensive and time-consuming interview protocols that exceed the practical limits required when working within a clinical setting. At the other end are brief patient self-report questionnaires which, while representing a less cumbersome approach to data collection, often leave unanswered the critical questions of instrument reliability and validity.

We report here the preliminary results of a study of the quality of life of lung cancer patients participating in clinical trials. Our initial goal was to construct measures of various dimensions of the quality of life construct that are reliable and valid, while remaining sufficiently brief to be of practical use in both routine treatment settings and clinical trial situations.

STUDY BACKGROUND

The present research represents a collaborative effort between the European Organization for Research and Treatment of Cancer (EORTC) Lung Cancer Coopera- tive Group and Study Group on Quality of Life. In October of 1982 a multicenter, cross-cultural, randomized clinical trial was begun to compare the relative effective- ness of five versus 12 courses of chemotherapy (cyclophosphamide, doxorubicin, and etoposide) in extending the disease-free interval and survival of patients with small-cell lung cancer (SCLC) and in maintaining or improving their quality of life. Details of the trial protocol are presented elsewhere (18). Briefly, patients with cytologically and/or histologically confirmed SCLC whose tumor has not progressed after five courses of chemotherapy are randomly assigned to receive either seven more courses of the same chemotherapy or follow-up (clinical evaluation without further chemotherapy). At the time of this analysis, more than 300 patients had been accrued into the trial.

In total, 30 hospitals from The Netherlands, France, Italy, England, Ireland, Switzerland, and Greece are contributing patients to the trial. Of these 30 hospitals, 10 are participating in the quality of life aspects of the trial. Thus in addition to collecting the required clinical data regarding tumor response, disease-free interval, and survival, these institutions are having their patients complete a quality of life questionnaire at entrance into the study (baseline), and at 12 weeks, 24 weeks, 33 weeks, and 1 year. These times correspond approximately to the end of the first five courses of chemotherapy, the middle of the second set of seven courses, and the end of the second set of courses, with a 1-year follow-up.

The current chapter presents data from the first 80 baseline questionnaires. Analy- sis of these data allows some judgment regarding the adequacy, from a psychometric perspective, of the hypothesized measures of quality of life included in the question- naire. Thus this psychometric analysis can be viewed as the necessary first step for examining the relative impact over time of the two treatment arms on the quality of life of SCLC patients.

CHARACTERISTICS OF THE STUDY SAMPLE

Most (87.1%) of the 80 SCLC patients for whom baseline quality of life data are available are men, with a mean age of 60 [standard deviation (SD) 8 years]. ECOG performance status ratings (a 5-point physician-rated measure of patients' physical activity level) range from 0 ("normal activity") to 3 ("needs to be in bed for more than 50% of normal daytime"), with a mean rating of 1 ("symptoms but nearly fully ambulatory"). The absence of patients with ECOG ratings of 4 ("unable to get out of bed") reflects one of the exclusion criteria employed in patient selection.

These sex, age, and ECOG score distributions for the quality of life baseline sample show an essential similarity with those of the total sample of patients

($n = 312$) accrued into the trial (87% men; mean age 66 with an SD of 11.5 years; mean ECOG rating of 1). This finding suggests that inclusion of patients in the quality of life aspects of the trial was not based on selected patient characteristics but, rather, on certain practical constraints that prohibited the collection of patient self-report data in some institutional settings (i.e., the lack of personnel to field the questionnaires, monitor the data collection, etc.).

OVERVIEW OF THE QUALITY OF LIFE QUESTIONNAIRE

The various dimensions of quality of life measured in the self-administered questionnaire are outlined in Table 1. Included are items tapping functional status (both personal functioning and role functioning), symptoms of lung cancer (coughing, shortness of breath, pain), side effects of treatment[1] (nausea, vomiting, and other effects of chemotherapy), fatigue and malaise (possibly reflecting both symptoms of lung cancer and side effects of treatment), psychological distress, sense of well-being, and social interaction (satisfaction and changes in interpersonal relationships, as well as perceived social support). For most of the questions, patients were asked to respond in terms of how they were feeling during the past 3 days (the exception being those items tapping functional status, where the time frame was left undefined).

TABLE 1. *Areas of quality of life measured in EORTC small-cell lung cancer trial 08825*

Concept	Type of measure	No. of items
Functional status		
Personal functioning	Guttman scale	6
Role functioning	Guttman scale	2
Symptoms of lung cancer		
Coughing, coughing blood	Single items	2
Shortness of breath	Likert scale	3
Pain and pain relief	Single items	5
Side effects of treatment		
Nausea and vomiting	Likert scale	3
Swallowing difficulties	Single item	1
Sore mouth, lips, or tongue	Single item	1
Tingling in hands or feet	Single item	1
Fatigue and malaise	Likert scale	5
Psychological distress	Likert scale	5
Sense of well-being/satisfaction	Likert scale	4
Social interaction		
Satisfaction with relationships	Likert scale	2
Change in relationships	Likert scale	2
Perceived social support	Likert scale	3

---

[1] Because the current analysis is restricted to the baseline questionnaire administered prior to administration of chemotherapy, data on side effects of treatment are not considered.

An effort was made to include at least several items hypothesized to tap each of the quality of life domains of interest. To the extent that such multiple items can be combined into summative ratings (i.e., scales or indices) they present a clear advantage over single-item measures. First, multiple-item measures reduce the number of scores necessary to define each variable while at the same time increasing the variability (i.e., the range) of responses. Thus instead of treating each item as a separate quality of life variable, a number of items can be combined to yield a summary score. Second, they increase score reliability by pooling the information that items have in common. Third, if items are carefully selected to provide a representative sample of information (e.g., attitudes, behavior) relevant to a particular dimension of quality of life, the resulting scales have increased validity (i.e., they are more likely to be measuring what is intended to be measured). Fourth, by employing both positively and negatively worded items, it is possible to reduce response bias introduced by the tendency of some individuals to endorse or reject items regardless of their content. Last, they can reduce the problem of missing data by providing the option, if individual item responses are missing, to estimate responses using other items in the measure.

METHODS OF ANALYSIS

Scale Construction

In order to test whether the individual items outlined in Table 1 could be combined into a more limited set of multiple-item scales, either Likert's method of summated ratings (30) or Guttman's Scalogram Analysis (24) was employed. For Likert scaling, item responses were first assigned numbers: 1, "not at all"; 2, "a little bit"; 3, "quite a bit"; and 4, "very much." Items in a hypothesized group (e.g., the five items hypothesized to measure psychological distress) were added together to form a total scale score. An item analysis was carried out in which each item was correlated with the total scale score but with the item score taken out of the total (i.e., the correlation is corrected for overlap). In order to be retained in the scale, each item had to correlate at least 0.40 with the total score (3).

Factor analysis[2] was used to confirm that only one scale should be constructed from such a set of items. Factor analysis is a statistical technique based on the correlation among items. It allows one to identify underlying dimensions or factors that a set of items have in common. A factor is essentially a cluster of items that are highly related to one another. With the use of this statistical procedure we can ensure the unidimensionality of the hypothesized scale (i.e., that the items comprising the scale measure only one concept).

Finally, the reliability of the Likert scale was assessed by calculating the internal consistency of the set of items. Reliability refers to the consistency of the score, or the extent to which the score is free of random error. The most commonly

---

[2] In all analyses principal components factor analysis with varimax rotation was employed (35).

employed measure of internal consistency is Cronbach's alpha coefficient (13,40). Internal consistency estimates were considered acceptable for group comparisons if they were of a magnitude of 0.50 or greater (26).

Guttman's Scalogram Analysis is an alternative method for combining items into a single score. A Guttman scale can be constructed if a set of items with dichotomous response choices (i.e., yes or no responses) represent a continuum of increasing levels of intensity, difficulty, or severity. For example, the three questions—Can you walk a block? Can you walk a mile? Can you run a mile?— represent a single dimension of increasingly strenuous physical activity. A Guttman scale score is essentially a count of positive responses to such a series of questions. Because of the cumulative nature of the items, the scale score describes rather precisely the logical pattern of responses to all of the items. Thus in the above example, if the patient reports being able to run a mile, it is a logical assumption that he or she can also walk a mile and can certainly walk one block.

In the current analysis the two statistics used to evaluate whether a set of items met the Guttman criteria for scalability were the coefficient of reproducibility (CR) and the coefficient of scalability (CS). Minimal standards of 0.90 for CR and 0.60 for CS were employed as evidence of scale reliability (35).

Construct Validity

For the final step in scale construction, a series of analyses were undertaken to examine the construct validity of the scales. Construct validity refers essentially to if the hypothesized scales are actually measuring the attitudes or behaviors (i.e., the underlying construct) they are intended to measure and, of equal importance, if they are *not* measuring some other underlying construct.

Three approaches were taken to assessing the construct validity of the quality of life scales. First, a series of factor analyses were carried out, each of which paired sets of items from different scales. Thus the items included in the malaise scale were factor-analyzed in combination with the items from the psychological distress scale, the items from the psychological distress scale were factor-analyzed in combination with those from the well-being scale, and so forth.[3] Evidence of construct validity was provided if the items representing the paired scales "loaded" on separate factors (e.g., if the items from the fatigue scale clustered together under one factor, and the items from the psychological distress scale clustered under a second factor).

Second, multitrait scaling techniques were employed to test for item-discriminant validity. A matrix of item-scale correlations was created such that each item was correlated with all the scales being constructed, including the scale to which it

---

[3] This "paired comparison" procedure was undertaken, rather than factor-analyzing all items for all scales simultaneously, primarily due to sample size constraints. It is recommended that the ratio of subjects to items in a factor analysis should be at least 10:1 (i.e., for every item included in the analysis there should be 10 subjects). In the current case, where the ratio of subjects to items was well below this criterion, the simultaneous analysis of all items was not possible.

was hypothesized to belong (corrected for overlap). According to the discriminant validity criterion, each item should correlate highest with its own scale.

Finally, a correlation matrix was constructed that included the various quality of life scales, as well as the ECOG performance rating for each subject. An examination of the direction and strength of relations among the scales provided evidence of construct validity. It was expected that those scales which were conceptually related would correlate significantly with one another, whereas those scales with less in common would exhibit lower correlations.

RESULTS

Functional Status

Functional status refers to the performance of (or the capacity to perform) a variety of activities that are normal for most people. Four categories of such activities commonly measured are (a) self-care activities (e.g., feeding, dressing, bathing, using the toilet); (b) mobility (i.e., ability to move around indoors, outdoors, in the community); (c) physical activities (e.g., walking, climbing stairs, lifting, bending); and (d) role activities (i.e., ability to carry out social roles associated with work, school, household activities) (46–48).

In the current study, two Guttman scales were developed to measure functional status. The first was a six-item measure of personal functioning, including items tapping self-care, mobility, and physical activity. The item content and hypothesized scale pattern is presented in Table 2. As is appropriate for Guttman scale items,

TABLE 2. *Guttman scale of personal functioning*

Scale score	Item 1	Item 2	Item 3	Item 4	Item 5	Item 6	Percent of patients
0	Yes	Yes	Yes	Yes	Yes	Yes	3.8
1	No	Yes	Yes	Yes	Yes	Yes	5.0
2	No	No	Yes	Yes	Yes	Yes	6.2
3	No	No	No	Yes	Yes	Yes	10.0
4	No	No	No	No	Yes	Yes	18.8
5	No	No	No	No	No	Yes	23.7
6	No	No	No	No	No	No	32.5

Coefficient of reproducibility = 0.93
Coefficient of scalability   = 0.71
Mean scale score   = 4.4
Standard deviation   = 1.7

Item 1: Do you need help with eating, dressing, washing, or using the toilet?
Item 2: Do you have to stay indoors most or all of the day?
Item 3: Are you in bed or a chair for most of the day?
Item 4: Do you have trouble either walking a short distance or climbing one flight of stairs?
Item 5: Do you have any trouble bending, lifting, or stooping?
Item 6: Do you have trouble either taking a walk or climbing a few flights of stairs?

the response choices were a simple "yes" or "no" dichotomy. The items are similar to those that have been extensively tested for scale validity and reliability in general healthy populations (27,46), in patients with arthritis (34), and among cancer patients (27,31,45). As can be seen, there are seven scale levels ranging from 0 ("unable to carry out even the most basic self-care activities") to 6 ("able to carry out all activities"). The coefficients of reproducibility and scalability were 0.93 and 0.71, respectively, indicating that the items conform to a Guttman scale pattern. The findings indicate that fewer than 5% of the sample were unable to undertake self-care activities, and approximately one-third of the sample were able to carry out all levels of activity represented in the scale. The mean scale score was 4.4, indicating a moderate level of functional limitation.

The second Guttman scale was composed of two items intended to measure the extent to which patients could perform their usual work and housework activities (i.e., role functioning). The item content and hypothesized scale pattern are presented in Table 3. As indicated, only three scale levels are possible, ranging from 0 ("unable to carry out work and housework activities") to 2 ("no limitation in carrying out these role activities"). This scale has been evaluated previously with general populations and cancer patients (31,45,48). The coefficient of reproducibility (0.95) and the coefficient of scalability (0.84) provide statistical evidence of the appropriateness of a Guttman scale. Approximately one-third of the sample reported no role function limitations, slightly fewer than one-half reported some limitation, and one-fifth indicated extensive limitations in carrying out normal role activities. The mean scale score was 1.1, with a standard deviation of 0.72.

Symptoms of Lung Cancer

Nine items asked patients to report cancer-related symptom experience (Table 4). All items employed a 4-point response scale, ranging from 1 ("not at all")

TABLE 3. *Guttman scale of role functioning*

Scale score	Item 1	Item 2	Percent of patients
0	Yes	Yes	20.0
1	No	Yes	46.2
2	No	No	33.7

Coefficient of reproducibility = 0.95
Coefficient of scalability   = 0.84
Mean scale score   = 1.1
Standard deviation   = 0.72

Item 1: Does your condition keep you from working at a job or doing household jobs?
Item 2: Are you limited in any way in doing your work or household jobs?

to 4 ("very much"). The items that assessed coughing, pain, and pain relief were treated as single variables. Frequent coughing (i.e., the categories "quite a bit" and "very much" combined) was reported by 38% of the sample, whereas coughing blood was evidenced only in a few patients.

With regard to pain experience, 14% of the sample reported frequent chest pain, 9% arm or shoulder pain, and 15% pain in other areas of their body. Although pain intensity was not measured directly, 28 (35%) of the patients were experiencing sufficient levels of pain to require medication. Of these 28 patients, 57% reported that their medication provided substantial pain relief.

Three items asked patients how often they experienced shortness of breath while resting, walking, and climbing stairs. These items were combined into a Likert scale, with scores ranging from 3 ("no shortness of breath") to 12 ("severe shortness of breath"). The mean score for the sample was 5.1, with a standard deviation of 2.1. The unidimensionality of the scale was demonstrated via a factor analysis that indicated that the three items loaded on a single factor. Furthermore, all item-scale correlations were above 0.50. The reliability of the scale, as measured by Cronbach's alpha, was found to be quite adequate for group comparisons (alpha coefficient = 0.75).

Fatigue and Malaise

General feelings of fatigue or malaise are common symptoms experienced by cancer patients. Such fatigue can be due to the cancer or its treatment, or it can represent a somatic manifestation of psychological distress (21,25,51).

Five items similar to those developed by Linssen et al. (31) were employed to assess fatigue/malaise. Response categories ranged on a 4-point scale from 1 ("not at all") to 4 ("very much"). Item content and score distributions are presented

TABLE 4. *Frequency distribution for items tapping symptoms of lung cancer*

Symptom	Frequency (%)			
	Not at all	A little	Quite a bit	Very much
Cough	14	49	29	9
Coughing blood	76	20	4	0
Shortness of breath				
Resting	71	20	8	1
Walking	57	25	17	1
Climbing stairs	40	25	24	11
Chest pain	66	20	13	1
Arm or shoulder pain	76	15	6	3
Other pain	72	13	10	5
Medication relieves pain[a]	11	32	46	11

[a] Percentages based on 28 patients who reported taking medication to relieve their pain.

in Table 5. These five items were combined into a Likert scale, with scores ranging from 5 to 20 (a higher score representing increasing levels of fatigue/malaise). The mean scale score was 11.9, with an SD of 3.5. Factor analysis supported the unidimensionality of the fatigue/malaise scale, with all items loading on a single factor. All item-scale correlations were above the 0.40 criterion for additive scales. The reliability of the scale, as determined by Cronbach's alpha coefficient, was 0.82.

Psychological Distress

A large number of studies have documented elevated levels of psychological distress among cancer patients compared with rates typically found among general medical and primary practice populations (1,12,14,41,43). Such distress can reflect the impact of the diagnosis of cancer, reaction to the progression of the disease, or side effects of treatment (2,23).

A variety of measures are available for assessing psychological distress or disorder, ranging from extensive psychiatric interviews to multidimensional self-report symptom inventories to unidimensional checklists. Although it would have been desirable to employ a standardized self-report measure of distress in the current study, several factors limited that possibility. First, although many of the available measures have been standardized on either healthy adult or psychiatric populations, very few have been tested for validity and reliability among cancer populations. Second, many of the available measures include items tapping somatic manifestations of psychological disturbance such as tiredness, decreased sexual drive, or appetite loss (17). This area becomes problematic when employing such measures among cancer patients (as well as those with other chronic physical diseases) in that it may not be possible to distinguish between symptoms of psychological disorder and symptoms of cancer, side effects of cancer treatments, or both. Third, even the most concise available instruments contain too many items to have been

TABLE 5. *Frequency distribution and summary statistics: fatigue and malaise scale*

	Frequency (%)			
Item	Not at all	A little	Quite a bit	Very much
Did you feel energetic?	11	32	46	11
Were you physically well?	28	36	32	4
Did you need rest?	14	44	25	17
Did you feel ill?	49	29	15	7
Were you tired?	19	44	26	11

Cronbach's alpha　= 0.82
Scale range　　　= 5–20
Scale mean　　　= 11.9
Standard deviation = 3.5

of practical use in the current clinical trial setting, where there were severe constraints on the *total* permissible length of the questionnaire.

For these reasons, in the current study we employed a set of five items similar to those used previously at The Netherlands Cancer Institute (32) which asked patients to report the extent to which they had felt tense, irritable, lonely, worried, and depressed during the previous 3-day period. Response categories ranged on a 4-point scale from 1 ("not at all") to 4 ("very much"). The advantages in employing this set of items were that: (a) preliminary psychometric analyses indicated that the items form a unidimensional scale (32); (b) the resulting scale yielded significant differences in psychological distress when comparing cancer patients with a normal group of healthy blood donors (31); (c) they exclude somatic complaints; and (d) they place minimum response burden on the patient.

Table 6 presents the item content and score distributions for the five psychological distress items. Combining the categories "quite a bit" and "very much," the most frequently cited symptoms were worrying and tension (reported by 44% and 45% of the sample, respectively), followed by depression (34%), irritability (21%), and loneliness (9%).

The five items were combined into a Likert scale, with scores ranging from 5 to 20 (a higher score representing more distress). The mean scale score was 9.9, with an SD of 3.5. The results of the various psychometric tests indicated that these items form a unidimensional scale: (a) in a factor analysis all items loaded on a single factor; (b) all item-scale correlations were above 0.40; and (c) the reliability of the scale was quite satisfactory for group comparisons (alpha coefficient of 0.79).

Well-Being/Satisfaction

Although most of the items included in the quality of life questionnaire were designed to tap problem areas in the patients' lives, there was also interest in

TABLE 6. *Frequency distribution and summary statistics: psychological distress scale*

Item	Frequency (%)			
	Not at all	A little	Quite a bit	Very much
Did you feel tense?	31	24	30	15
Did you feel irritable?	50	29	14	7
Did you feel lonely?	71	20	6	3
Did you worry?	21	35	26	18
Did you feel depressed?	35	31	23	11

Cronbach's alpha = 0.79
Scale range   = 5–20
Scale mean   = 9.9
Standard deviation = 3.5

assessing the effects of cancer and its treatment on overall feelings of well-being or life satisfaction. Although, to a limited degree, the absence of such symptoms as fatigue/malaise, pain, and psychological distress provides evidence of well-being, both theory and empirical data suggest that feelings of well-being and satisfaction represent an independent dimension of life quality (4,8,19,27).

In the literature, overall satisfaction is most often measured by a single global question (5,10,22), although examples of multi-item approaches can be found (29,45). Regardless of the specific measurement technique employed, there is general agreement that sense of well-being and life satisfaction represent related and complex subjective appraisals that embody both cognitive and emotional components.

Although we recognized that it would not be possible to question patients about the full range of issues that enter into judgments of well-being or satisfaction, there was an attempt to develop a multiple-item measure that could avoid many of the conceptual and psychometric limitations evidenced with single-item approaches. Four items were chosen to measure well-being/satisfaction: satisfaction with physical condition (single item), satisfaction with daily activities (single item), and global well-being/satisfaction (two items).

The content and score distributions of these four items are presented in Table 7. Response categories ranged from 1 (''not at all'') to 4 (''very much''). Combining the categories ''quite a bit'' and ''very much,'' we found that 46% of the sample reported satisfaction with their physical condition, 42% were satisfied with their daily activities, 34% felt that ''things were going their way,'' and 55% reported overall satisfaction.

A Likert scale of well-being/satisfaction was created by summing the scores for the four items. Scale scores ranged from 4 to 15, with a mean of 9.1 and an SD of 2.8. The results of the factor analysis indicated that all items loaded on a

TABLE 7. *Frequency distribution and summary statistics: well-being/satisfaction scale*

	Frequency (%)			
Item	Not at all	A little	Quite a bit	Very much
How satisfied were you with your physical condition?	28	26	35	11
Did you feel that things were going your way?	39	27	30	4
How satisfied were you with your daily activities?	33	25	36	6
Overall, how satisfied do you feel?	18	30	41	11

Cronbach's alpha = 0.76
Scale range = 4–15
Scale mean = 9.1
Standard deviation = 2.8

single factor. Additionally, all item-score correlations were above the 0.40 criterion. The scale reliability as assessed by Cronbach's alpha was 0.76.

Social Interaction

Both clinical observations and empirical research point to the importance of social contact and social support in the life of the cancer patient (53). In fact, it has been suggested by some that fears of social unacceptability, rejection, and isolation compete equally with fears of disease recurrence, pain, and death as sources of distress (50).

There are a number of ways in which cancer and cancer treatment can disrupt social relationships. Functional problems due to pain or fatigue may restrict the individual's ability to pursue normal social activities. Similarly, the demands of treatment regimens may place serious limitations and strains on the ability to maintain social contacts (9).

Psychological reactions of the cancer patient may also lead to restricted social interactions. Fear of being a burden to others, feelings of embarrassment about symptoms or disability, and fears of rejection may lead to avoidance of social contact and hesitancy in asking for social support (9,15,33,49).

Significant others (family, friends, and acquaintances) may also reduce the level of contact with the cancer patient or withdraw from the relationship entirely because of feelings of awkwardness, fear, or inadequacy (42,52). Lack of understanding of the nature of cancer and its treatment may also result in avoidance of contact (e.g., fear of contagion).

In the current study three approaches were taken to measuring the quality of and changes in social relationships. First, patients were asked two questions regarding the extent to which they found their relationships with their family and friends to be satisfying. Response categories ranged from 1 ("not at all") to 4 ("very much"). The distribution of responses to these two questions underscores the difficulty in assessing satisfaction with social relationships. Only 4% of the sample reported dissatisfaction with family relationships (combining the categories "not at all" and "a little" satisfied), and the comparable figure for relationships with friends was 10%. Although it is not inconceivable that these results reflect accurately the levels of (high) satisfaction with family and friends experienced by this group of lung cancer patients, an equally if not more compelling explanation is that patients have a difficult time responding directly to such questions regarding relational problems.

The second approach to assessing the effect of cancer and its treatment on the social well-being of patients also yielded little variance in responses. Patients were asked to rate, on a 5-point scale ranging from 1 ("much better") to 5 ("much worse"), the extent to which their health condition had affected their relationship with family and friends. Only 1% of the sample reported that their condition had made their relationship with their family worse, and only a slightly greater percentage (3%) reported increased difficulties with friends. Most patients reported no change in their family or friend relationships (51% and 59%, respectively), and many reported that their relationships had improved as a result of their condition (48% and 38%, respectively). Again, although one cannot preclude the possibility that these data reflect the actual social reality of these patients, it is more likely (given the available literature) that they point to the problem of social desirability in response patterns.

The final approach taken to measuring the quality of social relationships was to ask patients to report the frequency with which: (a) ''There was someone to talk to when I wanted''; (b) ''I felt close to someone''; and (c) ''People seemed to understand my problems.'' These three items, with response categories ranging on a 4-point scale from 1 (''never'') to 4 (''always''), were drawn from a more extensive set of items developed by Stewart (45). As can be noted in Table 8, the distribution of responses to this set of items was clearly more variable than in the previous two cases. Combining the categories ''never'' and ''sometimes,'' 14% of the sample reported the lack of availability of someone to talk to, 15% stated that they seldom had someone they felt close to, and 24% felt that people often did not understand their problems.

These items were summed to form a Likert scale, with scores ranging from 4 to 12. The mean scale score was 9.9, with an SD of 1.9. Both the factor analysis and item-scale correlation analysis indicated that it was appropriate to combine these items into a single social support scale (i.e., all items loaded on a single factor and all item-scale correlations were above 0.40). The reliability of the scale was acceptable for group comparisons (alpha coefficient of 0.69).

Evidence of Scale Validity

As described earlier, three approaches were taken to measuring the construct validity of the quality of life scales. First, a series of factor analyses were carried

TABLE 8. *Frequency distribution and summary statistics: social support scale*

Item	Frequency (%)			
	Never	Some-times	Most of the time	Always
There was someone to talk to when I wanted	4	10	24	62
I felt close to someone	3	12	23	62
People seemed to understand my problems	5	19	37	39

Cronbach's alpha = 0.69
Scale range   = 4–12
Scale mean   = 9.9
Standard deviation = 1.9

out, each of which paired sets of items from two hypothesized scales. Evidence of construct validity was provided if the items representing the paired scales "loaded" on separate factors.

Table 9 presents the results of this series of paired factor analyses for the fatigue/malaise scale, the psychological distress scale, the well-being/satisfaction scale, and the social support scale.[4] The consistency of results lends clear support to the construct validity of these scales. In each case the factor loadings fit the hypothesized pattern, with items belonging to each scale loading on separate factors. The only minor exception was the malaise/fatigue versus well-being/satisfaction contrast, where the item "Did you feel energetic?" loaded on both factors.

Second, multitrait scaling techniques were employed to test for item-discriminant validity.[4] A matrix of item-scale correlations was created such that each item in the fatigue/malaise scale, the psychological distress scale, the well-being/satisfaction scale, and the social support scale was correlated with each of the total scales (including its own scale, corrected for overlap). Across all scales there were 80 such tests of discriminant validity (data not presented in tabular form). Using the criteria suggested by Campbell and Fiske (11), no definite scaling errors were detected (i.e., there were no cases where the correlation of an item with another scale exceeded the correlation with its own scale by two standard errors), and only one test provided evidence of a probable scaling error (i.e., where the correlation of an item with another scale was within two standard errors of the correlation with its own scale). The low number of errors provides excellent empirical support for the distinctiveness of the quality of life constructs measured by the four scales.

Finally, a correlation matrix was constructed that included the personal and role functioning scales, the fatigue/malaise scale, the well-being/satisfaction scale, and the social support scale, as well as scores on the ECOG performance scale (Table 10). An examination of the direction and strength of relations among the scales provides additional evidence of construct validity. As noted: (a) the personal functioning and role functioning scales correlated significantly with each other, as well as with the ECOG scale[5]; (b) the fatigue/malaise scale exhibited a significant negative correlation with the personal and role functioning scales and the well-being/satisfaction scale, and a significant positive correlation with the psychological distress scale; and (c) the well-being/satisfaction scale had a significant positive correlation with the personal and role functioning scales and the social support scale, and a significant negative correlation with the psychological distress scale and the ECOG rating. It should be noted that these correlations, although statistically

---

[4] The personal functioning and role functioning Guttman scales were not included in this set of analyses. The items comprising these scales employed dichotomous response categories. The use of such dichotomous variables in principal components factor analysis and Pearson correlational analysis is not recommended, particularly not in combination with ordinal level variables such as those included in the remaining four scales.

[5] The negative sign for the correlation between the personal and role functioning scales and the ECOG rating is due to the directionality of the respective scale scores. A higher score on the personal and role functioning scales represents *higher* levels of functioning, whereas a higher score on the ECOG scale represents *lower* levels of functioning.

TABLE 9. Discriminant validity of quality of life scales: results of a series of paired factor analyses

Parameter	Fatigue × distress		Fatigue × well-being		Fatigue × support		Distress × well-being		Distress × support		Well-being × support	
	F1	F2	F1	F2	F1	F2	F1	F2	F1	F2	F1	F2
Fatigue/malaise												
Energetic	0.46		0.34	-0.47	0.47							
Physically well	0.68		0.53		0.65							
Need rest	0.76		0.79		0.83							
Feel ill	0.79		0.75		0.74							
Tired	0.70		0.72		0.74							
Psychological distress												
Tense		0.71					0.67		0.73			
Irritable		0.47					0.46		0.51			
Lonely		0.41					0.46		0.45			
Worry		0.74					0.67		0.73			
Depressed		0.86					0.84		0.86			
Well-being												
Physically well								0.69			0.73	
Going your way								0.52			0.52	
Daily activities								0.69			0.71	
Overall satisfied								0.65			0.71	
Social support												
Someone to talk						0.60				0.64		0.62
Felt close						0.80				0.79		0.86
Understood						0.55				0.56		0.50

TABLE 10. *Bivariate correlations between quality of life scales*

Scale	×1	×2	×3	×4	×5	×6	×7
Personal function (×1)	1.0						
Role function (×2)	0.42[a]	1.0					
Fatigue (×3)	−0.58[a]	−0.43[a]	1.0				
Distress (×4)	−0.07	−0.06	0.34[a]	1.0			
Well-being (×5)	0.29[a]	0.33[a]	−0.52[a]	−0.48[a]	1.0		
Support (×6)	0.02	0.01	−0.16	−0.02	0.21[a]	1.0	
ECOG (×7)	−0.36[a]	−0.24[a]	0.18	0.02	−0.23[a]	0.07	1.0

[a] $p < 0.05$.

significant, were of only moderate strength (ranging between 0.21 and 0.58). This finding suggests that, although they are related to one another in a predictable manner, the various scales are measuring distinct aspects of the quality of life construct.

CONCLUSION

We have reported on the development of a multidimensional quality of life questionnaire that is currently in use in a multicenter randomized clinical trial comparing the relative effectiveness of two chemotherapeutic strategies in the treatment of small-cell lung cancer patients. The questionnaire was designed with several goals in mind. First, because of the complexity of the quality of life construct and the varied ways in which cancer and its treatment can affect the life of the patient, it was desirable to assess a broad range of quality of life issues. Second, it was necessary to keep the questionnaire as brief as possible so as to minimize the demands placed on the trial participants. Finally, although recognizing the practical limitations imposed by a clinical trial setting, it was nevertheless essential to design a questionnaire that would yield quality of life scales exhibiting acceptable levels of instrument validity and reliability.

Results of the current analysis indicate that these goals have been achieved for the most part. The two-page questionnaire yielded, in addition to specific information about the nature and extent of physical symptoms of lung cancer (coughing, shortness of breath, and pain), valid and reliable scales of functional status (both personal and role functioning), fatigue and malaise, psychological distress, sense of well-being/satisfaction, and perceived social support. The only questions that failed to elicit useful information (i.e., did not exhibit score variability) were those intended to measure perceived satisfaction with and changes in interpersonal relationships. It appears that more subtle approaches to assessing the quality of such relationships than those employed in the current study are necessary to circumvent problems of social desirability in response patterns.

In the near future a number of additional studies are to be undertaken that will provide further evidence regarding the utility of this brief quality of life questionnaire. First, we are currently conducting a validity study in which patients who have completed the questionnaire are given a same-day semistructured interview that covers the same topics. By comparing the results obtained from these two methods of data collection we will develop further insight into the strengths and weaknesses of the questionnaire approach.

Second, as more quality of life data become available (from the questionnaires administered at 12 weeks, 24 weeks, 33 weeks, and 1 year), we will replicate the psychometric analyses that have been undertaken to date. To the extent that these future analyses yield similar results to those currently reported, we can increase our confidence in the validity and reliability of the quality of life measures.

Third, as medical data become available from the clinical trial, we will be able to compare changes in self-reported quality of life with observed changes in objective measures of physical health status (e.g., disease progression, weight change). To the extent that we hypothesize that subjective assessments of quality of life should covary with changes in physical health status, these analyses should yield valuable information regarding the validity of the questionnaire.

Ultimately, of course, our interest is in comparing the quality of life of patients in the two treatment arms of the trial. The current findings, combined with those to be obtained from the future studies outlined above, will provide the necessary groundwork for this more central task. Additionally, we hope that our findings will encourage other investigators regarding the feasibility of assessing quality of life outcomes as an integral part of their clinical research with cancer patients.

ACKNOWLEDGMENTS

This research was supported by grant 5R10 CA11488-11, awarded by the National Cancer Institute, DHHS, Bethesda, Maryland.

REFERENCES

1. Achute, K., and Vauhkonen, M. L. (1970): *Cancer and Psyche.* Kunnallispaino, Helsinki.
2. Adsett, C. A. (1963): Emotional reactions to disfigurement from cancer therapy. *Can. Med. Assoc. J.,* 89:391.
3. American Psychological Association (1974): *Standard for Educational and Psychological Tests.* APA, Washington, D.C.
4. Andrews, F. M., and McKennel, A. C. (1980): Measures of self-reported well-being: Their affective, cognitive and other components. *Soc. Indicators Res.,* 8:127–155.
5. Andrews, F. M., and Withey, S. B. (1976): *Social Indicators of Well-Being.* Plenum Press, New York.
6. Bakker, W., Nijhuis-Heddes, J. M. A., van Oosterom, A. T., Noordijk, E. M., Hermans, J., and Dijkman, J. H. (1984): Combined modality treatment of short duration in small cell lung cancer. *Eur. J. Cancer Clin. Oncol.,* 20:1033–1037.
7. Bardelli, D., and Saracci, R. (1978): Measuring the quality of life in cancer clinical trials: A sample survey of published trials. *UICC Technical Report Series,* Geneva.

8. Bradburn, N. (1969): *The Structure of Psychological Well-Being.* Aldine, Chicago.
9. Bury, M. (1982): Chronic illness as biographical disruption. *Sociology Health Illness,* 41:167–182.
10. Campbell, A., Converse, P. E., and Rodgers, W. L. (1976): *The Quality of American Life.* Russell Sage Foundation, New York.
11. Campbell, D. T., and Fiske, D. W. (1959): Convergent and discriminant validation by the multitrait-multimethod matrix. *Psychol. Bull.,* 56:81–105.
12. Craig, T. J., and Abeloff, M. D. (1974): Psychiatric symptomatology among hospitalized cancer patients. *Am. J. Psychiatry,* 141:1323–1327.
13. Cronbach, L. J. (1951): Coefficient alpha and the internal structure of tests. *Psychometrika,* 16:297–334.
14. Derogatis, L. R., Morrow, G. R., Fetting, J., and Penman, D. (1983): The prevalence of psychiatric disorders among cancer patients. *JAMA,* 249:751–757.
15. Eardley, A., George, W. D., and Davis, F. (1976): Colostomy: The consequences of surgery. *Clin. Oncol.,* 2:277–283.
16. Eklund, G., and Nou, E. (1979): Bronchial carcinoma. V. A methodological evaluation of the vitagram idex for measurements of quality of survival by means of the "MaxMin" correlation method. *Scand. J. Respir. Dis. [Supp.],* 104:173–208.
17. Endicott, J. (1984): Measurement of depression in patients with cancer. *Cancer,* 53:2243–2248.
18. EORTC Lung Cancer Cooperative Group (1982): *Protocol 08825: Induction Versus Induction Plus Maintenance Chemotherapy in Small Cell Lung Cancer.* EORTC Data Center, Brussels.
19. Fontana, A. F. (1980): Psychological impairment and psychological health in the psychological well-being of the physically ill. *Psychosom. Med.,* 42:279–288.
20. Fayers, P. M., and Jones, D. R. (1983): Measuring and analysing quality of life in cancer clinical trials: A review. *Stat. Med.,* 2:429–446.
21. Giel, R. (1977): De chirurg-oncoloog en de kwaliteit van het leven van zijn patienten. *Ned. Tijdschr. Geneeskd.,* 121:1315–1320.
22. Gough, I. R., Furnival, C. M., Schilder L., and Grove, W. (1983): Assessment of the quality of life of patients with advanced cancer. *Eur. J. Cancer Clin. Oncol.,* 19:1161–1165.
23. Greer, S., and Silberfarb, P. M. (1982): Psychological concomitants of cancer: Current state of research. *Psychol. Med.,* 12:563–573.
24. Guttman, L. A. (1944): A basis for scaling qualitative data. *Am. Soc. Rev.,* 9:139–150.
25. Haylock, P. J., and Hart, L. K. (1979): Fatigue in patients receiving localized radiation. *Cancer Nurs.,* 461–467.
26. Helmstadter, G. C. (1964): *Principles of Psychological Measurement.* Appleton-Century-Crofts, New York.
27. Huisman, S. (1982): Het Meten van Positieve Aspecten van Welzijn bij Kanker patienten. M.A. thesis, University of Amsterdam, Psychological Laboratory.
28. Karnofsky, D. A., and Burchenal, J. H. (1949): The clinical evaluation of chemotherapeutic agents in cancer. In: *Evaluation of Chemotherapeutic Agents,* edited by C. M. MacLeod. Columbia University Press, New York.
29. Lehman, A. F. (1982): The well-being of chronic mental patients: Assessing their quality of life. Unpublished manuscript. University of Rochester School of Medicine, Department of Psychiatry, Rochester, New York.
30. Likert, R. (1932): A technique for the measurement of attitudes. *Arch. Psychol.,* 140:1–55.
31. Linssen, A. C. G., Hanewald, G., Huisman, S. and van Dam, F. S. A. M. (1982): The development of a well-being (quality of life) questionnaire at The Netherlands Cancer Institute. In: *Proceedings of the 3rd EORTC Study Group on Quality of Life Workshop,* Paris.
32. Linssen, A. C. G., Hanewald, G. van Dam, F. and van Beek-Couzijn, A. L. (1981): The develop of the "complaint questionnaire" at The Netherlands Cancer Institute. In: *Proceedings of the 1st EORTC Study Group on Quality of Life Workshop,* Amsterdam.
33. Maguire, P. (1982): Psychological and social consequences of cancer. In: *Recent Advances in Clinical Oncology,* edited by C. J. Williams and J. M. A. Whitehouse. Churchill Livingstone, Edinburg.
34. Meenan, R. F. (1980): Measuring health status in arthritis: The arthritis impact measurement scale. *Arthritis Rheum.,* 23:146–152.
35. Nie, N. H., Hull, C. H., Jenkins, J. G., Steinbrenner, K., and Bent, D. H. (1970): *Statistical Package for the Social Sciences,* 2nd ed. McGraw-Hill, New York.

36. Nou, E. (1979): Bronchial carcinoma. II. Quantitative measurements of the quality of survival: A prospective randomized study of the result of therapy in inoperable patients with advanced disease. *Scand. J. Respir. Dis.,* 104:83–106.
37. Nou, E. (1979): Bronchial carcinoma. III. Quantitative measurements of the quality of survival: A prospective randomized study of the results of therapy in inoperable patients with localized disease. *Scand. J. Respir. Dis.,* 104:107–130.
38. Nou, E. (1979): Bronchial carcinoma. VI. Some aspects of the therapy of inoperable patients. *Scand. J. Respir. Dis.,* 104:209–225.
39. Nou, E., and Aberg, T. (1980): Quality of survival in patients with surgically treated bronchial carcinoma. *Thorax,* 35:255–263.
40. Nunnally, J. C. (1978): *Psychometric Theory,* 2nd ed. McGraw-Hill, New York.
41. Peck, A. (1972): Emotional reactions to having cancer. *AJR,* 114:591–599.
42. Peters-Golden, H. (1982): Breast cancer: Varied perceptions of social support in the illness experience. *Soc. Sci. Med.,* 16:483–491.
43. Plumb, M. M., and Holland, J. (1977): Comparative studies of psychological functions in patients with advanced cancer. I. Self-reported depressive symptoms. *Psychosom. Med.,* 39:264–276.
44. Silberfarb, P. M., Holland, J. C. B., Anbar, D., Bahna, G., Maurer, L. H., Chahinian, A. P., and Comis, R. (1983): Psychological response of patients receiving two drug regimens for lung carcinoma. *Am. J. Psychiatry,* 140:110–111.
45. Stewart, A. L. (1982): *Measuring the Ability to Cope with Serious Illness.* N-1907-GRS/RC. Rand Corporation, Santa Monica, California.
46. Stewart, A. L., Ware, J. E., Brook, R. H., and Davies-Avery, A. (1978): *Conceptualization and Measurement of Health for Adults in the Health Insurance Study, Vol. II: Physical Health in Terms of Functioning.* R-1987/2-HEW. Rand Corporation, Santa Monica, California.
47. Stewart, A. L., Ware, J. E., and Brook, R. H. (1981): Advances in the measurement of functional status: Construction of aggregate indexes. *Med. Care,* 19:473–488.
48. Stewart, A. L., Ware, J. E., and Brook, R. H. (1982): *Construction and Scoring of Aggregate Functional Status Measures,* Vol. I. R-2551-1-HHS. Rand Corporation, Santa Monica, California.
49. Strauss, H. M., and Glaser, B. G. (1975): *Chronic Illness and the Quality of Life.* Mosby, St. Louis.
50. Sutherland, A. M. (1960): *The Psychological Impact of Cancer.* American Cancer Society, New York.
51. Van Dam, F. S. A. M., Linssen, A. C. G., and Engelsman, E. (1980): Life with cytostatic drugs. In: *Breast Cancer: Experimental and Clinical Aspects,* edited by H. T. Mouridsen and T. Palshof. Pergamon Press, Oxford.
52. Wortman, C. B. (1983): Social support and the cancer patient: Conceptual and methodological issues. *Cancer,* 53:2217–2384.
53. Wortman, C. B., and Dunkel-Schetter, C. (1979): Interpersonal relationships and cancer: A theoretical analysis. *J. Soc. Issues,* 35:120–155.
54. Zubrod, C. G., Schneidermann, M., et al. (1960): Appraisal of methods for the study of chemotherapy of cancer in man: Comparative therapeutic trial of nitrogen mustard and triethylenethiophosphoramide. *J. Chronic Dis.,* 11:7–33.

The Quality of Life of Cancer Patients,
edited by N. K. Aaronson and J. Beckmann,
Raven Press, New York © 1987.

Comparison of Three Methods to Measure Quality of Life

Simon Schraub, *Diana D. Bransfield, Eric Monpetit,
and Jacqueline Fournier

*Service de Radiothérapie, Centre Hospitalier Regional de Besançon, F-25030 Besançon
Cedex, France; and *Division at Cancer Prevention and Control, National Institute,
Bethesda, Maryland 20892*

Cure of disease and prolongation of life are the major objectives in oncologic treatment. However, these goals need to be considered along with the psychosocial and somatic parameters of the patient or, more simply, the quality of life. As discussed in previous chapters, quality of life is a difficult concept to define and evaluate. Nevertheless, a tool that subjectively measures quality of life is needed to assist health providers in treatment decisions and rehabilitation planning (14,16). Although little agreement may exist regarding the constituents of quality of life, recurrent themes in the literature include: (a) the status of daily physical activities including professional and domestic duties; (b) the frequency of physical and psychological complaints (e.g., pain, anxiety, depression); (c) the ability to maintain one's usual sexual functioning; and (d) the subjective feeling of well-being.

Four types of measurement tools are available to explore these areas: open-ended interviews, questionnaires, linear analogues, and anamnestic comparative self-assessment scales. These modalities are briefly discussed followed by the results of a pilot project that compared the informative value and the feasibility of three quality of life measures in a French oncology setting. The first part of the project, which is presented, describes the development of the quality of life questionnaire (QOL-Q) and the simultaneous administration of the anamnestic comparative self-assessment scale (ACSA), the linear analogue scale (LA), and QOL-Q. The second part of the project, which will be reported at a later date, provides information about the ACSA, LA, and QOL-Q after two successive administrations, one at the beginning of treatment and one at the end.

TYPE OF EVALUATION

The open-ended interview is the most thorough method by which to explore the patient's perceptions of his quality of life. Using a nonstructured format, the interviewer questions the patient about the impact of the illness and the treatment on various aspects of his life. The interviewer then interprets, organizes, and codes the gathered information for either individual case studies, descriptive level, or experimental designs (17). The greatest limitation of the interviewer-rated measures is that the outcome data can be influenced by the perceptions and biases of the interviewer (5). Furthermore, interviews are time-consuming, often requiring 1 hr or more per patient, and rarely attain sufficient levels of reliability. For these reasons, this method has limited applicability in most oncology settings.

More recently, several questionnaires have been developed to assess the quality of life of the cancer patient, including self-administered scales (9,15) and interviewer rated measures (10). Because of their recency, the questionnaires, almost all of which are in English, are of unproved validity in cross-cultural settings. The advantages of questionnaires are that they are easily administered, they lend themselves to statistical interpretation, and they can be standardized more readily than the open-ended interview. The disadvantages are that the patient's life circumstances may not coincide with the selected items, thereby forcing the patient to reply to ill-suited questions, and that the patient's understanding of the items is partially related to such factors as educational background and previous testing experience.

Batteries of standardized psychological tests are available to provide a comprehensive profile of the patient's personality, mood state, and current level of psychopathology. However, with few exceptions, cross-cultural validity has not been established for most psychological tests, none of which were developed for or with cancer populations. Thus the use of the more familiar psychological tests in an oncology setting mandates a cautious interpretation of results, particularly in comparison to established test norms. Additionally, the latter point carries as its greatest risk the fact that test items which reflect somatic disturbance, e.g., nausea, vomiting, and fatigue, may be measuring the consequence of the disease and its treatment, not psychological status. It may be imperative to conduct a separate analysis of those items assessing physical symptoms and those assessing psychological ones.

Similarly, several linear analogue scales that rate subjective feelings are in existence (2), including linear analogue scales with cancer patients (12). Such scales were originally described by Freyd in 1923 and have been used to study various affective states (8). A visual linear analogue is a line, usually 10 or 20 cm long (18) with or without marked gradations that serves as a response continuum (13). The ends of the line are labeled with contrasting words or phrases, and the subject is asked to indicate where on the line he/she would place him/herself in relation to these extremes. An investigation that compared various types of linear analogue scales measuring pain intensity found that a horizontal line with gradations was preferred over vertical and curvilinear scales with or without gradations, and over a horizontal scale without gradations (18). Irrespective of the type of line, this measurement procedure yields ratio rather than interval level data (13), as one end of the line is treated as a true zero point, representing the total absence of the factor under question (e.g., I have *no* depression; I have *no* pain).

To date, visual analogue scales have been most heavily used in the measurement of pain. One pain study (7) has reported that the visual analogue scale is more difficult for patients to understand than are verbal scales. Patient comprehension of visual analogue scales appears to be related to the manner in which the scale is presented. Sriwatanakul et al. (18) and Price et al. (13) found that their pain subjects seldom had any problem using a visual linear analogue scale after it was adequately explained. Once the scale is understood, it can be administered quickly and produces more sensitive and precise measurements than scales that attempt to describe how the patient is feeling. The primary disadvantage of the visual linear analogue scale is that subjects idiosyncratically interpret the meaning of the end phrases, a situation that causes much variation between subjects. However, intrasubject variation is small, and thus linear analogue scales are particularly useful in research designs with repeated measures.

Another method by which to measure quality of life is the ACSA (1). In a slightly simplified version of the ACSA scale, subjects are asked to identify the "best" and the "worst" moments or periods in their life experience; the "best" moment is assigned a value of +5, the "worst" moment a −5, with 0 representing neither good nor bad. Using these two numerical reference points, the subject chooses a number that corresponds to his current state. The possibility also exists for the subject to score above +5 or below −5 if his/her current situation is perceived as surpassing those points. The chief advantages of the ACSA scale are that it allows the patient to define his own personal criteria, it is easily and quickly administered, and it lends itself readily to repeated-measures research designs. Simultaneously, the major drawback of the ACSA scale is that because quality of life is individually quantified the meaning of intersubject differences is difficult to ascertain. However, this problem can be overcome by considering not absolute scores but differences between the predisease ACSA score and the score during the disease, so as to determine the impact of disease and treatment on quality of life.

DESCRIPTION OF THE STUDY

The purpose of our investigation was to develop a quantifiable tool that would provide information about quality of life in addition to that obtained by the Karnofsky scale, a valid and reproducible instrument (4,6) currently used in our setting. Thus our first goal was to develop a questionnaire that could be used with French oncologic populations.

The secondary goal was to compare this scale with two other types of self-assessments, i.e., a LA method and the ACSA scale, in an effort to establish empirical validity. Among psychiatrists, the question of validity of self-report measures has been traditionally answered by establishing criteria based on their comparisons of the results of a self-report scale to their diagnostic findings from a psychiatric interview (3). This method of establishing the validity of a scale is frequently fraught with psychometric problems related to issues of objectivity and defining psychiatric symptoms. In the French setting, no full-time, trained interviewer was available, which mitigated against the establishment of such criterion validity. Instead, concurrent or empirical validity, which more closely approaches the highly desirable construct validity, was sought by comparing the QOL-Q with two other scales.

DEVELOPMENT OF THE MEASUREMENT TOOLS

Initially, a self-administered questionnaire with 67 items was developed after many discussions with patients and the staff about quality of life. From these discussions and a review of the literature, content factors were chosen and transposed into test items. Most of the content factors were represented by several items; some items were also selected to specifically test the impact of the illness versus the impact of the treatment modality.

Following this test construction, the questionnaire was administered to 50 outpatients in the Department of Radiation Therapy and Medical Oncology, Hospital St. Jacques, Besançon, France. Subjects were selected on the basis of their availability. For all subjects, sociodemographic information and data about their disease, its stage, and its treatment were recorded. All subjects were instructed to complete the questionnaire at home and return it to the researchers. Thirty patients complied with these instructions, giving a response rate of 60%.

The items were computer-analyzed using parametric statistics with the aid of the Statistical Package for Social Sciences (11). The items from each content factor were first examined. The items that had the most evenly distributed range of responses, relatively low positive correlations with items in other content factors, and a significantly positive correlation with the total score, and which contributed to a satisfactory alpha correlation coefficient for the total scale, were retained in the QOL-Q revised scale. Some of the items were reworded for easier comprehension, and the response categories were simplified and arranged unidirectionally. Because of the preliminary nature of the 67-item scale and the extent of the revision, no attempt was made to factor-analyze the items or content factors. The analysis that was completed resulted in construction of a 23-item scale, with each item response containing a 4-point Likert-type scale. The total score is obtained by summing the item response scores.

In addition to the QOL-Q, the LA scale was designed for use in the second part of our study. Five content areas that are frequently mentioned in relation to quality of life were selected: depression, fatigue, sense of well-being, pain, and self-confidence. For each content area, the endpoints of a 10-cm line were labeled with contrasting statements; the left statement represented the lowest quality of life, the right statement the highest. Each item score was determined by measuring in centimeters where the patient placed himself. The total score was obtained by summing the item scores.

COMPARISON OF QOL-Q, LA, AND ACSA

Between September 1983 and April 1984, 43 patients who had undergone radiation therapy for malignant disease were selected using a quota sampling technique. All subjects were administered the QOL-Q, LA, and ACSA scales by the same interviewer, a radiotherapist. Sociodemographic information and data related to the illness and treatment were collected for each subject.

Because the interviewer verbally read the scales and requested the patient's assistance in marking the appropriate responses, the response rate among the selected patients was 100%. It should be noted that the scale administration was incorporated into the medical consultation, not used as a separate, unique test procedure. The length of the administration time was approximately 15 min. Parametric statistics were used to analyze the relation between the three scales, specifically for intraitem and interitem analysis, and a comparison between patient characteristics and the test scores.

RESULTS

Information about subject age, marital status, location of the primary tumor, and treatment modality is displayed in Table 1. The average ACSA score was 0.463 with a range of -5 to $+4$ and a standard deviation (SD) of 2.325.

TABLE 1. *Subject sociodemographic and medical profiles*
(N = 43)

Age: average 57 years (range 19–85, SD 2.11)	
Marital status	
Married	58.1% (25)
Single	18.6% (8)
Widowed	16.3% (7)
Divorced	2.3% (1)
Unknown	4.7% (2)
Sex	
Male	39.5% (17)
Female	60.5% (25)
Tumor primary	
Breast	37.2% (16)
Head and neck	30.2% (13)
Gynecological	9.3% (4)
Gastrointestinal	7.0% (3)
Brain	4.7% (2)
Other	11.6% (5)
Treatment	
Irradiation	11.6% (5)
Irradiation + surgery	62.8% (27)
Irradiation + surgery + chemotherapy	23.3% (10)
Surgery + chemotherapy	2.3% (1)

The results of the linear analogue scale show that the average total score was 33.5 with a range of 11.5 to 48.0 and an SD of 8.53. The mean value for each of the items was as follows: depression 6.7, fatigue 5.4, "blues" 6.2, pain 7.2, and self-confidence 7.6. The alpha reliability coefficient for the scale was 0.712 with a standardized item alpha of 0.703. The item with the most correspondence ($r = 0.700$) with the total score was item 3, feeling "comfortable about myself" (*Je me sens bien dans ma peau*) to feeling "blue" (*J'ai le cafard*). The item with the least correspondence ($r = 0.205$) was item 4, about pain (*douleur*). In fact, the alpha correlation coefficient increased to 0.755 when the pain item was deleted from the reliability analysis.

The alpha reliability coefficient of the QOL-Q was found to be 0.754 with a standardized item alpha of 0.771. Intraitem analysis revealed that the item responses rarely attained a normal bell-shaped distribution and that fairly low correlations were found between the items. In regard to the distribution of responses, those items that were skewed in the direction of being least problematic included the items about everyday functioning: style of living, relations with family and friends, pain, appetite, and the untoward effects of treatment. The sole item that showed a similar skewing in the opposite direction was concerned with physical capacity. Moreover, a bimodal distribution was noted on the dimensions of nervousness and anxiety. Despite the uneven distribution of responses, the item scores were summated into a total score. This summation was done because it was unknown whether the skewed responses were accurate ones stemming from the characteristics of our outpatient population, or in fact the item responses were too narrowly conceived to permit subjects to indicate their actual situation. Because the QOL-Q was conceived for use with inpatient and outpatient populations who are in various stages of treatment, we have assumed that the results closely approximate the characteristics of our selected subjects. In regard to the low interitem correlations, the results were interpreted as reflecting the diversity of content factors, or dimensions, that were included in the scale.

Approximately one-third of the QOL-Q items had a significant positive correlation ($p < 0.05$) with the total score. The items that had the highest correlations with the total score (items 10, 11, 15, 16) are those with the same content factors as found on the LA scale, i.e., those items related to pain, fatigue, anxiety, and depression/feeling defeated. Conversely, the items with the least correlation (items 6, 20, 21, 23) were marital relationship, the depressing/defeating impact of chemotherapy, general interests, and leisure activities. As previously discussed, only 58.1% of the population were married, and about 25% had received chemotherapy; these items therefore were not applicable to the entire population. The alpha reliability coefficient, if each item was deleted, is shown in Table 2.

Person *r* correlation coefficients were used to compare the ACSA, LA, and QOL-Q. As presented in Table 3, positive relationships were found between the three scales.

TABLE 2. *Results of the quality of life questionnaire (N = 43): items means, SDs, variances, and alpha levels if the item score is deleted*

Items	Mean	SD	Variance	Alpha, score deleted
1. Everyday life	3.8	0.89	0.789	0.740
2. Professional life	2.1	1.15	1.331	0.735
3. Style of living	2.6	1.24	1.530	0.746
4. Family relations	3.8	0.47	0.217	0.747
5. Relations with friends	3.8	0.64	0.408	0.746
6. Marital relations	3.1	1.09	1.182	0.762
7. Marital relations	1.8	0.91	0.882	0.738
8. Sexual desire	1.8	1.33	1.759	0.753
9. Sexual activity	1.8	1.26	1.598	0.748
10. Pain	3.3	1.05	1.100	0.729
11. Tiredness	2.8	1.02	1.044	0.725
12. Appetite	3.5	0.91	0.827	0.742
13. Physical capacity	1.7	0.80	0.645	0.742
14. Nervousness	2.8	1.28	1.646	0.731
15. Anxiety	2.9	1.17	1.361	0.719
16. Depression	3.4	0.87	0.756	0.734
17. Crying	3.4	1.01	1.011	0.735
18. Surgical effects	3.0	1.12	1.261	0.755
19. Radiotherapy impact	3.1	1.08	1.162	0.751
20. Chemotherapy impact	2.1	0.73	0.534	0.760
21. General interests	2.4	1.02	1.049	0.784
22. Worry	2.3	0.77	0.587	0.748
23. Leisure	2.1	1.48	2.182	0.769

DISCUSSION

The present study was undertaken to evaluate and compare three measurement techniques for the assessment of psychosocial and somatic factors among cancer patients. This pilot investigation suggests that the QOL-Q may have some internal consistency and discriminant and concurrent validity, though this is a highly tentative conclusion based on preliminary data. Based on the presented results, the overall alpha reliability correlation coefficient of the QOL-Q suggests that the scale is a reliable measure, one deserving of more extensive analysis with larger populations.

TABLE 3. *Interscale comparisons*

Scale	ACSA	LA	QOL-Q
ACSA	1.000		
LA	0.468[a]	1.000	
QOL-Q	0.431[b]	0.484[a]	1.000

[a] $p < 0.001$.
[b] $p < 0.002$.

More specifically, the QOL-Q needs to be subjected to factor analyses and organized in a manner that permits the subtraction of various content factors from the test results, thereby yielding subscales that may be used with particular populations. For example, the questions about marital relationship and effect of illness on spouse may comprise one subscale that would be used with married subjects only. Also, the finding that the pain item detracted from overall alpha reliability suggests that this item must be factored out of the total score and placed on a subscale, particularly for well-functioning patients who report no pain.

The characteristics of the subjects, almost all of whom had social support, no pain, minimal fatigue, and satisfactory physical functioning, may have obscured some of the QOL-Q's ability to discriminate between subjects with high quality of life versus low quality of life. Administration of the QOL-Q to patients just beginning treatment, inpatients, or both should give more information about the scale's discriminative validity.

More extensive administration of the QOL-Q along with the ACSA and LA scales is also needed to better understand the interscale relations. The significant correlation found between the ACSA and the QOL-Q suggests that the QOL-Q has concurrent validity with the ACSA scale; i.e., the QOL-Q scores move in the same direction as those found in the ACSA scale. Important to consider, though, is the finding that the correlation between these two scales is low enough to assume that a duplicative function is not entirely being served by the QOL-Q. It is probable that the QOL-Q and the ACSA scales are measuring similar though not identical aspects of quality of life. As concerns the relation between the QOL-Q and the LA scales, there appears to be a high degree of concurrent validity. Indeed, this is not surprising as the QOL-Q items that were most highly correlated with the QOL-Q total score were virtually identical to the items measured on the LA scale. It seems then that one risks redundancy when the QOL-Q and the LA scales are given in tandem. If the same high levels of concurrent validity are found on subsequent administrations, one might recommend that the QOL-Q be used when more detailed information about quality of life is needed; the LA scale might be used as a general screening tool that alerts clinicians to patients having a poor quality of life. As found with the QOL-Q, the correlation between the LA and the ACSA scales suggests that the latter scale measures a different facet of quality of life, or that it defines quality of life differently than the LA and the QOL-Q scales. Thus it does not seem that the ACSA scale elicits the same information obtained on the other two scales. Future examinations of the association between the three scales need to employ analyses of variance to determine if the relation between the scales is due to variances of the scales or within the scales.

Apart from striving to establish the levels of reliability and validity for the QOL-Q, this pilot project proved to be clinically instructional for the health provider and beneficial for the patient. The oncologists gathered more information about their patients, information that could be integrated into their treatment plans. More importantly, physician–patient communication was facilitated, which often resulted in allayed patient anxiety and the sense that the physician cared about the whole person, not just the disease.

Because of cultural idiosyncrasies, an assumption had been made by the investigators that a French oncologic population would not be receptive to revealing information about marital, family, and economic concerns. This assumption was not borne out, as the subjects appeared willing and often eager to discuss highly personal matters with their oncologists. Part of this patient participation was undoubtedly due to the order in which the tests were administered. The ACSA scale appears to be an excellent tool to introduce the concept of quality of life. Though the conceptualization of the ''best'' and the ''worst'' moments was not always easy for the patient, most subjects openly discussed their happiest and saddest memories and were able to rate their current state according to their chosen indices. Likewise, the visual LA scale appeared to be readily understood by most subjects and provided an introduction to the lengthier QOL-Q. It is probable that had the patients been first presented with a 23-item test many would have been reluctant to respond.

SUMMARY

The QOL-Q and its concurrent use with the ACSA and LA scales needs to have larger administrations to oncologic populations to establish additional reliability and validity data, though it appears that the QOL-Q has a sufficient level of reliability. An investigation that assesses the QOL-Q's sensitivity to changes in the illness and treatment course is currently under way. Additionally, projects that segregate cancer type, stage of disease, and treatment modality are being considered for future administrations of the QOL-Q.

The ultimate goal of the development and the administration of the QOL-Q is to yield information about the effects of certain oncologic treatments, particularly randomized trials. Although the combination of the ACSA scale, LA scale, and the QOL-Q need further validation, these measures have the potential to fulfill this goal. They may assist clinicians and their patients to choose treatment programs that promote disease management while attending to the patient's quality of life.

REFERENCES

1. Bernheim, J. L., and Buyse, M. (1983): The anamnestic comparative self-assessment for measuring the subjective quality of life of cancer patients. *J. Psychosoc. Oncol.*, 1(4):25–38.
2. Bond, A. J., and Lader, M. H. (1974): The use of analogue scales in rating subjective feelings. *Br. J. Med. Psychol.*, 47:211–218.
3. Boyle, G. J. (1985): Self-report measures of depression: Some psychometric considerations. *Br. J. Clin. Psychol.*, 24:45–59.
4. Change, S. K., and Hawes, K. A. (1983): The adequacy of Karnofsky Rating and Global Adjustment to Illness Scale as outcome measures in cancer rehabilitation and continuing care. *Prog. Clin. Biol. Res.*, 120:429–433.
5. Green, C. J. (1982): Psychological assessment in medical settings. In: *Handbook of Clinical*

Health Psychology, edited by T. Millon, C. Green, and R. Meagher, pp. 339–375. Plenum Press, New York.

6. Grieco, A., and Long, C. J. (1984): Investigation of the Karnofsky Performance Status as a measure of quality of life. *Health Psychol.,* 3:129–142.

7. Kremer, E., Atkinson, J. H., and Ignelzi, R. J. (1981): Measurement of pain: Patient preference does not confound pain measurement. *Pain,* 10:241–248.

8. Mendelson, G., and Selwood, T. S. (1981): Measurement of chronic pain: A correlation study of verbal and nonverbal scales. *J. Behav. Assessment,* 3:263–269.

9. Mettlin, C., Cookfair, D. L., Lane, W., and Pickren, J. (1983): The quality of life in patients with cancer. *N.Y. State J. Med.,* 83:187–193.

10. Morrow, G. R., et al. (1981): Development of brief measures of psychosocial adjustment to medical illness applied to cancer patients. *Gen. Hosp. Psychiatry,* 3:79–88.

11. Nie, N. H., and Hull, C. H., eds. (1981): *SPSS Update 7-9: New Procedures and Facilities for Releases 7-9.* McGraw-Hill, New York.

12. Presant, C. A., Klahr, C., and Hogan, L. (1981): Evaluating quality-of-life in oncology patients: Pilot observations. *Oncol. Nurs. Forum,* 8(3):26–30.

13. Price, D. D., McGrath, P. A., Rafii, A., and Buckingham, B. (1983): The validation of visual analogue scales as ratio scale measures for chronic and experimental pain. *Pain,* 17:45–56.

14. Schipper, H. (1983): Why measure quality of life? *Can. Med. Assoc. J.,* 128:1367–1370.

15. Schipper, H., Clinch, J., McMurray, A., and Levitt, M. (1984): Measuring the quality of life of cancer patients: The Functional Living Index-Cancer: Development and validation. *J. Clin. Oncol.,* 2:472–483.

16. Schraub, S., Monpetit, E., Bransfield, D., and Zysman, H. (1984): Appreciation de la qualite de la vie. In: *Qualite de la Vie et Cancers (Progres en Cancerolgie 4, 1983),* edited by S. Schraub, J. Brugere, and B. Hoerni. Doin Editeurs, Paris.

17. Spitzer, W. O., et al. (1981): Measuring the quality of life of cancer patients: A concise QL-index for use by physicians. *J. Chronic Dis.,* 34:585–597.

18. Sriwatanakul, K., Kelvie, W., Lasagna, L., Calimlim, J. F., Weis, O. F., and Mehta, G. (1983): Studies with different types of visual analog scales for measurement of pain. *Clin. Pharmacol. Ther.,* 34:234–239.

The Quality of Life of Cancer Patients,
edited by N. K. Aaronson and J. Beckmann,
Raven Press, New York © 1987.

Assessment of Quality of Life: Scoring Performance Status in Cancer Patients

Everdina H. Klein Poelhuis, Augustinus A. M. Hart, Jeanette M.
V. Burgers, *Rudolphus J. J. Hermus, and Peter F. Bruning

*The Netherlands Cancer Institute, 1066 CX Amsterdam, The Netherlands; and *Institute
Civo-Toxicology and Nutrition TNO, 3700 AJ Zeist, The Netherlands*

Although experienced clinicians have a good general idea about the severity of cancer as a disease and of its therapy, they may also realize that the impact of cancer on individual patients is highly variable. Simple methods to assess the well-being of cancer patients are much needed. The increasing number of clinical trials requires assessment and comparison of the patient's quality of life.

Measures of patient's independence that have been widely used are the Karnofsky Performance Status scale (6) and the World Health Organization (WHO) scale (11). Generally, the scores on these scales are assigned by the attending physician. However, the physician is often unfamiliar with details of the patient's everyday life, and the nature of quality of life may be regarded as very subjective. It has been argued that only the patient himself is able to express how well he is feeling (1,4). To this purpose a complaint checklist that is completed by the patient himself has been developed in The Netherlands Cancer Institute (9). In this report we present a comparison of four methods of evaluation: the Karnofsky index, the WHO scale, a complaint checklist, and the opinion of experienced clinicians concerning the burden of radiotherapy to the patient.

Although the four methods differ somewhat by objective, they all aim at assessment of the patient's well-being. Consequently, one may expect similar information to be obtained by each method. By comparing them, a choice of the most appropriate method should be possible.

SUBJECTS AND METHODS

This study was part of a prospective quantitative analysis of the nutritional intake, nutritional status, and physical and mental fitness of cancer patients who underwent treatment with radiotherapy or combination chemotherapy (2). The patient sample selected for the present investigation consisted of 76 patients who were treated with radiotherapy only. The sample included 28 women who underwent irradiation for cervical or endometrial cancer after surgery and 48 men who were treated with irradiation of the lower abdomen for cancer of the urinary bladder or prostate. Four of the latter patients who took part in the original study were excluded because of missing data. The age of the subjects ranged from 27 to 84 years with an average age of 66.5 (SD 9.7).

Patient selection and treatment schedules have been described in detail elsewhere (2). All patients were assigned scores on the clinical scales according to Karnofsky (6) and the WHO (11). This was done five times during a 19-week period by one of two psychologist-investigators and one of three dietitian-investigators. The psychologists and dietitians had no previous experience with the use of the scales. The two investigators scored independently of each other. Karnofsky's 11-point rating scale ranges from normal functioning (100) to dead (0). The WHO 5-point rating scale ranges from normal functioning (0) to totally bedridden (4) (Table

TABLE 1. *Karnofsky Performance Status scale and WHO scale*

Karnofksy scale		WHO scale	
Status	Score	Status	Score
Normal, no complaints	100	Fully active, able to carry out all predisease activities without restriction.	0
Able to carry on normal activities. Minor signs or symptoms of disease.	90	Restricted in strenuous activity but ambulatory and able to carry out light work or pursue sedentary occupation.	1
Normal activity with effort.	80		
Cares for self. Unable to carry on normal activity or to do active work.	70	Ambulatory and capable of all self-care but unable to carry out any light work. Up and about more than 50% of waking hours.	2
Requires occasional assistance but able to care for most of his needs.	60		
Requires considerable assistance.	50	Capable of only limited self-care; confined to bed or chair more than 50% of waking hours.	3
Disabled. Requires special care and assistance.	40		
Severely disabled. Hospitalization indicated though death not imminent.	30	Completely disabled. Unable to carry out any self-care and confined totally to bed or chair.	4
Very sick. Hospitalization necessary. Active supportive treatment necessary.	20		
Moribund	10		
Dead	0		

TABLE 2. *Comparison of Karnofsky Performance Scale score and WHO score applied by two independent investigators to 76 patients*

	Psychologist			
Dietitian	100/0	90/1	80/2	70–0/3–4
100/0	6/8	3/13	1/0	0/0
90/1	5/5	27/34	10/4	2/1
80/2	1/0	1/3	6/3	7/1
70–0/3–4	0/0	0/0	0/1	7/3

The figures placed before the "/" represent the number of patients to whom corresponding Karnofsky scores were assigned. The figures placed after the "/" represent the number of patients to whom corresponding WHO scores were assigned. Kendall's tau = +0.63 and +0.53, respectively.

1). The ratings were based on contact with the patient just before or after a medical follow-up in the outpatient clinic. Ratings during the fourth week of observation were selected for the present study. Because all patients were either in their last week of therapy or in the week before an interval, the range of the scores was at its widest at this moment. It should be emphasized that the patients with cancer of the prostate had not completed their full course of irradiation. On the same occasion the patient completed a questionnaire. The checklist of complaints had been constructed and validated in a pilot study (7). The list consisted of 42 items, of which a cluster of four questions concerned "malaise." The cluster contained the following items: "Did you feel tired?" "Did you want to lie down?" "Did you feel as if you had no energy?" "Did you feel unwell?" The subjects were asked to express a complaint on a 4-point scale as "not at all" (0), "a little"

TABLE 3. *Comparison of the application of the Karnofsky scale and WHO scale to 76 patients*

	WHO score			
Karnofsky score	0	1	2	3–4
100	12	0	0	0
90	2	29	0	0
80	0	16	1	0
70–0	0	4	7	5

The figures represent the number of patients to whom corresponding scores were assigned. Kendall's tau = −0.77. The negative correlation is due to the direction of scoring on the two scales.

(1), "quite a bit" (2), or "very much" (3), yielding a total score on the malaise cluster that could range from 0 to 12. The questions were formulated in such a way that the patient was asked about his condition on the preceding day. Only the scores on the malaise cluster during the fourth week of observation were included in the current analysis.

Three experienced radiotherapists gave their opinion about the severity of the therapy on a 5-point scale ranging from "less severe" (1) to "very severe" (5), yielding a total score that could range from 3 to 15. The radiotherapists independently based their rating on the treatment as a whole, taking into account total tumor dose, number of fractions per week, field size, location, and the presence or absence of a break during therapy.

RESULTS

Table 2 shows the dietitians' and psychologists' Karnofsky ratings. In the same table the scores on the WHO scale, again with the two ratings for each patient, are given. As can be seen, there was fair agreement between the dietitians and psychologists, with the dietitians showing a tendency to score somewhat higher. For simplicity of presentation the scores of the psychologists were used for further analysis.

In Table 3 the Karnofsky ratings and the WHO scores can be compared. The results of the two methods appear to be in general agreement. The results of the comparison between Karnofsky and WHO scores and the scores on the malaise cluster are shown in Table 4. Both performance status measures correlated only moderately with the malaise cluster, suggesting that they represented somewhat

TABLE 4. *Comparison of malaise cluster score and Karnofsky score and of a malaise cluster score and WHO score of 76 patients*

Malaise cluster score	Karnofsky score/WHO score			
	100/0	90/1	80/2	70–0/3–4
0–1	7/8	14/14	2/0	0/0
2–3	3/4	9/11	2/0	2/1
4–5	1/1	5/0	4/0	0/0
6–7	0/0	4/12	8/5	6/0
8–12	0/0	1/4	1/3	7/4

The figures placed before the "/" represent the number of patients with corresponding malaise cluster scores and Karnofsky scores. The figures placed behind the "/" represent the number of patients with corresponding malaise cluster scores and WHO scores. Kendall's tau = −0.59 and +0.54, respectively.

TABLE 5. *Comparison of Karnofsky score and rating of treatment severity by radiotherapists and of WHO score and rating of treatment severity of 76 patients*

Treatment severity rating	Karnofsky score/WHO score			
	100/0	90/1	80/2	70–0/3–4
3–6	0/0	3/6	3/1	1/0
7–8	3/4	8/11	2/4	7/1
9–10	2/2	2/2	0/0	2/2
11–12	6/6	15/23	7/2	5/2
13–15	1/1	3/8	5/1	1/0

The figures placed before the "/" represent the number of patients with corresponding treatment severity ratings and Karnofsky scores. The figures placed behind the "/" represent the number of patients with corresponding treatment severity ratings and WHO scores. Kendall's tau = +0.03 and +0.01, respectively.

TABLE 6. *Comparison of malaise cluster score and rating of treatment severity by radiotherapists of 76 patients*

Treatment severity rating	Malaise cluster score				
	0–1	2–3	4–5	6–7	8–12
3–6	2	0	1	4	0
7–8	3	6	1	6	4
9–10	1	1	2	0	2
11–12	8	7	5	6	7
13–15	4	2	1	1	2

The figures represent the number of patients with corresponding scores. Kendall's tau = +0.09.

overlapping but nonetheless distinct areas of measurement. Table 5 gives a comparison between the Karnofsky scores assigned by the psychologists and the ratings of the treatment severity by the radiotherapists. A similar comparison between scores on the WHO scale and the radiotherapists' ratings is also represented in Table 5. Finally, the malaise cluster and radiotherapists' ratings are compared in Table 6. There was little relation between the clinicians' ratings and patients' scores on the malaise scale or the performance scores assigned by the investigators during week 4 of treatment.

DISCUSSION

The interrater reliability of the Karnofsky scale has been investigated in a number of studies (3,5,10,12) and has been found to be moderate. In the present study, both the Karnofsky index and the WHO scale were also found to have only a moderate interrater reliability. This may be due in part to the fact that the raters were relatively inexperienced.

A comparison of Karnofsky and WHO scores indicated that in the present study the two methods were in general agreement for the observed range. This conclusion was supported by the relation of each scale to the malaise cluster. Considering the similar results of comparison between malaise cluster scoring and the Karnofsky scale and the WHO scale, respectively, a practical choice between the latter two would be in favor of the WHO scale. Its simplicity makes it easy to apply even for health workers with no specific training. A comparison of the Karnofsky and WHO scales should be made in future prospective studies of patients scoring over a much wider range than in the present investigation. From our data a conclusion with regard to a definite choice between the malaise checklist completed by the patient himself and a score on a clinical scale assigned by an observer remains difficult. The administration of the clinical scales was easy and fast. The use of the checklist took more time, although it never presented great difficulties. With more ill patients the use of clinical scales may be preferable as their application relies less on the patient's ability to cooperate.

In the present study no relation was found between the radiotherapists' ratings of the total treatment's severity with the results of the three other methods. The clinicians based their opinions on technical data and their general clinical experience. Apparently, however, this general concept was not consistent with the individual patient's experience after 4 weeks of treatment as reported on the checklist or as assigned on the clinical scales by investigators having less clinical experience. This finding underscores the need for individual assessment of well-being when the merits of different treatment modalities are to be compared, as in clinical trials.

ACKNOWLEDGMENTS

This study was supported by a grant from the Queen Wilhelmina Cancer Research Fund and the Division for Nutrition and Food Research TNO, and is part of a research project concerning the nutrition of cancer patients. The authors are grateful to the radiotherapists for their cooperation and to dietitians Annet Giesbers, Ank Gooskens, and Anneke Huldij and to psychologist Ans Kobashi-Schoot for their help in collecting the data.

REFERENCES

1. Andrews, F. M., and Whitey, S. B. (1976): *Social Indicators of Wellbeing*. Plenum Press, New York.
2. Bruning, P. F., Egger, R. J., Gooskens, A. C., Hermus, R. J. J., Hulshof, K. F. A. M., Kistemaker, C., Klein Poelhuis, E. H., Kobashi-Schoot, A., Odink, J., Schreurs, W. H. P., and

Wedel, M. (1985): Dietary intake, nutritional status and well-being of cancer patients: A prospective study. *Eur, J. Cancer Clin. Oncol.,* 21:1449–1459.

3. Coscarelli Schag, C., and Heinrich, R. L. (1984): Karnofsky Performance Status revisited: Reliability, validity and guidelines. *J. Clin. Oncol.,* 2:193–197.

4. Fontana, A. F. (1980): Psychological impairment and psychological health in the psychological well-being of the physically ill. *Psychosom. Med.,* 42:279–288.

5. Hutchinson, T. A., Boyd, N. F., and Feinstein, A. R. (1979): Scientific problems in clinical scales, as demonstrated in the Karnofsky Index of Performance Status. *J. Chronic Dis.,* 32:661–666.

6. Karnofsky, D. A., and Burchenal, J. H. (1949): The clinical evaluation of chemotherapeutic agents in cancer. In: *Evaluation of Chemotherapeutic Agents,* edited by C. M. Macleod. Columbia University Press, New York.

7. Kobashi-Schoot, J. A. M., Hanewald, G. J. F. P., Van Dam, F. S. A. M., and Bruning, P. F. (1985): Assessment of malaise in cancer patients treated with radiotherapy. *Cancer Nurs.,* 8:306–31.

8. Deleted in proof.

9. Linssen, A. C. G., Hanewald, G. J. F. P., and Van Dam, F. S. A. M. (1981): The development of the complaint questionnaire at The Netherlands Cancer Institute. In: *Proceedings of the First Workshop on Quality of Life.* International Publication Study Group on Quality of Life, Amsterdam.

10. Mor, V., Laliberte, L., Morris, J. N., and Wiemann, M. (1984): The Karnofsky Performance Status Scale: An examination of its reliability and validity in a research setting. *Cancer,* 53:2002–2007.

11. *WHO Handbook for Reporting Results of Cancer Treatment* (1979): World Health Organization, Geneva.

12. Yates, J. W., Chalmer, B., and McKegney, F. P. (1980): Evaluation of patients with advanced cancer using the Karnofsky Performance Status. *Cancer,* 45:2220–2224.

The Quality of Life of Cancer Patients,
edited by N. K. Aaronson and J. Beckmann,
Raven Press, New York © 1987.

On Measuring Complaints of Cancer Patients: Some Remarks on the Time Span of the Question

Sjouke J. Huisman,* Frits S. A. M. van Dam,* Neil K. Aaronson, and Gerrit J. F. P. Hanewald

*Department of Clinical Psychology, University of Amsterdam, 1018 XA Amsterdam, The Netherlands; and *The Netherlands Cancer Institute, 1066 CX Amsterdam, The Netherlands*

When reviewing the literature on the consequences of cancer and cancer treatment, it becomes clear that most studies are concerned primarily with rates of recurrence and survival (15). Without challenging the primacy of such data, it is nevertheless disappointing to find that few systematic data are collected about the quality of life of cancer patients. At this moment we can fully subscribe to the position taken by Irwin et al. (11) when they stated: "We know that people survive, and how long they are likely to survive, but we do not know, in a systematic way, the quality of this survival, including social, economic, and psychological functioning."

There has been a growing interest, however, in the assessment of quality of life of cancer patients (21). One of the more important aspects of quality of life is the physical and psychological concomitants of cancer. It is therefore necessary to develop reliable and valid instruments to assess these physical and psychological symptoms or complaints.

One of the issues that has received relatively little attention in the development of such measures is the time span of the questions. When assessing the physical and psychological complaints of cancer patients, researchers have employed a variety of time frames, ranging from "at this moment" to "1 month." Often the time frame of the questions is left completely undefined. For example, Gill (5), measuring the subjective well-being of the chronically ill, asked about this moment ("right now"). The Hopkins Symptom Checklist (2), measuring five symptom dimensions, asks about the past 7 days, including "today." Bradburn's (1) Affect Balance Scale, measuring positive and negative affect, employs the last few weeks as a time frame. The Rand Health Insurance Study General Well-being Measure (17) focuses on a somewhat longer time period, i.e., 1 month. The Langner 22-item index of Mental Distress (13) and the Pain and Distress Scale (26), have no specified time frame. With the exception of Gill (5), none of these researchers has provided an explicit reason for choosing a specific questionnaire or interview time frame.

Particularly for the evaluation of cancer clinical trials, it may be essential to limit the time span of the questions to a relatively short period. For example, during almost every course of chemotherapy two periods can be distinguished: a period during which the immediate effects of the drug are at hand (e.g., nausea, fatigue) and a period of rest during which a patient recovers from these short-term effects (3). Thus if the time frame of the question is too long or undefined, the patient may be confused as to which period he should report: the rest period, the treatment period, or perhaps both (22). In order to evaluate toxicity it is therefore important to divide each trial according to these treatment periods and to structure questionnaire or interview items with a specific limited time frame in mind. A more general reason favoring a short time span has to do with memory effects. As Hofstee (9) has stated, one of the requirements for the use of self-ratings is that the subject is capable of fulfilling the role of an "objective observer." Clearly, such self-observation can be better accomplished when asking about the previous day than about the previous month. As an illustration, the reader is advised to undertake a brief experiment, i.e., to try to answer the question "Did you have a headache?" for each of the following time periods: "yesterday," "last week," and "last month."

In addition to these more practical issues, there is also a theoretical justification for limiting the time span of the questions about symptoms and side effects of treatment, one based on the distinction between state and trait measures. Trait measures, asking about how people feel or react in general (without time frame), are intended to measure the disposition of a person that predisposes him to perceive situations in particular ways and to react in a consistent manner in a wide variety of situations (20). Conversely, state measures, asking how people feel or react at a particular moment, are intended to assess the response pattern of a person in a specific situation. In other words, the very essence of a trait measure—its stability over time—prohibits its use as an index of behavioral change (24). State measures, on the other hand, are expected to fluctuate with conditions that affect the relevant constructs embodied in the tests. It is clear, then, that patient self-report instruments intended to be sensitive to treatment-related symptom experience must be designed in such a way as to minimize potential confounding by the trait dispositions of the individual. It is best accomplished by employing the shorter time frame found in state measures.

It remains unclear as to how short a time frame is necessary to yield a true state measure. Some evidence suggests that a time span of even 1 week is already too long. One of the characteristics of a state measure is its typical low retest reliability (25). When examining the retest reliability of the five scales of the Hopkins Symptom Check-List, with evaluations performed 1 week apart, we found retest correlations ranging from 0.75 to 0.84 (2). These rather high retest reliabilities are more representative of trait measures than state measures. Similarly, Ormel (16) performed an extensive analysis of the adequacy of a time span of 4 weeks for a state complaint list. His conclusion was that this state measure could not be differentiated from a trait complaint list. This analysis of Ormel was, in fact, the only study we could find on the adequacy of a certain time span for a state measure of complaints. Furthermore, we were surprised to find so few researchers who explicitly considered the distinction between state and trait measures when developing their study instruments.

In summary, when developing a reliable and valid instrument to measure the physical and psychological side effects of cancer treatments, it is necessary to investigate the influence of time span on measures of complaints. Toward this end, we carried out an investigation in which we used a complaint list with four time spans: 1 day, 3 days, 1 week, and 4 weeks. We contrasted these four ''state measures'' with a trait complaint list. Our expectation was that the longer the time span of the state measure, the stronger would be the relation with the trait measure.

METHOD

Subjects

Subjects were 963 blood donors (746 men, 217 women). The mean age for the men was 35.5 (SD 10.8) and for the women 26.4 (SD 5.0). The reason for not choosing cancer patients as the subjects for this study was primarily practical in nature. Because complaints of cancer patients are largely influenced by the state of the disease and the stage of therapy, it would have been necessary to employ a homogeneous patient group. It was not feasible, however, to find a sufficiently large group of cancer patients with a common diagnosis to meet the sample size requirements of this study.

Measures

The Neuroticism and Neurosomaticism scales of the ''Amsterdamse Biografische Vragenlijst'' (23) served as trait measures. The Neuroticism scale, based partly on the Maudsley Personality Inventory (12), is designed to measure the tendency to complain in psychological terms. The Neurosomaticism scale, based on the Two Part Personality Measure (7), is designed to measure the tendency to complain in somatic terms. Both measures have proved to be reliable indicators of neurotic lability (23). Results from a study by Ormel (16) indicated that both measures reflect personality traits, rather than a person's reaction to psychosocial stress. For practical reasons we chose the shorter version of these scales as used by Ormel. This shorter version consists of eight neuroticism questions (e.g., ''Do you often feel lonely?'') and 14 neurosomaticism questions (e.g., ''Do you feel dizzy sometimes?''). The three available response categories are: ''yes,'' ''no,'' or "uncertain." As a measure of state complaints we used a checklist with 37 physical (e.g., loss of appetite, nausea, dizziness) and psychological (e.g., depressed, tense, anxious) complaints. This checklist, with a time span of 1 day ("yesterday"), was developed at The Netherlands Cancer Institute for use with cancer patients. When employing the 1-day time frame, the checklist has been found to be a valid and reliable measure of cancer patients' symptom experience (14). Response categories for this checklist range on a 4-point scale from "not at all" to "very much."

Procedure

For purposes of the study, four versions of the state checklist were constructed, each employing a different time span. In addition to "yesterday" (state 1), we also used "the last 3 days" (state 3), "the last week" (state 7), and "the last 4 weeks" (state 28). Subjects were randomly assigned to one of these four versions of the state checklist. Together with one of these versions, subjects were asked to complete the trait measures of Neuroticism and Neurosomaticism. All questionnaires were filled out by the subjects after their blood donation.

RESULTS

In this study we have performed four Princals analyses (3,4), one for each of the four subgroups who completed a version of the state measure. Princals is more or less comparable to ordinary Principal Components Analysis. It is a method for extracting the underlying structure from a set of variables (i.e., to find the correspondence between variables). Princals was choosen over the conventional factor analysis method primarily because of its ability to handle ordinal level data. Our expectation was that in the Princals analysis of the state 1 data we could clearly differentiate state measures of complaints from both trait measures of Neuroticism and Neurosomaticism. We further expected that the longer the time span of our questions, the closer the correspondence would be between state and trait measures.

Prior to carrying out the multivariate analysis, several alterations of the data matrix were required. All items with more than 95% of the answers in the category "not at all" were deleted (four of the 37 items). Furthermore, because of the limited variability at the high end of the scale, the response categories "very much" and "fairly" were combined, thus yielding a 3-point response scale.

Before analyzing the relation between state and trait measures of complaints for each of the four time spans, we first examined the factor structure of the state 1 checklist. We expected this version to be the most clearly representative of a true state measure. Results of the Princals analysis were comparable to those obtained with ordinary factor analysis on samples of cancer patients (18) and blood donors (10), indicating that only the first two dimensions could be meaningfully interpreted. The first factor could be interpreted as a psychic factor with high loadings of seven items (worrying, depressed, nervous, desperate about the future, lonely, tense, anxious). The second factor had three high loading items (tired, spiritless, need to rest). This second factor was interpreted as a malaise factor. Most of the remaining items, representing primarily physical complaints, did not load on either factor.

On the basis of the first analysis we computed two additive subscales. The first scale, called the Psychological Complaint Scale (PCS), consisted of the total score on the seven psychological complaints. The second scale, called the Malaise Complaint Scale (MCS), consisted of the computed sum on the three malaise items. The reliability of both scales, indicated by Cronbach's alpha, was quite satisfactory (0.84 for the PCS and 0.78 for the MCS). To answer our central research question, i.e., the influence of time span on the relation between state and trait measures of complaints, we performed a series of four Princals analyses, one for each version of the state list. The analyzed variables were the 33 remaining items of the complaint list and the two scores on the Neuroticism (N) and Neurosomaticism (NS) scales. Because we expected the Psychological and Malaise complaint scales to be more reliable measures of complaints than their constituent items, we also included both complaint scales in the analysis. This addition may have a small effect on the results, but the advantage was a clearer interpretation of the Princals analyses. To make all four scales more comparable to the 33 items, each scale was recoded into three categories, with approximately one-third of the subjects per category.

Results of these four analyses are plotted in Figs. 1 through 4. Plotted in these figures are the component loadings of the four scale scores on the first two dimensions. Component loadings are comparable to factor loadings in factor analysis. A component loading represents the computed correlation between a factor and a variable. In other words, the higher the component loadings of a variable, the more this variable is representative of that factor. For ease of comparison we rotated the loadings so that the component loading of the PCS on the first dimension was maximal.

Furthermore, the length of an arrow is determined by the component loading of a variable on either dimension. Within our two-dimensional model, the cosine of the angle between two arrows corresponds approximately to the correlation between two measures.

As can be seen in Fig. 1 (analyzing state 1), two rather independent factors, PCS and MCS, can be distinguished. As expected, N as well as NS can be differentiated from both PCS and MCS. When Fig. 2 (analyzing state 3) is examined, some changes can already be observed. First, we see that the angle between PCS and N has narrowed considerably, indicating that these two constructs are more closely related than was the case in Fig. 1. Additionally, N is somewhat longer than in Fig. 1, providing further evidence of the greater similarity of these two measures. Figure 3 (analyzing state 7) and especially Fig. 4 (analyzing state 28)

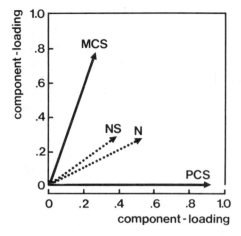

FIG. 1. Princals analysis: the relation between 1-day complaint checklist and trait measures.

FIG. 2. Princals analysis: the relation between 3-day complaint checklist and trait measures.

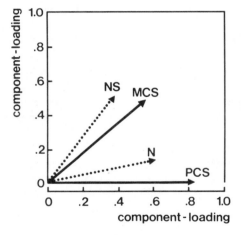

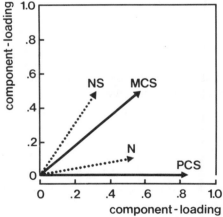

FIG. 3. Princals analysis: the relation between 1-week complaint checklist and trait measures.

FIG. 4. Princals analysis: the relation between 4-week complaint checklist and trait measures.

shows that the angle between PCS and N is nearly zero, indicating the close correspondence between these measures.

More or less the same pattern emerges with the MCS and NS measures. Although they can be clearly differentiated in Fig. 1, it is less apparent in Fig. 2. The heightened correspondence between the MCS and NS measures can be most clearly observed in Figs. 3 and 4. From Figs. 3 and 4, it also appears that the angle between MCS and PCS has decreased, indicating that with a longer time span it becomes more difficult to differentiate psychological complaints from malaise complaints. Although not evident in these simplified plots, another interesting change could be observed in the actual results. As stated before, the Princals analysis of the state 1 checklist indicated that no relation could be observed among the physical complaint items. On the other hand, the analyses of state 7 and especially state 28 showed the emergence of a new factor consisting of the physical complaints. More interesting, however, is the finding that this "physical factor" had a clear relation with NS. In other words, when long time spans were used in measuring these complaints a close correspondence could be observed between people's reported physical symptoms and their tendency to complain in somatic terms. This emergence of a physical factor in the state 7 and state 28 analyses is also the reason for the shift upward of NS in Figs. 3 and 4.

DISCUSSION

Summarizing the results, it can be stated that the time span of questions had a rather clear impact on the relation between our state complaint questionnaire and both trait measures of complaints. Specifically, when subjects were asked about their complaints with "yesterday" as the time frame, their responses to these state questions could be clearly differentiated from their answers to the trait questions included in the Neuroticism and Neurosomaticism scales.

When this time span was enlarged from 1 day to 3 days, responses to the psychological complaint items could not clearly be differentiated from the trait measure of Neuroticism, which is purported to measure a general tendency to complain in psychological terms. Moving from the "last 3 days" to the "last week," we found that the questions about malaise complaints were more or less measuring the same thing as the trait measures of Neurosomaticism, i.e., the tendency to complain in somatic terms. Also, when asking about the last week, subjects had more difficulty differentiating psychological complaints from malaise complaints. When looking at the answers on questions framed in terms of the "last 4 weeks," we found that the aforementioned shifts were even more pronounced.

It is clear, then, that the closer relation between the "state measures" and the trait measures (N and NS) was already evident when expanding the time frame from 1 day to 3 days. This relation became more pronounced when still longer time periods were used. In other words, the longer the time span of a complaint questionnaire, the more it appears to be measuring the tendency of people to complain and the less it seems to measure their actual symptom experience.

As argued before, when evaluating symptoms and side effects of cancer and cancer therapies we are not interested in measuring the tendency to complain, as this tendency, being a more stable characteristic of persons, is not influenced by changing conditions. What we do want to measure is the way a person actually feels in a situation, e.g., the number and seriousness of complaints due to a treatment. The results of our study suggest that framing questionnaire items in terms of the previous day (or "today") may be better suited for evaluating side effects of cancer treatments than measures pertaining to longer time periods.

We think, however, that some important caveats should be introduced. First, when such a narrow time frame is used there is a real danger that questionnaire responses may not be representative of the patient's recent experiences. For example, a systematic sampling error was found in a previous study (10) in which subjects had significantly fewer complaints on Monday than on other days of the week. In this case it was clear that asking on Monday about "yesterday" (i.e., Sunday, a work-free day for most people) was the source of this difference. An example of random sampling error could be found when some of the respondents simply had experienced a "bad," but atypical day. This last pitfall could be circumvented by using sufficiently large groups, so that this kind of random error could be reduced. Given these caveats, we recommend using as short a time frame as is feasible given the specific research question at hand. Clearly, our findings indicate that asking patients to report complaints relating to a time period longer than 1 week may be ill-advised.

It should also be cautioned that our sample of blood donors was not drawn from a cancer population and may not even be representative of a more general healthy population. Thus although our findings point to a serious measurement problem that should be addressed in any research undertaken to evaluate patients' symptom experience, there is need for replication of our findings among cancer and other chronic disease patients.

REFERENCES

1. Bradburn, N. (1969): *The Structure of Psychological Well-Being.* Aldine, Chicago.
2. Derogates, L. R., Lipman, R. S., Rickels, K., Uhlenhuth, E. H., and Covi, L. (1974): The Hopkins Symptom Checklist (HSCL): A self report inventory. *Behav. Sci.,* 19:1–15.
3. Gifi, A. (1981): Non-Linear Multivariate Analysis. Department of Data Theory, Faculty of Social Sciences, University of Leiden, The Netherlands.
4. Gifi, A. (1983): Princals users guide. Department of Data Theory, Faculty of Social Sciences, University of Leiden, The Netherlands.
5. Gill, W. M. (1984): Subjective well-being: Properties of an instrument for measuring this (in the chronically ill). *Soc. Sci. Med.,* 18:563–573.
6. Deleted on proof.
7. Heron, A. (1956): A two-part personality measure for use as a research criterion. *Br. J. Psychol.,* 47:243.
8. Herson, J. (1980): Evaluations of toxicity: Statistical considerations. *Cancer Treat. Rep.,* 64(2–3).
9. Hofstee, W. K. B. (1965): De vragenlijstsituatie. *Ned. Tijdschr. Psychol.,* 20:592–602.
10. Huisman, S. J. (1982): De ontwikkeling van een zelf-beoordelingsschaal voor welbevinden en dagelijkse Aktiviteiten. Ph.D. dissertation, University of Amsterdam.
11. Irwin, P. H., Gottlieb, A., Kramer, S., and Danoff, B. (1982): Quality of life after radiation therapy: A study of 309 cancer survivors. *Soc. Indicators Res.,* 10:187–210.
12. Jensen, A. (1958): The Maudsley Personality Inventory. *Acta Psychol.* (*Amst.*), 14:314.
13. Langner, T. S. (1962): A twenty-two item screening score of psychiatric symptoms indicating impairment. *J. Health Hum. Behav.,* 3:269–276.
14. Linssen, A. C. G., van Dam, F. S. A. M., Engelsman, E., van Benthem, J., and Hanewald, G. J. F. P. (1979): Leven met cytostatica. *Pharm. Weekbl.* [*Sci.*], 114:501–515.
15. McPeck, B., Gilbert, J. P., and Mosteller, F. (1977): The end result quality of life. In: *Costs, Risks and Benefits of Surgery,* edited by J. P. Bunker, B. A. Barnes, and F. Mosteller. Oxford University Press, New York.

16. Ormel, J. (1980): Over neuroticisme gemeten met de vragenlijst: Een persoonlijkheidskenmerk of een maat voor psychosociale belasting. *Ned. Tijdschr. Psychol.*, 35:223–241.
17. Schmale, A. H., Morrow, G. R., Schmitt, M. H., Adler, L. M., Emelow, A., Murawski, B. J., and Cates, L. (1983): Well-being of cancer survivors. *Psychosom. Med.*, 45:163–169.
18. Schoot, A. (1981): Malaise bij kankerpatiënten. Ph.D. dissertation, University of Amsterdam.
19. Silberfarb, P., Holland, J. C., Bahna, G. F., Anbor, D., Mourer, H., and Comis, R. (1981): Differences in psychological response on two treatment regimes for localized small cell lung carcinoma. *Proc. Am. Soc. Cancer Res.*, 158.
20. Spielberger, C. D. (1966): Theory and research on anxiety. In: *Anxiety and Behavior*, edited by C. D. Spielberger. Academic Press, New York.
21. Spitzer, W. D., Dobson, A. J., Hall, J., et al. (1981): Measuring the quality of life of cancer patients. *J. Chronic Dis.*, 34:585–597.
22. Van Dam, F. S. A. M., Linssen, A. C. G., and Couzijn, A. L. (1984): Evaluating quality of life: Behavioral measures in clinical trials. In: *Cancer Clinical Trials: Methods and Practice*, edited by M. E. Buyse, M. J. Staquet, and R. J. Sylvester, Oxford University Press, New York.
23. Wilde, G. J. S. (1970): *Neurotische Labiliteit Gemeten Volgens de Vragenlijstmethode*. Van Rossum, Amsterdam.
24. Zuckerman, M. (1976): General and situation-specific traits and states: New approaches to assessment of anxiety and other constructs. In: *Emotions and Anxiety*, edited by M. Zuckerman and C. D. Spielberger. Erlbaum, Hillsdale, New Jersey.
25. Zuckerman, M. (1979): Traits, states, situations and uncertainty. *J. Behav. Assess.*, 1:43–54.
26. Zung, W. W. K. (1983): A self-rating pain and distress scale. *Psychosomatics*, 24:887–894.

The Quality of Life of Cancer Patients,
edited by N. K. Aaronson and J. Beckmann,
Raven Press, New York © 1987.

Practical Problems in Conducting Cancer-Related Psychosocial Research

Frits S. A. M. van Dam and Neil K. Aaronson

The Netherlands Cancer Institute, 1066 CX Amsterdam, The Netherlands

Application of psychosocial measures in cancer research is a relatively new enterprise. Much of the extant literature has focused on issues surrounding the development of valid and reliable instruments tapping the various psychosocial outcomes relevant to cancer and its treatment. Relatively little attention has been paid to the host of practical or logistical problems confronting researchers in this area (14,15). Yet it is our experience that it is the practical issues surrounding the collection of psychosocial data, rather than the psychometric issues involved in instrument development, that represent the greatest obstacle to the conduct of research in psychosocial oncology. In this chapter we concentrate on the more common practical problems of collecting psychosocial data and offer some broad guidelines that may facilitate the successful management of such data in cancer research settings.

The use of psychosocial measures is by no means common in clinical cancer research. Those responsible for conducting such clinical research—doctors, nurses, and data managers—often view psychosocial data collection as burdensome to themselves and their patients. Whereas such perceived burden may be due in part to a basic lack of familiarity with the nature and intent of assessing psychosocial outcomes, it may also reflect a degree of naïvité on the part of social scientists with regard to what is feasible in clinical settings. Often the procedures for collecting psychosocial data require the use of lengthy questionnaires to be filled out by patients during the rush of outpatient clinic visits. Although such procedures may be optimal in an abstract sense (i.e., they potentially yield the greatest amount of data), they do not reconcile the practical constraints operating in most clinical settings.

Thus social scientists wishing to conduct psychosocial research in the cancer field must be cognizant of the attitudinal and practical barriers that may inhibit the successful implementation of their research. On the one hand, they should anticipate that psychosocial research questions are typically met with a degree of skepticism by medical personnel. It is essential that the research topic be selected with an eye toward answering questions relevant to the clinician rather than the academic scientist. On the other hand, the methods and procedures selected for collection of psychosocial data must be compatible with the practical demands and limits of a clinical setting. This selection requires a thorough understanding of the range of clinical procedures, both diagnostic and therapeutic, around which the cancer clinic operates. Without such an understanding it is likely that the wrong questions will be asked at the wrong times.

PATIENT BURDEN

Psychosocial data collection should be acceptable to the patient in terms of the form and manner of application of the instrument used, the content areas it covers, and the effort required (11). Before describing possible difficulties in these areas, it must be noted that patients are generally willing to answer questions about how they feel and what they do (9). Within our health care systems (whether European or American) patients are frequently denied the opportunity to express their feelings and problems. For example, as many as 86% of cancer patients in one study wished they could discuss their situation more fully (7). Thus many cancer patients may welcome the opportunity to discuss their experiences and concerns, even within the format of a research project (12). They may also be interested in contributing to cancer knowledge, perhaps with the hope that such knowledge may contribute to their medical treatment and care (4). On the other hand, serious consideration should be given to the amount of burden placed on patients who are seriously ill and undergoing cancer therapies. Every effort should be made to design studies that minimize such burden through careful selection of methods and procedures.

Form and Manner of Application of Instrument

It is important to consider what patients are comfortable with when deciding on a method of data collection. Methods requiring the completion of written questionnaires may be unfamiliar to many patients and may not be feasible. If the sample includes patients of different cultures or of lower socioeconomic status or patients who are unaccustomed to "paper and pencil" tests, they may have difficulty reading or understanding the questions and may thus be unable to complete them accurately (11).

Patients may mask their inability to understand the questions or may simply mark the questionnaires in an arbitrary manner. For example, T. J. Priestman (*personal communication*) told of one patient who, during clinic visits when a questionnaire was to be filled out, stated that she had forgotten to bring her eyeglasses. After some probing it was discovered that the patient was illiterate and was embarrassed to admit that she could not read the questions.

This kind of problem may be overcome by providing someone to assist patients with the questionnaires. Such help can range from full assistance when needed (someone to read and explain each question) to having a person available to answer specific questions. Because patients may be reluctant to ask for help, however, the latter solution may not be effective.

If interviews are being conducted, it is wise to determine if there are certain cultural or class characteristics of interviewers that are more acceptable to patients. This point may be especially important if the population comprises different cultures. For example, Spinetta (13) found that less well educated Mexican families were uncomfortable when an interviewer came from a "well-to-do" Mexican family but responded well to an interviewer more similar to themselves. It should be of great concern to researchers in psychosocial oncology to understand the ways patients perceive their investigators. Do they see them as a part of the medical system? Do they see them as patients' advocates or as people who are totally outside the medical system with no power to influence their situation?

Content Area

All agree that questions should not distress the patient unnecessarily. However, what is distressing to a patient is subject to much debate. Some argue that questions regarding prognosis or death are especially distressing and should be avoided. Others argue that such issues are foremost in the minds of cancer patients and to avoid them indicates an unwillingness of researchers to pursue relevant topics. Unfortunately, little systematic information is available about which topics are threatening to patients and the extent of the threat. Therefore, assumptions about unacceptability of questions should be tested by means of feasibility studies. Undoubtedly, there is also variation in patients' reactions to various questions, and research is needed to describe the distribution of such reactions. In any case, questions should be phrased carefully to avoid undue anxiety. This point applies particularly to questions regarding perceived prognosis. There are clearly vast differences in the way patients have been informed about their disease and treatment. For example, in the United States there is more disclosure about the diagnosis than in France, the USSR, or Japan. Any measurement should take this cultural difference into account. The word "cancer" should be used cautiously to allow those patients who wish to deny that they have cancer (or who may not actually know) to continue to do so. Thus one can refer to their illness or condition rather than their cancer. When repeated questionnaires are used and patients are deteriorating, they sometimes report being distressed at having to answer questions that call attention to this fact. For example, patients may notice that, where they previously reported feeling well, they now must report feeling quite ill. This change may cause some patients to refuse to complete follow-up questionnaires.

Effort Required

The length of time a patient can tolerate spending in an interview or filling out a questionnaire may vary depending on how he or she is feeling at the time. It is important to consider this factor in the planning stages of the research. If patients must wait until they feel better to complete the instrument, results are biased in the direction of more positive feelings and fewer complaints. Indeed it is our experience that dropout due to disease progression is a quite common event. In a pilot study for a lung cancer project it was found that about 25% of the patients did not fill out a questionnaire simply because they felt too ill (3). Similarly, in a survey among behavioral scientists working with cancer patients, approximately 30% of the respondents reported problems when collecting data from seriously ill patients (1). It is of utmost importance that precise records be kept of reasons for missing data. Without knowing why patients drop out of a study, we cannot say much about the generalizability of the results.

Patients who are not experiencing extensive symptoms or fatigue and who have agreed to participate in a study are usually interested enough that they are willing to spend up to an hour in an interview (5,6,8,9). Although a questionnaire is less interesting (i.e., there is minimal personal contact), patients are nevertheless generally willing to spend up to about one-half hour to complete it. If patients are feeling tired or not well, their tolerance may go down. If repeated questionnaires/interviews are used, as in most clinical trials, the length of time patients are willing to spend is typically much less. In our experience at The Netherlands Cancer Institute, frequently applied tests should take no longer than 15 to 20 min. In prospective studies or clinical trials, one may want to ask participants to complete the same questionnaire or interview at several points in time. The time span between these administrations should be selected to be relevant to the study design yet not be burdensome to the patient. Our experience is that once every 4 to 5 weeks is feasible. Even so, some way of motivating patients to continue completing repeated questionnaires may be necessary. For example, a newsletter could be sent with each repeat questionnaire acknowledging the burden and reassuring patients that their efforts are still appreciated. Another possibility is to do the follow-up by telephone. In countries where 90 to 100% of the population has a telephone this choice is a real possibility.

Selection and Training of Psychosocial Data Managers[1]

"The successful conduct of a clinical trial relies heavily on each individual participant being fully informed and able to carry out his responsibilities. Both clinical and nursing staff have to understand protocol procedure as regards to the treatment and evaluation of each patient" (10). This applies of course to psychosocial data managers who have a central role in the collection and quality control of the data. Their training should be as precise and thorough as that of other medical personnel.

The selection and training of psychosocial data managers depends on a variety of factors including the complexity and level of standardization of the assessment method used, the similarity between cultures in which the investigation is carried out, the likely duration of the study, and the expectations of the subjects who are

---

[1] We mean by psychosocial data managers those workers in the medical setting who are responsible for collecting the psychosocial data, doing the interviewing, handing out the questionnaires, etc. In most cases the psychosocial data managers are also responsible for preparing the data for computer analysis.

to be examined. Some patients may view the data manager as someone with whom they can talk about their problems, whereas others may view him or her as a technician.

If extensive interviews are not feasible, as is the case in most multicenter trials, the demands placed on the interviewers can be reduced. The interviewers should, however, have a good understanding of the purpose and design of the study and of the composition of the questionnaire in order to answer questions from the patients or the medical personnel.

Observations by interviewers are often not recorded in their entirety in the schedules used in the study. Unless actively encouraged, interviewers tend to neglect giving narrative accounts of observations they could not rate in the schedule. Such narratives and regular discussions about interviews can provide valuable information for improving the technique used and for assessing and selecting the interviewers. Discussions about the interviews also serve the important function of maintaining the motivation of interviewers and improving their performance through the development of team spirit and identity.

The training of interviewers should also include instruction about frequent sources of bias that have their origin in the relation between interviewer and respondent. Some of these sources are easy to identify and demonstrate in training sessions, whereas others can be discovered only in the course of the study. More frequent sources of bias include:

1. Differences in the respondents' perception of the interviewer and the interview. Better educated subjects are often more accustomed to being interviewed and have seen interviews performed or have read about them. They perceive the interviewer's inquisitiveness and his intrusion in their private life differently from subjects who do not have such prior experience.

2. In some cultural settings the respondents try to guess what the interviewer wants and give the answer they think will please him.

3. Some of the biases known to occur in attitude assessment can also affect the interview. Subjects often tend to give answers that make them (or their family members) appear in a socially desirable light. This kind of bias is particularly evidenced in cultures where it is not uncommon for the interview to be carried out in the presence of family members who insist on attending the interview and being helpful to the interviewer.

MEDICAL STAFF BURDEN

The data collection should not excessively burden the staff or the medical setting in which the research is being conducted. In a survey of problems encountered by members of the EORTC Study Group on Quality of Life (1), the most prevalent problem encountered was difficulty in obtaining cooperation of medical staff. Hyland et al. (2) noted that the introduction of a clinical research project into a medical setting can arouse anxiety, opposition, and disruption. It may be viewed as intrusive and demanding of the time of existing staff, thereby interfering with the quality of care provided to patients. When describing their experiences, they noted that the medical staff did not always view the project as being of benefit to patients or staff. In view of the possibly laborious and unusual task the medical and nursing staff is confronted with, it is essential that behavioral scientists explain clearly what the measures and procedures encompass. It might mean that simple courses should be given in measurement and discussions held regarding the kind of results that can be expected from psychosocial measures. It is always a good idea to identify key figures in the hospital who can foresee problems in the implementation of the study. If a hospital has a tradition of conducting clinical trials, a medical data manager, research nurses, and research oncologists are usually available. If this is not the case, time should be devoted to motivating other workers in the hospital to take on this task. If this program is not feasible, one should consider whether that particular hospital should cooperate in a trial that includes research on psychosocial and behavioral outcomes.

Another important issue is the place where the data collection takes place. The situation (at home, in the clinic) in which self-report data are collected can exert a strong influence on the way patients respond to questions. Thus one should try to avoid varying the data collection setting within a single study.

If interviews are being conducted in a hospital, the time and place should be coordinated with the staff. If staff members are being asked to conduct the interviews, the time needed should be agreeable to the staff and the interview schedule easy to complete. Researchers must keep in mind that patient care comes first. If data collection is not designed to fit both the work schedules and abilities of the staff, it may not be completed at all. Once the trial is under way, interview appointments must be scheduled to conform to the prescribed treatment follow-up dates.

If questionnaires are being mailed, someone must be available to note when each follow-up questionnaire is to be mailed out to ensure that it is completed on the prescribed follow-up dates. Unreturned questionnaires must be obtained by contacting patients, and incomplete questionnaires must be followed up.

Because many studies have limited resources for these tasks, they must often be undertaken by existing staff (e.g., medical secretaries, social workers, nurses). It is extremely important that such tasks be feasible in terms of the abilities and time requirements of those to whom they are assigned. If psychosocial research is not possible because of the lack of personnel or an inadequate infrastructure, the hospital should be discouraged from taking part in the study. In some cases a hospital may be able to cooperate in only a part of the study (e.g., fielding questionnaires but not interviews).

CROSS-CULTURAL ISSUES IN MULTICENTER TRIALS

Most research within the EORTC is carried out in different countries, with varying cultural norms and values. This factor poses particular problems for psychosocial research. Whereas it is not necessary to consider cultural differences in blood counts, biochemical assays, or remission rates, such differences should be considered with the psychosocial sequelae of the therapies. Thus either one should use instruments that have been tested in various cultures, or considerable effort should be made to achieve as close to cross-cultural equivalence as possible (14). Even within a single "culture" or "language" setting one may encounter cultural differences. For example, questions on sexuality or the expression of emotions may be quite acceptable to a young, urban population but quite unacceptable to an elderly, rural population. The problem may lie both in the refusal of certain patients to answer questions and the unwillingness of certain medical staff to ask them.

COOPERATION IN MULTICENTER TRIALS

A crucial element in the management of a multicenter psychosocial cancer clinical trial is regular contact among the collaborating investigators. In addition to usual meetings of all the chief collaborators, exchanges of visits should be organized, bringing together smaller groups of investigators.

During these meetings it should be possible to:

1. Discuss technical and organizational problems within the study
2. Continue joint training in the use of research instruments and carry out reliability exercises
3. Formulate protocols for additional studies
4. Ensure that investigators become thoroughly familiar with the different centers' activities
5. Discuss and jointly interpret results of preliminary data analyses
6. Review drafts of papers and reports and agree on their conclusions

Most importantly, however, the exchange of visits contributes to the team spirit and strengthening of personal links among the participants in the study. The participation in decision-making about important aspects of the study increases feelings of involvement and significantly contributes to the value of the study as a whole.

CONCLUSION

If psychosocial oncology is to be more than an ephemera, the numerous problems of practicality must be resolved. It is one thing to decide to implement psychosocial measures in clinical trials; it is quite another to see that this part of the research is properly executed according to the study design. If we do not appreciate the demands of psychosocial research, the area will end up with many disappointed medical researchers, psychologists, and data managers who can only clear away the debris. To get such psychosocial research off the ground requires the development of a research infrastructure in which psychosocial oncology has its own place.

REFERENCES

1. Aaronson, N. K., van Dam, F. S. A. M., Polak, C. E., and Zittoun, R. (1986): Prospects and problems in European psychosocial oncology: Survey of the E.O.R.T.C. study group on quality of life. *J. Psychosoc. Oncol. (in press)*.
2. Hyland, J. M., Novotny, E., and Coyne, L. (1982): Psychosocial aspects of oncology: Challenges and problems of research in a radiotherapy center of a community hospital. *Int. J. Psychiatry Med.*, 11:341–351.
3. Kooy, A., and Snel, R. (1983): Het is net alsof je in een trein zit, je moet maar mee en je kunt er niet uit. Psychosociaal onderzoek bij longkankerpatiënten en hun partners. M.A. thesis, Psychological Laboratory, University of Amsterdam.
4. Luce, J. K., and Dawson, J. J. (1975): Quality of life. *Semin. Oncol.*, 2:323–327.
5. Mages, N. L., Castro, J. R., Fobair, P., et al. (1981): Patterns of psychosocial response to cancer: Can affective adaption be predicted. *Int. J. Radiat. Oncol.*, 7:385–393.
6. McCorkle, R. (1981): Social support and symptom distress in two samples with life-threatening diseases. Paper presented at American Cancer Society Second Conference on Cancer Nursing Research, Seattle, Washington.
7. Mitchell, G. W., and Glicksman, H. S. (1977): Cancer patients: Knowledge and attitudes. *Cancer*, 40:61–66.
8. Nerenz, D. R., Leventhal, H., and Love, R. R. (1982): Factors contributing to emotional distress during cancer chemotherapy. *Cancer*, 50:1020–1027.
9. Peck, A. (1972): Emotional reactions to having cancer. *AJR*, 114:591–599.
10. Pocock, S. J. (1983): *Clinical Trials: A Practical Approach*. Wiley, New York.
11. Sartorius, N. (1979): *Crosscultural Psychiatry*. Springer-Verlag, Berlin.
12. Silver, R. L., and Wortman, C. B. (1980): Coping with undesirable life-events. In: *Human Helplessness*, edited by J. Garber and M. E. P. Seligman. Academic Press, New York.
13. Spinetta, J. J. (1983): Measurement of family function, communication and cultural effects. Paper presented at American Cancer Society Conference on Methodology in Behavioral and Psychosocial Cancer Research, St. Petersburg, Florida.
14. Van Dam, F. S. A. M., Linssen, A. C. G., and Couzijn, A. L. (1984): Evaluating quality of life: Behavioral measures in clinical trials. In: *Cancer Clinical Trials: Methods and Practice*, edited by M. E. Buyse, M. J. Staquet, and R. J. Sylvester, Oxford University Press, New York.
15. Yates, J. W., and Edwards, B. (1984): Practical concerns and pitfalls in measurement methodology. *Cancer*, 53:2376–2379.

The Quality of Life of Cancer Patients,
edited by N. K. Aaronson and J. Beckmann,
Raven Press, New York © 1987.

Evaluation of Psychosocial Intervention in Oncology

Diana D. Bransfield

*Division of Cancer Prevention and Control, National Cancer Institute,
Bethesda, Maryland 20892*

The evaluation of psychosocial intervention in oncology populations is an important component of any clinical program designed to promote the quality of life for the patient and his family. The assessment of a particular psychosocial intervention is essential to discern its strengths and weaknesses, its cost-effectiveness and cost-benefits, and to appraise the efficacy of an intervention strategy. Conversely, the absence of evaluation research severely limits the application of the therapeutic intervention to other patient populations and other clinical settings. More succinctly, without evaluation there is no way to determine whether an intervention is "good" or "bad," regardless of the well-meaning intentions of the clinician.

As intervention strategies in the area of psychosocial oncology proliferate (10,29), an important question is, "How will the program be evaluated?" Undoubtedly, the allocation of grant funding from private and public sources is tied partially to the strength of the evaluation research design. Therefore the evaluation of psychosocial interventions is not only vital to foster optimal clinical service, it is also imperative if psychosocial oncology expects to successfully compete for limited financial resources.

To acquaint those clinicians who have little experience in systematically assessing their therapeutic efforts, some basic tenets and theoretical issues of evaluation research are presented below. The reader should note that the text outline closely follows the familiar hypothesis testing format. This organization was chosen because thorough evaluation of clinical intervention is synonymous with research; that is, one must be prepared to conceptualize and operationalize a research program if one expects to measure therapeutic outcomes. Furthermore, the evaluation research design, as with most scientific experiments, should be constructed *before* the clinical intervention takes place, not afterward. Evaluation research requires careful foreplanning, not hindsighted scrambling to justify one's therapeutic efforts.

RESEARCH DESIGN

The evaluation of psychosocial intervention may be conducted through nonexperimental, experimental, or quasiexperimental research designs. Nonexperimental designs refer to situations in which neither the independent variables (e.g., the type of clinical intervention, the number of sessions) nor the dependent variables (e.g., the patient's rating of well-being, the number of patient requests for pain medication) are under the control of the researcher. In nonexperimental studies, the assignment of variables to independent or dependent categories is often arbitrary. The identification of independent variables (IVs) and dependent variables (DVs) is based on the research objectives or purpose of the study. Frequently nonexperimental designs are referred to as survey or correlational studies. A survey implies that descriptive data have been collected and analyzed to provide information on specific populations. A correlational design measures two or more identified variables of a population and examines the relation between these variables. In a nonexperimental study a correlation coefficient (a statistical technique originally developed and used in, but not limited to, nonexperimental studies) may be used to compare the relation between an IV and a DV. Changes in the DV, however, cannot be attributed to or said to be caused by the IV; only an association between the variables may be reported. The major difference between nonexperimental and experimental designs is that in experimental research the investigator has strict control over one or more IVs. Ideally, there would also be control over confounding or extraneous variables, the number of research subjects and/or the number of study groups, and the timing and duration of the exposure to the IV (7). In a true experiment each individual in the sample has an equal chance of being assigned to the experimental or control conditions. Such a process, called randomization, helps ensure that all subjects are relatively alike on the DVs before the IV is introduced. Thus when significant differences are found after exposure to the IV, the experimenter can conclude that the intervention *caused* the difference.

Traditionally, an experimental design uses one or more experimental groups and a control group. The experimental group is exposed to the IV; the control group is not. Subjects are randomly assigned to either the experimental group(s) or the control group with the assumption that equality on all extraneous variables exists before the IV is manipulated. When no comparison groups are used, as in single group or single case study designs, the study is sometimes referred to as preexperimental (21).

Often the researcher cannot randomly assign subjects or control for when or how long the subjects are exposed to the IV. Even though the investigation may be identical to a true experiment in all other respects, the term quasiexperimental is used because of this lack of control (7,18). "Quasi" implies that it is "as if" the research is experimental. Often the same procedures and statistical analyses found in experimental designs are used in quasiexperimental ones. With rare exception, most experimental research in psychosocial oncology is of a quasiexperimental nature; social scientists cannot control for which individuals in the population develop cancer or decide when or where the individual will be medically treated.

HYPOTHESIS

Whether the research is nonexperimental, experimental, or quasiexperimental, it needs to begin with a hypothesis. A hypothesis is a conjecture or an assumption deduced from theory, clinical impressions, or observations that can be tested empirically (24). A null hypothesis proposes that there will be no significant difference between the experimental and control groups after exposure to the IV. An alternative hypothesis predicts that a significant difference between groups will be found. Alternative hypotheses may also predict the direction of that difference, proposing that one group will have higher or lower scores than another group. In evaluation research a hypothesis most often derives from clinical experience; psychosocial oncology clinicians frequently have a suspicion that one type of treatment is preferred to another or one group of patients needs more psychotherapeutic intervention than another group. Such suspicions lend themselves to the development of a workable hypothesis—a hypothesis that generates measurable independent and dependent variables.

DEFINING THE INDEPENDENT AND DEPENDENT VARIABLES

In experimental research several variables, or factors, are simultaneously studied. As stated above, the variable manipulated by the experimenter is the IV. It has the potential of effecting the dependent variable(s) under question. In some studies of psychotherapeutic intervention with oncology patients, the type of treatment may serve as the IV. The literature is replete with examples of different types of intervention: psychoanalytically oriented psychotherapy (17,26), short-term dynamic psychotherapy (11,12,16), crisis intervention (8,13), behavioral therapy (1,6,14,15,19,20,31) including behavioral relaxation techniques (5) and cognitive therapy (28), and other treatment approaches such as music therapy (4), group therapy (3,30), family interventions (9), and psychopharmacologic therapy (27).

The researcher must select or design one or several intervention approaches to assess their comparative effectiveness in improving the targeted behavior or emotional status. As elucidated by Ryle (22), the comparison of treatment approaches has been unsuccessful in the past. For example, psychoanalysis typically addresses issues of the integration of unconscious and conscious factors and defense mechanisms while focusing on broadly defined life plans and relationships. Conversely, behavioral therapy disavows the presence of unconscious mediators, including defense mechanisms, and focuses on discrete, observable behaviors. With such divergent theoretical frameworks, it is essential that psychosocial interventions be operationally defined as best as possible, and that from these definitions measurable variables be used in their evaluations (2).

In the oncology setting, it would be preferable for less experienced researchers to investigate the effect of just one treatment procedure against, for example, a nontreatment control group. The use of a control group poses particular concerns. Many clinicians perceive *any* psychotherapeutic interventions with cancer patients as beneficial, and understandably there is often a reluctance to withhold treatment. However, because the availability of psychological counseling in oncology settings is rather scarce, randomly assigning patients to treatment versus nontreatment control groups is not inappropriate or unethical; most subjects in the control group would not be receiving psychological intervention in any case, with or without the research program.

Complex treatments that necessitate extensive training in the research procedure are less likely to achieve treatment integrity, which is defined as the extent to which the intervention conditions are carried out as planned. Poor treatment integrity causes a threat to the internal validity of the research design and hinders replication studies or application of the presumed treatment approach in other settings (23). Thus the treatment evaluator needs not only to choose and clearly define the intervention procedures but to do this in a manner that facilitates its use by other clinicians.

The behavior or psychological status that is measured and attributed to variations in the IV is referred to as the DV. Compared to medical science, the behavioral and social sciences have a more formidable task in the measurement of their DVs. Quality of life or affective states are abstract, highly personal concepts that are difficult to observe and objectively measure. The researcher must first define the DVs and then decide whether subjective or objective measurements, or both, will be taken. Ideally, the measurement of the DV in psychological studies includes *both* types of evaluation. Objective assessment refers to the measure of observable behavior or physiological indices; subjective assessment requires a cognitive interpretation by either a rater or the subject, or both. If a subjective assessment is completed by someone other than the patient, it is highly recommended that an independent rater (not the researcher) be used to assess posttherapeutic outcome to minimize an experimenter bias. Even more desirable is the use of two or more independent raters, for whom interrater reliability levels can be determined. Another approach is to include multiple assessments from raters pooled from various sources, such as the family, health team, or community members.

The tool for measuring the DV(s) must have demonstrated levels of reliability and validity that indicate its capability of measuring the psychological construct under question. The chosen tool must "fit" or reflect the dependent variable(s) under investigation. If these conditions for choosing the measurement instrument are not met, the validity of the research results is highly questionable. In many instances appropriate scales do not exist for measuring the quality of survival or specific affective states among cancer patients. This situation means that the investigator must develop and adequately pretest a new scale for use with the intended population. Well-defined and measured DVs allow the researcher to more confidently assert that changes were caused by exposure to the intervention (IV).

SELECTING A SAMPLE

A sample is a group of individuals drawn from a population who ideally are representative of that population. The number of individuals selected for a study is based on several factors. First, the researcher needs a sufficient number of subjects in order to minimize the chance of failing to reject the null hypothesis when in fact it is false (beta or type II error). That is, the researcher needs *power,* or strength, in a statistical analysis that detects differences between groups of subjects. Too few subjects minimizes the ability to identify differences, or decreases statistical power.

Second, if the anticipated *effect* (amount of detectable difference between groups after exposure to the IV) is small, more subjects are needed to demonstrate the impact of the experimental intervention. Conversely, if a large anticipated effect is expected, fewer subjects are needed. Frequently the researcher has some preconceived notion about effect size based on clinical experience or past research findings. Hence if few subjects are known to produce a large, noticeable change as the result of the intervention, fewer subjects are needed to show that same effect.

A third consideration is *measurement error.* Measurement error refers to a lack of reliability, validity, or both in the techniques used to measure the DVs. If a measurement procedure does not have sufficiently high levels of reliability, larger numbers of subjects are necessary (25). Lastly, both practical and economic considerations should be operative in determining sample size. A guiding principle in setting sample size is to weigh the benefits of increasing the number of subjects against its costs. If no new information is gleaned from an increased sample size, the effort expended to collect more data is unmerited.

Once sample size has been determined, the type of sampling procedure must be identified. Examples of sampling procedures include (a) systematic sampling in which every n^{th} member is chosen from the population; (b) stratified sampling, the selection of subjects by chance within levels of different attributes; (c) cluster sampling, which collects data on subject groups in the same location; (d) sequential sampling, which examines the data as it is collected and ceases data collection when enough information has been obtained; (e) simple random selection, which makes use of tables of random numbers; and (f) convenience sampling, which selects subjects based on their availability to the researcher (24).

As stated above, true random selection is rarely possible in psychosocial oncology research; instead, a nonrandom sample of the population is used. A sample that is nonrandom may not be representative of the larger population and restricts the generalization of the research findings to groups or individuals who share the same characteristics as the research subjects. Thus if an intervention is introduced to patients with breast cancer, the research findings cannot be extrapolated to patients with Hodgkin's disease.

PLANNING THE STATISTICAL SCHEME

After the variables are defined and operationalized, and the subjects are selected, the next step in evaluation research is determining how the data will be statistically analyzed. Some of the objectives of using statistical tests are to: (a) decide whether a difference between sets of scores, e.g., scores on a depression scale, is due to the effect of the experimental treatment or to chance factors; (b) infer whether differences among the intervention procedures are reliable; and (c) aid in decision-making, e.g., whether the intervention should be recommended in other settings. In experimental designs, inferential statistics permit one to *infer* what those missing parameters are (24) and to draw conclusions from the data about the total population, not just the sample. Examples of inferential statistics are Student's *t*-test, analysis of variance, the Wilcoxon matched-pairs signed-rank test, the Mann-Whitney U-test, and the Pearson *r* correlation coefficient.

It is unacceptable practice in evaluation research to analyze experimental research results by using descriptive statistics only. Although frequencies, means, ranges, standard deviations, and variances provide interesting information, such statistics do not test an interactive effect between multiple variables, nor do they detect barely perceptible differences.

INTERPRETING THE RESULTS

Except in a true experimental design, the researcher rarely claims that the IV *caused* a change in the DV. Instead, the IVs and DVs are more often reported as being statistically *associated*. This relation is particularly true in social science research where many unknown or hidden "third factors," or confounding variables, may account for the change in the DV.

Frequently the results of a study are used to predict what will occur in the future given a similar set of circumstances. However, one can only make a prediction about the future associations between variables if one believes that the future sample will be drawn from the same population. Prediction also assumes that the sample on which the results are inferred is unbiased, or representative of the larger population (24). Thus because such representativeness is usually unattainable in psychosocial oncology research, predictions are made cautiously in studies that examine psychotherapeutic intervention.

Alternatively, if the broader meaning and implications of the research are not sufficiently exposed (that includes comparing the results with previous findings and existing theories), valuable interventions may not become actualized in the cancer setting. The prudent researcher walks a fine judgment line that divides underinterpreting the results on the one hand and overinterpreting them on the other. With increased research experience this line becomes more clearly demarcated.

CONCLUSION

The only way to evaluate the efficacy of a psychosocial intervention in oncology is to design and implement a valid research program. It requires an *a priori* research approach that closely adheres to the traditional outline of scientific inquiry. The "stronger" the research design and its statistical interpretation, the more inferences can be drawn from the intervention experience and applied in other settings or to other intervention strategies within the same population and setting. It is through such a research process that advances in psychosocial intervention with cancer patients can be made.

REFERENCES

1. Ahles, T. A., Cohen, R. E., and Blanchard, E. B. (1984): Difficulties inherent in conducting behavioral research with cancer patients. *Behav. Therapist*, 7(4):69–70.
2. American Psychiatric Association Commission on Psychotherapies (1982): *Psychotherapy Research: Methodological and Efficacy Issues*. American Psychiatric Association, Washington, D.C.
3. Arnowitz, E., Brunswick, L., and Kaplan, B. H. (1983): Group therapy with patients in the waiting room of an oncology clinic. *Soc. Work*, 28:395–397.
4. Bailey, L. M. (1983): The effects of live music versus tape-recorded music on hospitalized cancer patients. *Music Ther.*, 3:17–28.
5. Burish, T. G., Carey, M. P., Redd, W. H., and Krozely, M. G. (1983): Behavioral relaxation techniques in reducing the distress of cancer chemotherapy patients. *Oncol. Nurs. Forum*, 10(3).
6. Burish, T. G., Redd, W. H., and Casey, M. P. (1985): Conditioned nausea and vomiting in cancer chemotherapy: Treatment approaches. In: *Cancer, Nutrition, and Eating Behavior: A Biobehavioral Perspective*, edited by T. G. Burish, S. M. Levy, and B. E. Meyerowitz, pp. 205–224. Erlbaum, Hillsdale, New Jersey.
7. Campbell, D. T., and Stanley, J. C. (1963): *Experimental and Quasi-Experimental Designs for Research*. Houghton Mifflin, Boston.
8. Capone, M. A., Westie, R. S., Chitwood, J. S., Feigenbaum, D., and Good, R. S. (1979): Crisis intervention: A functional model for hospitalized cancer patients. *Am. J. Orthopsychiatry*, 49:598–607.
9. Cohen, M., and Wellisch, D. (1978): Living in limbo: Psychosocial intervention in families with a cancer patient. *Am. J. Psychother.*, 32:561–571.
10. Feinstein, A. D. (1983): Psychological interventions in the treatment of cancer. *Clin. Psychol. Rev.*, 3:1–14.
11. Forester, B., Kornfeld, D. S., and Fleiss, J. L. (1985): Psychotherapy during radiotherapy: Effects on emotional and physical distress. *Am. J. Psychiatry*, 142:22–27.
12. Goldberg, R. J., Wool, M., Tull, R., and Boor, M. (1984): Teaching brief psychotherapy for spouses of cancer patients: Use of a codable supervision format. *Psychother. Psychosom.*, 41:12–19.
13. Hyland, J. M., Novotny, E., and Coyne, L. (1980): Counseling interventions in cancer patients with emotional adjustment difficulties. Presented at The National Forum on Comprehensive Cancer Rehabilitation and Its Vocational Implications, November 13–15, Williamsburg, Virginia.
14. Levy, S. M. (1982): Biobehavioral interventions in behavioral medicine: An overview. *Cancer*, 9(Suppl.):1928–1935.
15. Levy, S. M., and Morrow, G. (1982): Workshop report: Biobehavioral interventions in behavioral medicine. *Cancer*, 9(Suppl.):1936–1938.
16. Lonnqvist, J., et al. (1981): Adaptation to cancer. *Psychiatr. Fenn. [Suppl.]*, 179–188.
17. Maguire, P. (1984): The recognition and treatment of affective disorders in cancer patients. *Int. Rev. Appl. Psychol.*, 33:479–491.
18. Plutchik, R. (1983): *Foundations of Experimental Research*, 3rd ed. Random House, New York.
19. Redd, W. H., and Hendler, C. S. (1983): Behavioral medicine in comprehensive cancer treatment. *J. Psychosoc. Oncol.*, 1(2):3–17.
20. Redd, W. H., Burish, T. G., and Andrykowski, M. A. (1985): Aversive conditioning and cancer chemotherapy. In: *Cancer, Nutrition, and Eating Behavior: A Biobehavioral Perspective*, edited by T. G. Burish, S. M. Levy, and B. E. Meyerowitz, pp. 117–132. Erlbaum, Hillsdale, New Jersey.

21. Robinson, P. W. (1981): *Fundamentals of Experimental Psychology,* 2nd ed. Prentice-Hall, Englewood Cliffs, New Jersey.
22. Ryle, A. (1984): How can we compare different psychotherapies? Why are they all effective? *Br. J. Med. Psychol.,* 57:261–264.
23. Salend, S. J. (1984): Therapy outcome research: Threats to treatment integrity. *Behav. Modif.,* 8:211–222.
24. Tabachnick, B. G., and Fidell, L. S. (1983): *Using Multivariate Statistics.* Harper & Row, New York.
25. Tarnover, W. (1984): Psychotherapy with cancer patients. *Bull. Menninger Clin.,* 48:342–350.
26. Tarrier, N., and Maguire, P. (1984): Treatment of psychological distress following mastectomy: An initial report. *Behav. Res. Ther.,* 22:81–84.
27. Tarrier, N., Maguire, P., and Kincey, J. (1983): Locus of control and cognitive behavior therapy with mastectomy patients: A pilot study. *Br. J. Med. Psychol.,* 53:265–270.
28. Watson, M. (1983): Psychosocial intervention with cancer patients: A review. *Psychol. Med.,* 13:839–846.
29. Wood, J. D., and Tambrink, J. (1983): Impact of cancer on sexuality and self-image: A group program for patients and partners. *Soc. Work Health Care,* 8(4):45–54.
30. Wood, P. E. (1978): Group counseling for cancer patients in a community hospital. *Psychosomatics,* 19:555–561.
31. Zeiter, L., and LeBaron, S. (1983): Behavioral intervention for children and adolescents with cancer. *Behav. Med. Update,* 5(203):17–22.

The Quality of Life of Cancer Patients,
edited by N. K. Aaronson and J. Beckmann,
Raven Press, New York © 1987.

Psychosocial Research in Childhood Cancer

Bob F. Last and Anne M. H. van Veldheuzen

*Children's Oncology Center, Emma Children's Hospital,
1018 HJ Amsterdam, The Netherlands*

Only a few decades ago the literature about emotional reactions of children suffering from cancer and their parents comprised a description of experiences and impressions of the authors. Friedman et al. (9) comprise one of the first investigator groups who systematically gathered data about the behavior and feelings of the parents during the hospitalization of the child. The title of the study "Behavioral observations on parents anticipating the death of a child" shows that, in those early days, attention was focused on coping with the fatally ill and dying child.

The diagnosis of childhood cancer carried with it, in nearly all cases, a fatal prognosis. Thus articles about the psychosocial aspects of the child with cancer focused on the notion the child can have of his own fate (17), on the parental process of anticipatory mourning, and on hospital staff coping with the reactions of the parents and the child (8).

A striking change has taken place as a consequence of the improved prognosis for children suffering from cancer. Attention has shifted to the effects of the disease and the treatment on the quality of life of the child and the family. Attention is focused not only on the possible effects on the social life of the child and the family (10,14,25) but also on the impact on emotional life (1,21,26), on intelligence (4,22,24), and on functioning in school (3).

The aim of such research is threefold. First, there is interest in gaining insight into the problems characteristic of the total population of juvenile cancer patients as well as into the problems of specific groups of children with cancer and their families. With systematically gathered data it may be possible to develop more effective psychosocial care for the child and the family. Second, psychosocial studies on quality of life can contribute to medical regimens so that harmful side effects can be minimized. In clinical trials, quality of life assessment instruments can provide data of importance for decision-making about medical treatment. Third, research on quality of life issues with respect to childhood cancer can contribute to the development of psychological theory.

DESCRIPTIVE, EXPLORATIVE, AND
HYPOTHESIS-TESTING RESEARCH

Certainly, descriptive studies about the impact of the disease and the treatment on the life of the child and the family are valuable. Descriptive studies are desirable for showing what is relevant in a certain field of study in order to develop a theory or the instrumental realization of concepts. Koocher and O'Malley (10) typified the descriptive literature as follows: "There is a considerable body of literature on the psychosocial and emotional aspects of childhood cancer. Although rigorous research is lacking and the work is largely descriptive and anecdotal, it nevertheless reveals a fairly clear and detailed picture of the 'cancer experience' for the children and their families." The implications of the disease and its treatment on the daily life of the child and the family are, generally speaking, well known. At this moment it is of interest to investigate the relations among the various factors affecting the quality of life of children with cancer.

Explorative studies represent an intermediate form of research between descriptive studies on the one hand and hypothesis-testing research on the other. The aim of the investigator in explorative studies is to formulate and select hypotheses. The investigator has certain expectations and is keen on finding certain correlations in the research material, but he is not yet able to formulate exact hypotheses. An example of such research is that of Eiser and Landsdown (7), which was concerned with the intellectual development of children treated for acute leukemia. Eiser examined the correlation between age at which a child undergoes cranial irradiation and further performance on intelligence tests. In a follow-up study, Eiser (5) tested her preliminary findings with a precisely defined hypothesis that was confirmed. Other investigators (15,16,18,22) also concluded that cranial irradiation has a greater negative effect on the intellectual functioning of the child under the age of 7 than on those above this age.

Another example of such a study is that of Lansky et al. (11). In this study it was hypothesized that couples having a child with cancer run a greater risk of getting divorced than the rest of the population. This hypothesis was formulated on the basis of findings in stress research about families having a child suffering from another chronic disease. In a large sample study Lansky et al. rejected this hypothesis.

THREE LEVELS OF RESEARCH

Research on aspects of the quality of life of the child with cancer and his family can be done on three levels (Fig. 1): on the level of the child (micro level), on the level of the family (meso level), and on the level of the environment (macro level).

On the first level we find the *child* himself. Research can be directed to handicaps that can occur as a woeful effect of the disease, the treatment, or both. It is important to know what the effects are on the physical development of the child (e.g., increase in length and weight, motor capability), cognitive development

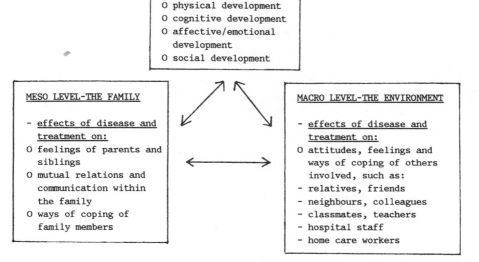

FIG. 1. Three levels of research on the aspects of quality of life of a child with cancer and the family.

(e.g., intelligence, capacity to concentrate, perception), affective-emotional development (e.g., capacity to cope with and express feelings), and acquisition of social abilities (e.g., adequate functioning in a group of peers). When we know more precisely the effects of the disease and the treatment on the various areas of development we are better able to take measures in the field of caretaking and medical treatment.

A second level of research is found within the *family*. The development of the child with cancer does not take place in isolation; the child is part of the family system. The mutual relations between the members of the family influence the child, his adaptation to the disease, and his development. Gaining insight into the effects of patterns of family coping on the adaptation and the development of the child with cancer may yield methods of intervention with regard to the quality of life of the child and the family.

The third level of research concerns the larger, social *environment*. The reactions of people more or less close to the family are of significance with regard to the coping ability and the feelings of the child, his parents, and his siblings. Most people are still frightened when confronted with cancer. They associate it with a quick downhill course and certain death.

It is also of importance to investigate the relations between the hospital staff, the home care workers, the child, and the family. The attitude of the doctors, nurses, general practitioner, and district nurse influence the feelings and the attitudes of the child and the other members of the family toward the disease. With empiric-scientific knowledge about the reactions of those in the immediate social environment, we can take more appropriate measures to organize the provision of care in a way that is beneficial to the quality of life of the child with cancer and the family.

The levels of research indicated above are not independent of one another. When we design a study at one level we have to take into account possible interactions with another level. For example, in a study of the impact on physical and emotional development of children with osteosarcoma who have undergone an amputation, we must think of the possible impact of reactions of the family (meso level) and the environment (macro level), especially with regard to the visibility of the mutilation.

PROBLEM OR CHANGE-ORIENTED MODEL

In most studies of the effects of childhood cancer it is assumed that the disease and its treatment will lead to a certain pathology in the development of the child. The main focus, then, is on documenting the nature of such pathology so that appropriate interventions can follow.

Susman et al. (23) suggested an alternative model which assumes that emotional, social, and cognitive development may be altered by a diagnosis of cancer because of its life-threatening nature and because of the nature of treatment regimens. It is therefore important to assess how cancer affects psychological development. However, reactions to such an illness need not be synonymous with problems of adjustment. "An assumption of this model is that individuals progress along a developmental course and, although such a course may be altered by major medical crises, basic processes of psychological development still occur. Two corollaries of this assumption are (a) physiological, social, and cognitive development will proceed in spite of illness and hospitalization and (b) the reactions to illness and hospitalization, although stressful, need not be pathological and are likely to be oriented to age-related developmental concerns."

This model offers fruitful ideas. It is indeed important to realize when designing a study of aspects of the quality of life of juvenile cancer patients that, apart from the identification of problem areas, the disease and treatment period may also have positive effects on the development of the child. Physical limitations, for example, can change the child's cognitive and emotional development in such a way that the child becomes more interested in intellectual and/or cultural activities.

HOMOGENEITY AND HETEROGENEITY OF THE GROUP

There is a tendency to see children with cancer as a homogeneous group. They certainly have a number of characteristics in common. The uncertainty of survival, the chronic life-threatening nature of the disease, the special position of the child in the family because of his illness, and the confrontation with the reactions of the outside world are important features of children with cancer. Yet, as a group, children with cancer also have a number of heterogeneous characteristics. Essential differences in development between various age groups account for qualitatively and quantitatively different effects of disease and treatment. For example, negative effects of disease or treatment on the physical functioning of the child may manifest in the young child by regression of still insufficiently developed body functions (enuresis, encopresis). In the older child it may be expressed in an inability to participate in sports, which in turn can have consequences for his social standing among peers and for his self-esteem.

In the area of cognitive development, concentration problems and learning disabilities have been demonstrated in children with acute lymphoblastic leukemia in several studies (6,12,18). The schoolchild, however, is confronted much more with these defects than the child who is not yet at school age or the child who has already finished school.

The age and the allied cognitive developmental stage of the child is also related to the meaning the child gives to the illness. At a very young age children can already realize the serious nature of their illness (1,20), but the child may have to reach the stage of formal thinking (approximately 12 years of age) to realize the more future-oriented implications of the disease.

A quantitative difference can be seen in the greater impact of a prolonged hospital stay on children below the age of 5 or 6 (2). As the young child is more dependent on his parents, we can expect him to experience greater separation anxiety and resulting emotional disturbance than older children.

Age differences have consequences for the research design and the choice of research instruments. For children under the age of 8 it is generally not possible to use questionnaires and interviews. Observational measures and projective tests are more appropriate but have the disadvantage that, even if their reliability is demonstrated, their validity is difficult to assess.

Next to the age of the child, disease and treatment factors constitute heterogeneous characteristics of children with cancer. Cancer is a collective noun for a number of diseases that vary in symptoms, length of treatment, treatment procedures, temporal or permanent side effects, response to treatment, prognosis, and so on. Moreover, some forms of cancer have peak age incidences.

In the research design and data analysis it is necessary to isolate these factors of disease and treatment and to analyze their possible interaction with the age of the child. Koocher and O'Malley (10) concluded from their study that relapsed patients and those with second tumors or recurrences run a substantially greater psychological risk, even though they can be treated successfully. They also investigated psychosocial adjustment in relation to diagnosis and found more adjustment problems among survivors of Hodgkin's disease and acute lymphoblastic leukemia than among survivors of neuroblastoma and Wilms' tumor. As the average age at diagnosis in the sample was 18 months for the neuroblastoma survivors and

46 months for the Wilms' tumor survivors, the authors reasoned that extreme youth at the time of diagnosis and a prolonged continuous remission of disease are important factors in long-term psychosocial adjustment. This conclusion seems to us unwarranted. First, the peak age incidence of acute lymphoblastic leukemia is also during early childhood. Second, although Koocher and O'Malley noted the more prolonged treatment for the leukemia patients, they did not statistically analyze the weight of the three factors involved: diagnosis, age at the time of diagnosis, and duration of treatment. Thus their conclusion about the relation between age at the time of diagnosis and future psychosocial adjustment is not yet demonstrated. It remains an interesting hypothesis for future research.

To determine the relative influence of age, illness, and treatment variables statistically, the size of a research sample has to be sufficient. Most of the time this factor poses a problem because the total number of children with cancer is relatively small, and variations in age, illness, and treatment variables are relatively large. For example, investigating neurological and intellectual functioning of children treated for medulloblastoma would be interesting because (clinical) findings in these areas differ greatly (e.g., 4,19). The number of children available for such an investigation, however, is very small. In The Netherlands, for example, only 10 to 15 children in the ages between 0 and 15 are being treated for this disease in cancer centers per year. In this supposedly homogeneous group, however, we can expect substantial differences in brain damage caused by differences in the size of the tumor before surgical excision and other symptoms before and during the treatment such as intracranial pressure. These expected differences in such a small group of patients make a statistical analysis of effects of the variables virtually impossible.

SIMPLICITY OR COMPLEXITY OF RESEARCH

Thus far we have mentioned a few problems in conducting research into the quality of life of the child with cancer and his family. Other problems arise in the area of availability of research instruments. The use of an instrument of one's own design is often necessary to answer certain specific questions about the child with cancer or his family. Assessment of the reliability and validity of such an instrument is necessary but usually requires a research effort that is beyond the scope of most projects. Furthermore, there is the problem of adequate control groups.

Some of these problems are not unique to research into childhood cancer. The problem of isolation and systematic variation of some variables and the problem of controlling for other relevant variables is a major one in the social sciences. The sheer number of interacting variables in cancer research makes this task an extremely difficult one. For this reason an investigation into the effects of variables is not always possible. In that case one must confine oneself to an investigation of relations between variables. A correlational study need not be qualified as being inferior, especially when such a study has been designed to organize psychosocial care more adequately. An example of research that serves this purpose is the study of Last et al. (13). In this study the care delivered by district nurses and general practitioners to the family of a child with cancer was evaluated. We found a declining frequency of visits of these workers to the family as the prognosis of the child grew worse. Without knowing the particular causes of this phenomenon, efforts were directed at changing this tendency to avoid the family when the condition of the child deteriorates.

Apart from such practical purposes, correlational research can serve a theoretical purpose. It can stimulate ideas and further the development of theory in the area of childhood cancer when empiric-scientific data are lacking.

It is our opinion that research into the quality of life of children with cancer and their families can best be done by people working in the centers where children with cancer are treated. Not every center has the necessary conditions to carry out large research projects. Nevertheless, whenever the essential conditions of scientific inquiry have been met, even an investigation confined to a small research area, needing only a minimum of organization and manpower, can be of value in increasing insight into the quality of life of the child with cancer and his family.

REFERENCES

1. Bluebond-Langner, M. (1977): Meanings of death to children. In: *New Meanings of Death,* edited by H. Feifel. McGraw-Hill, New York.
2. Bowlby, J. (1973): *Attachment and Loss, Vol. II: Separation and Anger.* Basic Books, New York.
3. Deasy-Spinetta, P. (1981): The school and the child with cancer. In: *Living with Childhood Cancer,* edited by J. J. Spinetta and P. Deasy-Spinetta. Mosby, St. Louis.
4. Duffner, P. K., Cohen, M. E., and Thomas, P. (1983): Late effects of treatment on the intelligence of children with posterior fossa tumors. *Cancer,* 51:233–237.
5. Eiser, C. (1978): Intellectual abilities among survivors of childhood leukaemia as a function of irradiation. *Arch. Dis. Child.,* 53:391–395.
6. Eiser, C. (1980): How leukaemia affects a child's schooling. *Br. J. Soc. Clin. Psychol.,* 19:365–368.
7. Eiser, C., and Landsdown, R. (1977): Retrospective study of intellectual development in children treated for acute lymphoblastic leukemia. *Arch. Dis. Child.,* 52:525–529.
8. Friedman, S. B. (1967): Care of the family of the child with cancer. *Pediatrics,* 40:498–504.
9. Friedman, S. B., Chodoff, P., Mason, J. W., and Hamburg, D. A. (1963): Behavioral observations on parents anticipating the death of a child. *Pediatrics,* 32:600–625.
10. Koocher, G. P., and O'Malley, J. E. (1981): *Psychosocial Consequences of Surviving Childhood Cancer.* McGraw-Hill, New York.
11. Lansky, S. B., Chairns, N. U., Hassanein, R., Wehr, J., and Lowman, J. T. (1978): Childhood cancer: Parental discord and divorce. *Pediatrics,* 62(2):184–188.
12. Last, B. F., van Veldhuizen, A. M. H. and de Ridder-Sluiter, J. G. (1982): Intelligentie en concentratievermogen van kinderen met leukemie en hun aanpassing op school. *Tijdschr. Kindergeneeskd.,* 50(3):76–82.
13. Last, B. F., van Veldhuizen, A. M. H., Koopman, H., and Roelofsen, J. F. (1982): Thuiszorg bij het kind met kanker. *Maatschappelijke Gezondheidszorg,* 10(10):8–12.
14. Márky, I. (1982): Children with malignant disorders and their families: A study of the implications of the disease and its treatment on everyday life. *Acta Paediatr. Scand. [Suppl.],* 303:1–82.
15. Meadows, A. T., Massari, D. J., Fergusson, J., Gordon, J., Littman, P., and Moss, K. (1981):

Declines in IQ scores and cognitive dysfunctions in children with acute lymphocytic leukaemia treated with cranial irradiation. *Lancet,* 7:1015–1018.

16. Moss, H. A., Nannis, E. D., and Poolack, D. G. (1981): The effects of prophylactic treatment of the central nervous system on the intellectual functioning of children with acute lymphocytic leukemia. *Am. J. Med.,* 71:47–52.

17. Natterson, J. M., and Knudson, A. G. (1960): Observations concerning fear of death in fatally ill children and their mothers. *Psychosom. Med.,* 22(6):456–465.

18. Pavlovsky, S., Fisman, N., Arizaga, R., Castano, J., Chamoles, N., Leiguardo, R., and Moreno, R. (1983): Neuropsychological study in patients with ALL. *Am. J. Pediatr. Hematol. Oncol.,* 5(1):79–86.

19. Sheline, G. E. (1975): Radiation therapy of tumors of the central nervous system in childhood. *Cancer,* 35:957–964.

20. Spinetta, J. J. (1974): The dying child's awareness of death. *Psychol. Bull.,* 81(4):256–260.

21. Spinetta, J. J., Rigler, D., and Karon, M. (1973): Anxiety in the dying child. *Pediatrics,* 52(6):841–845.

22. Stehbens, J. A., Kisker, C. T., and Wilson, B. K. (1983): Achievement and intelligence test-retest performance in pediatric cancer patients at diagnosis and one year later. *J. Pediatr. Psychol.,* 8(1):47–56.

23. Susman, E. J., Hollenbeck, A. R., Strope, B. E., Hersch, S. P., Levine, A. S., and Pizzo, P. A. (1980): Separation-deprivation and childhood cancer: A conceptual re-evaluation. In: *Psychological Aspects of Childhood Cancer,* edited by J. Kellermann. Charles C Thomas, Springfield, Illinois.

24. Tamaroff, M., Miller, D. R., Murphy, M. L., Salwen, R., Ghavimi, F., and Nyr, Y. (1982): Immediate and long-term posttherapy neuropsychologic performance in children with acute lymphoblastic leukemia treated without central nervous system irradiation. *J. Pediatr.,* 101(4):524–529.

25. Van Eys, J. (1977): *The Truly Cured Child: The New Challenge in Pediatric Cancer Care.* University Park Press, Baltimore.

26. Waechter, E. H. (1971): Children's awareness of fatal illness. *Am. J. Nurs.,* 71:1168–1172.

The Quality of Life of Cancer Patients,
edited by N. K. Aaronson and J. Beckmann,
Raven Press, New York © 1987.

Psychosocial Aspects of Leukemia and Other Cancers During Childhood

Jillian R. Mann

Birmingham Children's Hospital, Birmingham B16 8ET, England

The psychological and social aspects of leukemia and other cancers during childhood are reviewed here, with particular emphasis on some of the studies undertaken in the United Kingdom.

It is evident that many individuals may be affected by the stresses associated with the diagnosis and treatment of childhood cancer, including the patient him/ herself, the parents, siblings, grandparents, other relatives, and friends. Persons involved in the day-to-day care of the child are also vulnerable, especially nurses, doctors, laboratory technicians, and social workers.

The nature of the distress varies with the stage of the child's illness and the response to treatment. When the diagnosis is first made the parents usually display shock and disbelief. They often express guilt, fearing that their child's illness may have arisen from lack of vigilance or some other failure of parenting; these feelings are heightened if diagnosis was delayed. Feelings of anger and inability to cope with the child's illness are also common and are made worse if the child shows physical or emotional distress, aggressive or otherwise disturbed behavior.

For many young children the admission to hospital may be their first separation from home and family, and they may appear to blame their parents for allowing it and the unpleasant tests and treatment. The child notices and reacts to the parents' shock and distress. Little is known about what children really do understand about their illnesses and what worries them. Even when great care has been taken to explain in simple terms that they are "seriously ill"—have "a bad blood disease," leukemia, or cancer—they may find it difficult to accept that the unpleasant treatments are making them get better, and they often continue to fear and dislike injections and drugs that cause vomiting and loss of hair. Other children accept their illness and support other members of the family who cannot cope. Alopecia is a particularly distressing experience for older children, some of whom feel that they cannot face friends and schoolmates after they have become bald, even when they are provided with a good wig. The emotional effects of mutilating surgery, such as amputation, are also profound.

Despite the initial angry and fearful reactions, most children do come to terms with having frequent blood tests and treatments, although some exhibit disturbed behavior, such as aggression, excessive dependence on their parents, and school phobia. Many of these early problems can be lessened by swift diagnosis and treatment, sympathetic and detailed explanatory interviews with parents, and the support of the whole oncology team, particularly doctors, nurses, and social worker. The latter can provide much practical help as well as skilled counseling. The child also benefits from gentle and accurate explanation of the illness and its treatment, within his capacity to understand.

When the child goes home parents often feel insecure and can be helped by having easy telephone access to members of the hospital team for advice. Few family doctors are familiar with childhood cancer and its treatment; therefore although they may provide practical and moral support, parents still tend to rely on hospital staff for detailed advice.

During outpatient treatment continuity of care by familiar doctors and nurses reduces the distress of hospital visits, as do measures such as anesthesia for painful procedures and good play facilities in clinics. During this time parents may develop exaggerated hopes of cure while also harboring fears of relapse. They experience the conflict that results from attempts to resume normality, including usual discipline, while fearing that the child may die. Overprotective and indulgent behavior toward the child is thus commonplace. The siblings may feel neglected because of the attention lavished on the sick child.

After relapse and during the terminal phases of the illness the emphasis changes toward keeping the child comfortable and happy while preparing for his death. Although community health services are important, it remains necessary for the personnel of the hospital to continue to take an active role. Their advice is required for practical measures, especially medication, as few family doctors have ever cared for a dying child, and the child and his family need their support. Home visits by members of the hospital team are invaluable. With adequate help most families can care for their dying children at home. Continuing support for some time after the bereavement is also often welcomed.

A substantial proportion (more than 50%) of children with cancer are now cured, and they and their families need to make the appropriate psychological and social adjustments in order to achieve a good education and a normal adult life style.

PSYCHOLOGICAL AND SOCIAL PROBLEMS IN FAMILIES OF CHILDREN WITH LEUKEMIA

Sixty children with leukemia and 60 controls who had been treated for minor surgical problems were studied in Manchester (1); their parents were interviewed 6 months after the diagnosis and about a year later. Approximately one-third of the mothers of children with leukemia were suffering from severe anxiety, depression, or both, whereas similar symptoms affected only about one in 20 of the mothers of the controls. The children with leukemia more frequently showed disturbed behavior than did the controls, and many brothers and sisters of the leukemic children were emotionally disturbed. Factors that increased the likelihood of a mother breaking down included additional stresses such as housing or financial problems, severe side effects of treatment, behavior problems in the child, lack of support from relatives and friends, and failure to resolve feelings of guilt about the child's leukemia. Only very rarely had the true depression been recognized by the child's doctor or by the mother's general practitioner.

SCHOOL PROBLEMS

School attendance was studied in 41 children aged 5 to 11 years in remission of acute lymphoblastic leukemia treated at the Hospital for Sick Children in London (2). Absence rates were 64% during the first 0 to 6 months after diagnosis, 34% at 6 to 24 months, 27% during treatment 2 years or more after diagnosis, and 22% after all treatment had been completed. Three children were not attending school at all but were having home tutoring. The absence rate for siblings was 15%. Teachers thought that about 50% of children with leukemia and 25% of siblings were having problems with their education. Nevertheless, the childrens' achievements were similar to their classmates', although 22% of children with leukemia were getting extra help. Teachers commented that they would like more information about prognosis, the length of treatment, and how much could be expected of the child.

Further studies on 129 children treated in seven centers in the United Kingdom (3) have indicated that most functioned within the average range of intelligence several years after completing treatment but that they had significantly lower intelligence quotients (IQs) than their siblings (Average British Ability Scales IQ 101.3 in the patients and 111.8 in their siblings). Patients treated under the age of 3 years had lower IQs than those who received treatment when older.

Similar results were obtained in 23 children with lymphoblastic leukemia evaluated in Newcastle (4), but 19 children with solid tumors showed few intellectual deficits. The deficits seen in the lymphoblastic leukemia patients were probably caused by the prophylactic treatment of the central nervous system with cranial irradiation and intrathecal methotrexate.

FINANCIAL PROBLEMS

In Birmingham a study of 59 families of children with leukemias and other cancers showed that during the first inpatient week of treatment the sum of income lost plus additional expenditure exceeded 50% of total income in more than 45% of families (5). During a subsequent week of outpatient treatment, loss of income plus additional expenditure amounted to more than 20% of income in more than half the families. These findings were similar to those of the nonmedical costs of illness in America (6).

The problems affected all groups studied and were not confined to the lowest paid or those living furthest from the center. Financial help was available from charitable sources and the Department of Health and Social Security toward travel, extra nourishment, and heating but could not be obtained to compensate for loss of earnings. The families of children who died had difficulty meeting the cost of funerals.

LONG-TERM SURVIVORS

In Liverpool families of 24 children with lymphoblastic leukemia or Wilms' tumor were studied at least 2 years after completion of treatment (7). Parental anxiety was still present, particularly over the possibility of relapse and death. Other fears concerned whether the children would reach adulthood, marry, and produce normal, healthy offspring.

Parents' marriages had been placed under strain by their childrens' illnesses, and many of the siblings had had problems. Parents would have liked more information about their children's illnesses. Other areas also needed more attention, such as better communication with schoolteachers, grandparents, and other relatives, financial help for parents, and marital counseling.

BEREAVEMENT

Families of 59 children who had died after treatment for leukemia in Liverpool, Sheffield, Leeds, and Birmingham were interviewed (8). The period of grief and adjustment commonly lasted more than 3 years, and in 47% of families at least one member had needed psychiatric help. Mothers had been especially seriously affected, and 8% had attempted suicide. In many families the parents had experienced marital difficulties, and the other children had shown emotional disturbance. Whereas most parents had turned chiefly to hospital staff and relatives for support during their children's illnesses, after their deaths the hospital contacts were usually abruptly severed. Many parents would have welcomed continuing contact with the hospital staff during their period of mourning. Some units had special bereavement groups to help parents. Other helpful factors included mothers taking employment, having another baby, temporary involvement in fund raising, the needs of surviving siblings, moving house, strong religious beliefs, vacations during the first year of bereavement, and having friends available to listen.

CONCLUSION

Much progress has been made in the treatment of leukemia and other cancers. Attention has been focused on new advances in management and on the clinical trials and other research endeavors that are greatly improving the prospects for cure. However, the treatments remain rigorous for both the patient and the relatives. Nearly all children and their parents suffer at some stage from emotional distress, even when the child is doing well, and it is clear that a price must be paid for the better chances of cure. This price may include severe disruption of family life and much emotional, financial, and other distress to the child and his relatives.

REFERENCES

1. Maguire, G. P., Comaroff, J., Ramsell, P. J., and Morris Jones, P. H. (1979): Psychological and social problems in families of children with leukaemia. In: *Topics of Paediatrics, Vol. 1: Haematology and Oncology,* edited by P. H. Morris Jones. Pitman Press, Bath.
2. Eiser, C. (1980): How leukaemia affects a child's schooling. *Br. J. Soc. Clin. Psychol.,* 19:365–368.
3. Jannoun, L. (1983): Are cognitive and educational development affected by age at which prophylactic therapy is given in acute lymphoblastic leukaemia? *Arch. Dis. Child.,* 58:953–958.
4. Twaddle, V., Britton, P. G., Craft, A. C., Noble, T. C., and Kernahan, J. (1983): Intellectual function after treatment for leukaemia or solid tumours. *Arch. Dis. Child.,* 58:949–952.
5. Bodkin, C. M., Pigott, T. J., and Mann, J. R. (1982): Financial burden of childhood cancer. *Br. Med. J.,* 284:1542–1544.
6. Lansky, S. B., Cairns, N. U., Clark, G. M., Lowman, J., Miller, L., and Trueworthy, R. (1979): Childhood cancer: Non-medical costs of the illness. *Cancer,* 43:403–408.
7. Peck, B. (1979): Effects of childhood cancer on long-term survivors and their families. *Br. Med. J.,* 1:1327–1329.
8. Peck, B., Martin, J., and Pinkerton, P. (1983): Bereavement following the death of a child from leukaemia. Presented to the XV Annual Conference of the Societe Internationale d'Oncologie Pediatrique, York.

The Quality of Life of Cancer Patients,
edited by N. K. Aaronson and J. Beckmann,
Raven Press, New York © 1987.

The Concept of Quality of Life in Pediatric Oncology

Robert P. Kamphuis

Department of Pediatrics, University Hospital, 2333 AA Leiden, The Netherlands

As in medicine in general, progress has also been seen in pediatrics. Improvements in diagnostic and therapeutic methods have led to cure for many children who, only some decades ago, would certainly have died. There seems to be no end to medical possibilities. There is, however, another side to the coin. Especially in children with a severe disease, serious psychological and social sequelae to the treatment are often encountered—immediately as well as in the long run. The patient's way of life can be affected quite drastically (5).

Physical consequences of medical interventions can be observed rather easily. Vomiting, weariness, and loss of appetite are well known symptoms after chemotherapy. Effects of irradiation can be measured without much difficulty in many cases. Results of surgery are visible most of the time. The meaning of these phenomena for the patient and his family is not as clear-cut as the easy visibility suggests, however. Even when treatment is the same, one patient suffers more than another. Unpredictable changes in the situation at home can occur when customary roles cannot be taken up in the same way as before. Reactions of friends and relatives influence the behavior of the patient. Somatic inconveniences can interfere with intellectual, affective, and social functioning. Personality characteristics play an important role in each individual's way of coping (22).

The interest in these effects of a disease and its treatment is not new and has been strongly stimulated by the rapid developments in medicine. The term "quality of life" has been coined as an eclectic compilation of a variety of notions relevant to widely different aspects (physical, emotional, mental, behavioral, social) of an individual's well-being. However, the assemblage of so many aspects under one heading inevitably leads to vagueness and therefore to the necessity for clarification. Only when a concept is clearly defined can measurement become possible. During the process of medical decision-making quantification is a precondition to blending these elements in a meaningful way with the often more accurately measurable somatic effects. In pediatric oncology special problems arise because the patient is a child.

Obviously, this problem has consequences for their outlook on the quality of life, whatever the definition of the concept. A child is a person in development.

His perceptions, attitudes, and judgments change continuously. Moreover, as a rule, adults make decisions, including medical decisions, for the child. These differences between adult and pediatric patients are discussed in this chapter, and a number of conceptual and methodological points are addressed.

GENERAL DIFFERENCES BETWEEN ADULTS AND CHILDREN AS PATIENTS

A characteristic of the child is his orientation toward the facts directly perceivable. He lives in the present and focuses on the directly observable. His reactions are very concrete. He wants to know what happens now, whether it will hurt, and what he will experience. This situation is particularly so when a child has such a damaging and threatening disease as cancer (5). Of course, the behavior of the child with regard to his illness correlates with his age, his level of development, the medical consequences of his disease, and the degree of anxiety and fear that goes with it (14). In order to better capitalize on these factors it is important to look closely at those aspects of the illness that are important to the child.

Nature of the Disease

In a study of 264 children 6 to 13 years old, Campbell (3) investigated the development of the concept "illness." He found that children associate this concept primarily with specific bodily feelings like "not feeling quite fit."
Differentiation of the concept came about at age 11 and was not related to sex or socioeconomic background. Even then, however, the diagnostic specificity remained a relatively unimportant element. Of much more interest for the child were such questions as: Is the disease a lasting one, or will it pass? Will the illness come back [as with leukemia]?

Complaints

It is very important for the child to know whether the disease will lead to any impediments or handicaps and if daily activities will be hampered. Obviously, subjective complaints condition the child to a far greater extent to his being ill than when there are no or practically no such disadvantages. Goldberg (6) stressed the point about the visibility of a handicap. After interviewing children 11 to 15 years of age, he concluded that an invisible disease with severe physical handicaps (e.g., a complicated congenital heart disease) has a less harmful effect on social adjustment than a visible handicap without physical complaints (e.g., facial burns).

Restrictive Rules for Behavior

Sometimes the child is not allowed to exert himself freely. Occasionally restrictions come from the physician, as when the child is not allowed to go to the cinema because of his lowered immunological defence capacity caused by aggressive cytostatic therapy. The child suffers when he is not permitted to do the same things as other children (e.g., restricted physical education at school). Restrictions from outside, time after time, function as a reminder of the disease. The unpleasant effect is that the child feels different from other children. In this way the child is put in an exceptional position. Most children do not like this and want some sort of explanation.

Beginning of the Disease

When a child is born with a disease he does not know the difference between the situation with and without the illness. In children with cancer, however, the illness most often appears suddenly. The confrontation is acute, and the impact on daily life is more violent. Depending on his age, there are more recollections of life before the disease, which makes it much more difficult to accept the present situation. Symptoms such as feeling ill, pain, and nausea often lead to regression and increased dependency. In young children these symptoms may be interpreted as punishment and revenge. In the child's world magic can play an important role. The child of 6 years and older may look on his disease as responsible for his incapacities, although this perception varies depending on the nature of the disease and the extent to which information is provided to the child.

Medical Consequences

The nature of the diagnostic and therapeutic procedures can also cause the child to focus his attention on his disease. A hematological illness, for instance, requires many needle punctures, which represents a clear burden to a child. Almost all children are afraid, especially when a bone marrow puncture is necessary (9). On the other hand, noninvasive investigations lead less often to negative feelings. As a rule, a disease with only a few hospital admissions (e.g., congenital heart disease) has less impact than an illness with frequent admissions (e.g., leukemia). Many treatments, such as hemodialysis, confront the child to a greater extent with his illness than do less demanding forms of treatment.

Prognosis

Probably the most important point for the child is to know if he will be cured and, if so, when. Presumably there are few children who on becoming ill think they will not recover. When the prognosis is uncertain or unfavorable, it can lead to a problem in communication between the child and the adults involved. On the one hand, there is a right to know. On the other hand, there are the emotional consequences of knowing. In some American centers for bone marrow transplantation it is customary to tell children from the age of 4 onward all possible risks and complications of treatment before the therapy begins. In such situations anxiety, even death anxiety, and depression are common (10). In Leiden (The Netherlands) these symptoms are observed in young children only now and then (7). There the information is more confined to what the child wants to know at any particular moment. The provision of details is attuned to the behavior of the child and the current medical situation. Although other centers may explain the results as well, it is suggested that it may be better not to tell children everything all at once. This is not to say that an open communication between children and their families, as advocated by Spinetta et al. (17,19), has to be discouraged. However, it is evident that the timing and level of information about the prognosis is an important point to consider when studying the reactions of the child to the treatment.

The differences in appraisal of a malignancy between adult and child patients are presented in Table 1. The purpose of this approach is to stimulate an analysis of the disease process from the viewpoint of the child. In pediatric oncology this approach seems to be an essential condition when one agrees that the quality of life concept has to be formulated in highly individualized terms.

In Table 1 the average course of events in a disease is shown in the left column, and in the right columns some frequently occurring behavioral reactions are indicated. A guiding principle is that the attention of the child, as a rule, is drawn sharply toward the immediately perceivable consequences of his disease and its treatment rather than toward the diagnosis itself.

TABLE 1. *Differences in illness behavior between adult and pediatric patients*

Development of the disease and medical consequences	Frequently expected reactions	
	Adults	Children
First symptoms	Recognition defines emotional color	Unsuspecting
Medical investigations	Reluctant but gradual acceptance of medical situation	Continuously adverse reactions to unpleasant medical procedures
Diagnosis	Affectively colored reactions, especially in case of malignancy	Often not mentioned; usually not evoking special associations
Treatment	Realization of inevitability with individual differences in coping behavior	Adjustment to the situation as a whole but strong emotional reactions to medical treatment
Results and prognosis	Strong emotional reactions	Negative outcome often not mentioned directly; behavior not alway predictable

In most cases, this pattern remains up to the age of 12 years and may be valid even after that age. For adults the etiology and, of course, the prognosis often dictate the color of the reactions. In many respects this situation also is true for the parents. Their emotional and pedagogic course of action is a very important factor for the behavior of the child. Even without words the child perceives something of the way in which the parents react. Therefore the behavior of the child cannot be seen apart from that of the adults around him. As a patient, however, the child often adjusts rather quickly to the medical situation as a whole. The distinction between diagnostic and therapeutic procedures often remains diffuse.

It must be emphasized that the terminology used here serves only as a rather vague starting point for studying the impact of disease variables on the quality of life of the pediatric patient. Depending on the specific group of patients under study, more detailed issues have to be formulated (2). Side effects such as difficulty with nausea, loss of hair, impairment of mobility and activity, periods of isolation, and a constant bombardment with interventions and procedures may present problems in adjustment that are as great as those caused by the illness itself. Social relationships are often greatly altered by disease, hospitalization, and treatment. Thus the interaction with other oncology patients deserves special attention.

METHODOLOGICAL PROBLEMS

When thinking about the concept quality of life, many questions need to be asked. Most of these apply equally to adults and children. Nevertheless, the fact that a child is concerned influences the possible answers.

Why Should One Measure Quality of Life?

When a child is confronted with a serious and life-threatening illness such as cancer, a long period of treatment awaits him. The impact on his life and sense of well-being is tremendous (11,16,18). In many respects it means an assault on the daily life of the child. In order to help him to cope effectively with the situation, a registration of the medical outcome of the treatment is not sufficient. Moreover, decisions must be made as to the treatment to be given, bearing in mind the psychological and social side effects for the child. Especially when two or more treatments are available, qualitative criteria can play an important role in making a choice. This also holds for policy-making, when the allocation of resources is under discussion.

What Is Quality of Life?

Quality of life is a very complex concept that cannot be formulated in a unified sense for all persons and all situations. It refers to a highly individualized notion of what makes sense for a person, related to his values, preferences, and ideals. A great number of interacting variables are involved (13).

General circumscriptions are vague and do not meet the requirements for operationalization. A solution to this problem can be reached, at least in part, when aspects of the concept are identified and are related to the kind of disease and treatment and the group of patients under study. Those components should include physical, social, and emotional functioning, implications of the medical procedures as seen by the child, his conceptualization of the illness, the consequences for his daily life and education, his attitude toward the illness, and the effect of illness and treatment on family interactions. Sometimes it is possible to use objective indicators such as school performance, but even these may be unrelated to what the child himself is experiencing. Subjective indicators such as satisfaction with school life probably are more of value to the child.

Who Makes the Assessment?

Whoever is judging certain aspects of the quality of life brings in his or her own frame of reference, despite specific instructions to the contrary. Physicians, for instance, are apt to use criteria other than those of parents when evaluating the possible effects of a treatment. Pain as a result of a puncture can be seen as nearly insurmountable by the child but does not bring about any hesitation by the doctor in carrying out the procedure. Response bias may be noteworthy when parents answer for their children (4).

Parental attitudes toward their children may systematically raise or lower their assessments. Problems with understanding what is asked may influence the answers of the child himself. A schoolteacher is likely to compare the patient with his healthy peers. Nurses see the children only in the hospital where the immediate reactions to the treatment overshadow all else. The degree of the illness may be the standard of judgment for them. Several solutions to this assessment problem are possible. As a starting point the areas of interest to the child himself can be studied, and then the opinion of "significant others" can be sampled: parents, schoolteacher, physician, nurses. Thus a system of values can be developed.

When Does the Measurement Take Place?

As has been said before, the behavior of the child depends to a large extent on what is happening to him at a particular moment. Thus an assessment during treatment says little or nothing about what he experiences during a later period, and the late effects of the disease and the treatment have to be taken into account. Although this is true for all patients, it is particularly relevant in the study of children who are undergoing rapid development and maturation. Repeated measurements may be relevant in order to tap transient effects. Even the same outcome of a therapeutic regimen, e.g., infertility after total body irradiation, carries a different weight for the sense of well-being when the patient is 6 years old than when he is an adolescent. On the other hand, the present may become more decisive than the future when the child's condition deteriorates. The impact of medical care and technology may then become overwhelming. Young children may associate pain with punishment. Their appraisal of the situation can diverge dramatically from that of the adults around them. Appalling and acute unhappiness can cause an alteration of the judgment about the ultimate satisfaction with life. Therefore it seems reasonable to expect changes in the relative importance and the content of certain quality of life variables in relation to the moment they are evaluated. Interwoven with this point of view, the influence of the surroundings on the measurement process must be considered.

Where Is the Assessment Made?

The current functional, intellectual, and emotional status of the child cannot be seen apart from the circumstances of the moment of the investigation. The child develops his behavior as part of a continuous interaction with his environment. The way he adapts to the hospital setting may influence his outlook on life as a whole. In school other qualities come to the fore. A short visit to the outpatient department at regular times may have a different impact on the child than a stay in hospital for a longer time, even with the same kind of treatment. At home the implication of symptoms such as hair loss and skin discoloration is different from those in the situation at school or in the neighborhood. Issues relative to fatality can become less menacing in an interval between treatments than during the time of diagnosis and initial treatment.

Comment

Many areas of concern have been delineated. Results depend on the form of the instrument, the context and wording of the interview, and the questionnaire or the rating scales used. Other prerequisites for good measurement, e.g., applicability, acceptability, variability, reliability, and validity, must be mentioned as well (1). However, these requirements for data-gathering instruments are more or less common to all approaches to the quality of life problem, irrespective of the age of the subject (20).

Almost all questions raised imply subjective decisions as to what kind of solution is to be chosen. Moreover, most of them are interdependent. Thus it is essential to develop a procedure as explicit as possible to arrive at a research design suitable for a specified group of patients based on an adequate selection of conceptual aspects in relation to the aim of the study. In order to look for possibilities to combine efforts in this field, a questionnaire about quality of life projects with children as subjects was sent to the European centers involved in the Society Internationale d'Oncologie Pediatrique (SIOP) (8,12).

QUALITY OF LIFE STUDIES IN PEDIATRIC PATIENTS WITH CANCER

A questionnaire was sent to 76 centers in Europe involved in the treatment of children with oncological and hematological diseases. Responses were obtained from 22 centers (28.9%), all interested in doing research in this area. Most of these centers (*n* = 18) had already done some work on quality of life.

On the question "Which points should be stressed in defining the concept quality of life with regard to pediatric patients?" the answers could be summarized under the following headings: (a) what to measure; (b) goals concerning the patients; and (c) how to help the patients. Suggested medical data to be gathered were growth, development, nature of the disease, short-term effects, number of traumatic events, disfigurement, time spent in hospital, and time spent away from normal activities. Nonmedical data to be studied included physical functioning, intellectual functioning, schooling, education, social functioning, affective/emotional behavior, coping mechanisms, family functioning and reactions, socioeconomic aspects, points of support for the patient, confidence in the treatment, and the capacity to maintain a normal life. With regard to goals, the following were mentioned: normal life and participation in activities appropriate to the age of the child.

Several respondents expressed interest in investigating ways of helping the patients: the best methods of providing support, active contribution to defense mechanisms against disease, avoidance/alleviation of side effects, how to cope with daily problems, relief of suffering (medical, social, and psychological support), how to maintain quality of life during and after cessation of treatment, and terminal care.

It seemed difficult to combine all of these aspects in a single project. When asked about this, most of the centers expressed a willingness to participate in a multicenter study. Mainly because of cultural and language problems some centers doubted the suitability of an international investigation. Eighteen centers were already involved in projects on a local-regional level.

Further specifications regarding areas of research interest expressed by the various respondents (more than one area could be checked) are given in Table 2. Most areas are thought to be useful, but no clear-cut preference stands out for a specific area to be studied. In the studies already under way or finished, many investigators make use of the interview method, together with checklists, tests, observation scales, or a combination of methods. In most projects the child himself is the subject together with the mother, father, or both.

The investigations took place with approximately equal frequency during an outpatient visit, during a stay in the hospital, or at home. Relatively often a case study model was used, although in some studies a systematic registration of the functioning of a larger number of individual patients was scheduled. Differentiation

TABLE 2. *Specification of areas of interest to the respondents of the inquiry*

Research area	Useful	Willing to participate	Already involved in a project
Intellectual/cognitive functioning	15	5	10
Affective/emotional behavior	17	5	8
Social behavior	13	5	3
Physical performances	14	4	5
Coping mechanisms	13	4	1
Interaction within the family	17	6	4
Socioeconomic aspects	13	3	3
Other	4	2	4

among the answers categorized in Table 2 does not show any clear pattern of substantive areas measured.

CONCLUDING REMARKS

The boundaries of medicine are ever extending. The problem arises as to the cost of such expansion, psychologically and otherwise. The position of the child with a life-threatening disease deserves special attention. His sense of well-being may be seriously affected by the treatment and the medical side effects. The process whereby his personal values and those of his family are to be incorporated into the medical decision-making is colored by the fact that he is an individual in development, in most cases dependent on the decisions of the adults involved. This dependency complicates the definition of the concept of quality of life in pediatric oncology. It has been argued that the way in which a child looks at his illness is different from the manner in which an adult patient experiences his situation. This view holds true from the onset of the first complaints until the ultimate result of the treatment, with or without incapacitating symptoms somewhere along this route. This difference in orientation may influence the behavior of the parents and the medical and nursing staff. They run the risk of basing their decisions on their own frame of reference as adults, not realizing what the meaning is for the child. Such decision-making can have essential consequences for the study of the quality of life of the pediatric patient.

Bearing in mind other methodological difficulties as well, it must be stated that *the* quality of life does not exist. What aspects are most indicative for a certain group of children? What criteria have to be taken into account? Which frame of reference and which reference groups have to be chosen at which moment during or after the treatment and by whom? Choices have to be made in all these areas. Each choice will result in a different quality of life assessment. Subjectivity seems to be an unavoidable determinant in the decisions the investigator must make.

A small survey among the pediatric oncology centers in Europe indicated the difficulty in reaching a consensus about the outline for further research in this field. A strategy is required in which the children themselves, the parents, and the treatment staff play a role to guarantee a controlled intersubjectivity by carefully weighing all factors involved.

For the particular category of children to be studied the aim should be to identify relevant areas of concern based on information about the medical and nonmedical consequences for the child of the specific form of the disease and its treatment. The meaning of these aspects for the life of the child and his need for support have to be taken into account at home, at school, during leisure time, now and in the future, specified with regard to his physical, intellectual, emotional, and social development.

Subjective as well as objective indicators of general well-being should be developed. The instruments for assessment specific to the problems being investigated can then be designed. Finally, their application ought to be attuned to the support given to the child.

In the end, data relevant to the criteria used should be included in the evaluation of the outcome of the medical treatment of the juvenile cancer patient. The evidence with adult patients so far (15) suggests that this process may be complicated and difficult.

However, striving toward this goal may be crucial for the happiness of the child with a malignancy. Implementing this kind of measure in the medical decision-making process can give a more realistic base to the search for as normal a life as possible for these children.

REFERENCES

1. Boyle, M. H., and Chambers, L. W. (1981): Indices of social well-being applicable to children— a review. *Soc. Sci. Med.,* 15E:161–171.
2. Brunnquell, D., and Hall, M. D. (1982): Issues in the psychological care of pediatric oncology patients. *Am. J. Orthopsychiatry,* 52(1):32–44.
3. Campbell, J. D. (1975): Illness is a point of view: The development of children's concepts of illness. *Child Dev.,* 46:92–100.
4. Eisen, M., Donald, C. A., Ware, J. E., and Brook, R. H. (1980): *Conceptualization and Measurement of Health for Children in the Health Insurance Study.* Rand Corporation, Santa Monica, California.
5. Gogan, J. L., O'Malley, J. E., and Foster, D. J. (1977): Treating the pediatric cancer patient: A review. *J. Pediatr. Psychol.,* 2:42–49.
6. Goldberg, R. T. (1974): Adjustment of children with invisible and visible handicaps: Congenital heart disease and facial burns. *J. Consult. Psychol.,* 21:242–248.
7. Kamphuis, R. P. (1979): Psychological and ethical considerations in the use of germfree treatment. In: *Clinical and Experimental Gnotobiotics.* Fischer Verlag, Stuttgart.
8. Kamphuis, R. P., and Last, B. F. (1981): Inquiry into the concept "quality of life" with regard to child patients suffering from cancer. In: *Proceedings Second EORTC Quality of Life Workshop,* pp. 40–51, internal report.

9. Katz, E. R., Kellerman, J., and Siegel, S. E. (1980): Behavioral distress in children with cancer undergoing medical procedures: Developmental considerations. *J. Consult. Clin. Psychol.*, 48:356–365.

10. Kellerman, J., Rigler, D., Siegel, S. E., McCue, K., Pospisil, J., and Uno, R. (1976): Psychological evaluation and management of pediatric oncology patients in protected environments. *Med. Pediatr. Oncol.*, 2:353–360.

11. Koocher, G. P., and O'Malley, J. E. (1981): *The Damocles Syndrome: Psychosocial Consequences of Surviving Childhood Cancer*. McGraw-Hill, New York.

12. Last, B. F., and Kamphuis, R. P. (1982): Psychosocial research in childhood cancer: Some preliminary remarks on further research. In: *Proceedings Third EORTC Quality of Life Workshop*, pp. 23–34, internal report.

13. Lehman, A. F. (1983): The well-being of chronic mental patients; assessing their quality of life. *Arch. Gen. Psychiatry*, 40(4):369–373.

14. Nagera, H. (1978): Children's reactions to hospitalization and illness. *Child Psychiatr. Hum. Dev.*, 9:3–19.

15. Najman, J. M., and Levine, S. (1981): Evaluating the impact of medical care and technologies on the quality of life: A review and critique. *Soc. Sci. Med.*, 15E:107–115.

16. Schulman, J. L., and Kupst, M. J., eds. (1980): *The Child with Cancer: Clinical Approaches to Psychosocial Care: Research in Psychological Aspects*. Charles C Thomas, Springfield, Illinois.

17. Spinetta, J. J. (1982): Behavioral and psychological research in childhood cancer: An overview. *Cancer*, 50(Suppl.):1939–1943.

18. Spinetta, J. J., and Deasy-Spinetta, P., eds. (1981): *Living with Childhood Cancer*. Mosby, St. Louis.

19. Spinetta, J. J., and Maloney, L. J. (1978): The child with cancer: Patterns of communication and denial. *J. Consult. Clin. Psychol.*, 46:1540–1541.

20. Spitzer, W. O., Dobson, A. J., Hall, J., Chesterman, E., Levi, J., Shepherd, R., Battista, R. N., and Catchlove, B. R. (1981): Measuring the quality of life of cancer patients. *J. Chronic Dis.*, 34:585–597.

21. Van Eys, J. (1983): *Psychosocial Care of Pediatric and Adolescent Cancer Patients* (selected abstracts). ICRDB, National Cancer Institute, Bethesda.

22. Zeitlin, S. (1980): Assessing coping behavior. *Am. J. Orthopsychiatry*, 50:139–144.

The Quality of Life of Cancer Patients,
edited by N. K. Aaronson and J. Beckmann,
Raven Press, New York © 1987.

Neuropsychological Abilities of Long-Term Survivors of Childhood Leukemia

Pim Brouwers

Clinical Center, National Institutes of Health, Bethesda, Maryland 20205

Most psychological care for children with cancer has been focused on acute rather than long-term effects of the disease and its treatment, largely because these cancers were associated with very low survival rates and short life expectancy. The main psychosocial concern was thus on the emotional impact of the fatal disease and in providing supportive therapy and counseling for the dying children and their families.

However, major advances have been made in the treatment of most childhood cancers but in particular of acute lymphoblastic leukemia (ALL), the most frequent childhood cancer. The introduction of combination chemotherapy and central nervous system (CNS) preventive therapy has resulted in prolonged disease-free survival for most children with ALL (32). However, there is an increasing body of data suggesting that this formidable improvement in treatment has been associated in some children with adverse long-term sequelae as a presumed consequence of CNS preventive therapy with cranial irradiation and intrathecal chemotherapy (23). Psychosocial research and care have thus partially shifted to issues of quality of life after cure. Researchers are now attempting to determine the variables that may identify patients who are "at risk" for adverse behavioral sequelae.

FACTORS INFLUENCING BEHAVIOR CHANGE

The social and personality changes as well as the cognitive and intellectual defects observed in a number of long-term survivors of leukemia may result from a number of factors (Fig. 1). These factors are called behavior modifiers. In turn, behavior modifiers are related to certain aspects of the disease and its treatment. Two broad categories may be distinguished (13): One consists in psychosocial factors and the other in organic components. The psychosocial category includes, for example, emotional stress caused by the uncertainty of living with a potentially fatal disease. Stress can also be produced by repeated returns to the clinic for painful medical procedures and treatment. In addition, these repeated trips may cause school absence and psychoeducational difficulties. The organic category is

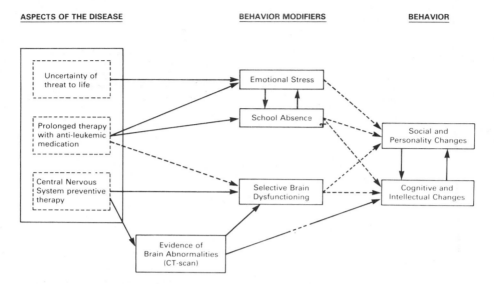

FIG. 1. Behavioral sequelae of childhood leukemia may result in changes in both personality and social behavior as well as in cognitive and intellectual functioning. These changes may be caused by two types of behavior modifiers: psychosocial factors (e.g., emotional stress and school absence) and organic factors (e.g., selective brain dysfunctioning). These behavior modifiers in turn are related to certain aspects of childhood leukemia and its treatment. Also illustrated is how CT brain scan abnormalities, because of their relation to selective brain dysfunctioning, can be used to provide evidence of the link between the organic factors and behavioral sequelae.

related to selective brain dysfunctioning, which may be caused by the effect of delayed neurotoxicities of the systemic chemotherapy or, more likely, by the CNS preventive therapy.

In this chapter it is argued that the observed behavioral sequelae in long-term survivors can be related to CNS abnormalities and thus may be largely of organic nature. Although the influence of psychosocial factors should not be neglected, it is believed that their effects have more impact and are more likely to occur during the acute stages of the disease. We turn first to the evidence for adverse organic sequelae and then to the psychological sequelae that may be related to these organic abnormalities.

ADVERSE ORGANIC SEQUELAE

Adverse sequelae that involve the CNS have been reported largely as acute side effects of concurrent therapy and mostly associated with the presence of CNS leukemia (14,37). A number of investigations have identified CNS abnormalities in asymptomatic long-term survivors who may be off all chemotherapy (31).

Three types of abnormality, each of which has neuropathological and neuroradiological expressions, have been demonstrated. Even though the incidence of these abnormalities is higher in patients who have had CNS leukemia, meningeal involvement is not a necessary condition for the development of these brain abnormalities.

Neuropathological Findings

Autopsy investigations by Price and co-workers (33,34) and Crosley et al. (8) have distinguished the following three types of brain abnormality in patients with ALL after CNS therapy: (a) subacute leukoencephalopathy, a white matter disorder with necrosis of the myelin sheets and neuronal processes; (b) mineralizing microangiopathy, a degenerative and mineralizing disorder of small vessels accompanied by dystrophic calcifications of adjacent cortex; and (c) cortical atrophy, a gray matter disorder with irregular neuronal loss involving all six layers of the cortex.

Furthermore, these investigators have reported that a number of factors influence the risk of developing these brain abnormalities. Age at diagnosis was an important factor; younger patients, particularly those under 6 years of age at diagnosis, were more likely to develop brain abnormalities. Second, time since treatment was found to influence the incidence of mineralizing microangiopathy: the longer the interval, the higher the risk. Finally, the number of relapses, particularly in the CNS, influenced the incidence of brain abnormalities.

Neuroradiological Abnormalities

Abnormal computed tomography (CT) brain scan findings were initially described in children with ALL who had clinically evident necrotizing encephalopathy (30). Subsequently, similar findings have been described in asymptomatic children with ALL who had received CNS preventive therapy with cranial irradiation and intrathecal chemotherapy (31). In that study one or more of four types of CT scan abnormality that may be related to the previously described neuropathological abnormalities were observed in 53% of the patients: (a) areas of parenchymal decreased attenuation coefficient, indicating white matter hypodensity that may be representative of subacute leukoencephalopathy; (b) evidence of mineralizing microangiopathy in the form of pathological intracerebral calcifications on CT brain scan; and finally (c) ventricular dilatation and (d) subarachnoid space dilatation, which are compatible with cortical atrophy. Since that initial report, a number of subsequent studies have described varying incidences of CT brain scan abnormalities in asymptomatic patients following CNS preventive therapy (29). Moreover, we (35) have shown that abnormal CT brain scan findings may appear for the first time several years after the initiation of CNS preventive therapy. Specifically, 22% of our patients developed intracerebral calcifications that became evident only 5 to 7 years after the initiation of CNS preventive therapy. Our results indicated that long-term follow-up with CT brain scans is essential to adequately assess the adverse sequelae associated with CNS preventive therapy. The exact nature and evolution of these abnormalities remains unclear. An association between the presence of intracerebral calcifications and cranial irradiation (35) as well as the cumulative dose of methotrexate have been made (25). Furthermore, we (35) found a significant negative correlation between the incidence of calcifications and age at diagnosis, confirming previously reported neuropathological findings (33). These CT scan findings have stimulated efforts to identify equally effective but less toxic forms of CNS prophylaxis. Current treatment protocols have reduced the amount of cranial irradiation or refrain from irradiation altogether (1).

ADVERSE PSYCHOLOGICAL SEQUELAE

Intellectual and Cognitive Deficits

Initial studies of survivors of childhood leukemia treated with CNS preventive therapy did not reveal any permanent behavioral or intellectual impairment. Other than the observation of transient electroencephalographic (EEG) abnormalities and the somnolence syndrome (15), which occur during or immediately after the CNS treatment, no generalized behavioral sequelae were noted (17,21,38,42). However, subsequent and more sophisticated studies have reported significant functional defects, particularly in patients who were younger at the time of diagnosis and exhibited more marked cognitive defects than older patients (7,11,13,27,28). Furthermore, some British studies (18,41) have indicated that cognitive deficits may become evident only many years after diagnosis and treatment. Most of these studies have used the Wechsler intelligence tests (44,45) as the main instruments of measurement. Because intelligence quotient (IQ) is a reliable predictor of academic achievement, these results suggest the likelihood of school problems in a number of children and the need for specific remedial assistance. However, the Verbal, Performance, and Full Scale IQs (VIQ, PIQ, FSIQ) and the subtests that comprise these measures are not uniquely defined in terms of cognitive functioning or with respect to cerebral localization of function. Thus although IQ deficits in these patients are well documented, these studies provide little understanding about the nature of the neuropsychological deficits that may underlie these IQ abnormalities and on which specific remedial attention may have to be focused. The various stages of psychological functioning that may be affected are discussed later.

Psychosocial and Personality Changes

Few studies directly have addressed the psychological and social status of long-term survivors of childhood leukemia. Although acute problems such as school phobia, anxiety, and depression have frequently been reported, these problems tend to be largely reversible. Some of the most extensive studies on psychiatric sequelae of childhood cancer are the investigations of Koocher and O'Malley (19). These authors studied a variety of aspects of the quality of life in long-term survivors. It should be noted, however, that their population of 475 patients, from whom they obtained a sample of 117 patients, contained only 27 (5.7%) who were originally diagnosed with leukemia, reflecting the long-term survival rates of the various types of childhood cancer prior to the 1970s. The overall outcome of these studies may therefore not be representative for leukemia survivors. Still, a number of general trends in these studies are highly interesting, specifically the predictors of the incidence of problems in psychiatric adjustment. The authors reported that age at diagnosis was significantly related to the incidence of maladjustment; those younger at diagnosis were less likely to have difficulties. Furthermore, these psychiatric abnormalities tended to have a transient character, and a negative correlation was found between time elapsed since diagnosis and the incidence of abnormalities.

Another important variable in their studies was the presence of physical changes. These changes, due to the disease and its treatment, may result in a fear of social rejection or ridicule as well as feelings of being different. Because of these apprehensions, physical changes can lead to extended school absence, even school phobia and social isolation. Regular school attendance is of great importance for these children, as lack of it may affect their psychosocial and psychoeducational development. It must be noted, however, that school-related factors largely affect the older patients, i.e., those who started school before or shortly after their diagnosis (13). Moreover, these physical changes, particularly hair loss, tend to be reversible in leukemia. Furthermore, the trauma of hair loss is most pronounced for the adolescent group and seems to have little impact on the very young patient.

UNDERLYING DEFICITS

In this section we discuss stages of psychological functioning that may have been implicated in the reported IQ deficits. Identification of the affected stages may suggest appropriate remedial courses of action and could facilitate rehabilitation.

Attention

A critical, initial component of cognitive processing involves attention to stimuli from the internal and external environments. Therefore a first step, when systematically evaluating which components of human behavior are affected in long-term survivors of cancer, is to study attentional processes. In a previous study (5) we used simple alerted auditory reaction time (SRT) with various fore-periods to objectively study these processes. Concurrent CT brain scanning made it possible to divide the ALL patients into three groups: those with normal CT scans, those with evidence of cortical atrophy, and those with intracerebral calcifications. The SRT results indicated significant differences between patients with normal and abnormal CT scans. Specifically, patients with abnormal CT scans reacted more slowly, and this latency was exaggerated by increasing the length of the preparatory interval. They also reacted with larger variability, which increased over the duration of testing, suggesting the presence of an atypical "fatigue effect." Moreover, the severity of impairment was related to the type of CT scan abnormality; patients with calcifications performed more poorly than patients with cortical atrophy. These findings confirmed and extended other reports that suggested the presence of a pattern of attentional deficits in long-term ALL survivors on the basis of discrepancies in the IQ subtest profile (6,7). Furthermore, because attentional processes are altered, interpretation of the nature and severity of other neuropsychological deficits as well as the observed IQ abnormalities should take into account the presence of attentional defects in long-term leukemia survivors.

Language

The years between 4 and 16 are formative in the child's full language development. Almost without effort the child or adolescent accumulates a broader and more differentiated vocabulary and develops more complex syntactical abilities. It is the incidental character of this learning process that might be instrumental in the observed language poverty in a number of long-term survivors (26). Furthermore, as is reported later, in a number of patients evaluated to assess long-term adverse sequelae, a specific language deficit (anomia) related to a breakdown in semantic knowledge (22) could be demonstrated.

As mentioned before, these survivors may exhibit attentional deficits, particularly patients with intracerebral calcifications. Attentional abnormalities may cause these patients to retain and incorporate language information only when attention is specifically focused on it. For example, Eiser (12) used a paired-associate learning task with both easy and difficult associates. Easy associates are based on "overlearned" semantic relations such as hammer–nail, and the difficult ones are novel associations, such as mountain–pot. She reported that long-term ALL survivors were impaired on the easy associates, whereas control subjects might have been able to utilize their superior, incidentally obtained, semantic knowledge. In contrast, for the difficult, new associates no difference was found, probably because both groups had to learn these new associations, and sufficient attention was focused on the task and its material.

Furthermore, a number of investigators have reported that younger patients tend to have more depressed VIQs compared to PIQs (28,39) owing in large part to low scores on vocabulary, similarities, and information subtests (7). Finally, it has been assumed that the ability to remember information is related to the extent to which it is initially encoded. The described language deficits may therefore affect the depth of initial encoding and lead to impoverished memory.

Memory

Some indications that memory processes might be affected were already found in the first study in this area (38), where it was noted that ALL patients did not benefit from previous test experiences whereas control subjects did. Subsequent studies (7,12,13,43) have also suggested impaired memory and learning performance in long-term survivors, but systematic studies are generally lacking.

In another study (4) we investigated the relation between CT brain scan abnormalities and patterns of neuropsychological functioning. Using standard tests of verbal and nonverbal memory and learning as well as tests of concept formation and concept shifting, verbal fluency, and shifting of attention, we were able to correctly predict CT scan results for 87% of the patients utilizing discriminant analysis. This study thus established a strong relation between patterns of neuropsychological functioning and cerebral integrity.

In addition, we studied which neuropsychological functions most powerfully differentiated patients with calcifications from those with cortical atrophy or without abnormalities. We found that patients with calcifications experience a global memory deficit, with poor recall of both verbal and nonverbal material, although the deficit was larger for verbal material. Furthermore, long-term retention was more affected than immediate recall. These patients showed a larger decrease in the amount of verbal information retained between immediate and delayed recall than the other patients; this decrease was found both in absolute terms and when percentage information loss was calculated. Finally, they showed a severe word-finding problem, indicated by impaired performance on a word fluency test. This deficit may be related to poor semantic knowledge (22), described earlier, or to the lack of verbal spontaneity, which may be associated with frontal lobe abnormalities (40).

QUESTION OF ORGANICITY IN BEHAVIORAL SEQUELAE

As discussed previously, our studies of long-term asymptomatic survivors of leukemia have shown strong correlations between the presence and type of brain abnormality demonstrated by CT scan findings and patterns of neuropsychological dysfunction. We were able to reliably predict CT brain scan findings of patients on the basis of their neuropsychological test scores. In addition, we showed reliable differences in attentional processes between the groups with cortical atrophy, with intracerebral calcifications, and without CT scan abnormalities.

In addition, one can also relate some of the observed social and personality changes to patterns of cerebral dysfunctioning. Specifically, most of the intracerebral calcifications are located in the region of the basal ganglia, an area, particularly the caudate, with extensive connections to the frontal lobes (16). Damage to the basal ganglia area may produce neuropsychological profiles similar to those seen in patients with frontal lobe abnormalities (3). Indeed for the patients we studied, tests that are sensitive to frontal lobe dysfunctioning (e.g., word fluency and Wisconsin card sorting) showed large discrepancies between patients with calcifications and patients with atrophy or no abnormalities. Frontal lobe lesions have often been associated with changes in behavior such as lack of initiative, loss of motivation, increased distractibility, flat affect, and irritability (40). These traits have also been described among the personality changes observed in some long-term leukemia survivors (10,20,36).

In summary, a number of factors may be responsible for the observed behavioral sequelae in long-term, asymptomatic survivors of childhood leukemia. As illustrated in Fig. 1, these factors can be classified into two categories: psychosocial factors and organic factors. We have presented evidence that a number of factors which may play an important role in affecting outcome produce opposite predictions. These factors are age at diagnosis and time since diagnosis. Research on delayed neurotoxicities of CNS preventive therapy, using histological and radiological techniques, has shown that a higher incidence of abnormalities is associated with younger age and longer time since diagnosis. A similar relation has repeatedly been found for intellectual and cognitive deficits. In contrast, the literature on psychiatric sequelae of childhood cancer has shown that extreme youth at the time of diagnosis and prolonged continuous remission are important factors in long-term psychological adjustment. It may thus be concluded that the observed neuropsychological sequelae in long-term survivors of childhood leukemia are largely of an organic nature.

LONG-TERM SURVIVORS WITH EDUCATIONAL COMPLAINTS

In the previous sections we have dealt with psychological research on asymptomatic long-term survivors of childhood leukemia. These patients were in continuous first remission and had never experienced overt CNS involvement of the disease. Most of them belonged to groups that were studied as part of a research project or protocol. We now turn to the individual long-term survivor and discuss the more clinical neuropsychological aspects of patients seen in the clinic for long-term follow-up evaluation.

Patients with long-term adverse sequelae present in a number of ways. Many children, considered normal on routine medical follow-up examination, may have started to show poor school performance as a first indication of their developing difficulties. Some children are very aware of the inconsistencies in their school performance and express concerns about this problem (27). However, thorough interviewing is sometimes required to uncover these matters as a number of patients and their parents do not volunteer this information. In fact, some may be reluctant to admit such problems and even deny they exist, possibly because they see the changes as a precursor to relapse (7).

To investigate and assess the late sequelae and to provide guidance and counseling for patients and their parents, the Pediatric Branch of the National Cancer Institute

(NCI) has instituted a "Late Effects Team." This group is composed of skilled professionals from a number of disciplines with the aim to comprehensively assess the patients' problems and suggest appropriate remedial courses of action to them or responsible persons in their environment (24). In the assessment special emphasis is placed on the patient's current medical and psychological status, on evidence of improvement or deterioration in their condition, and on the appropriateness of the current work or educational situation.

Most of these patients can be classified as having one of two types of neuropsychological impairment with a different profile and degree of severity (2). One group of patients are impaired compared to their siblings, but on standard psychological tests they still score within normal limits. Patients in the second group are more severely impaired and score below the average range.

Less Affected Patients

The less affected patients have suffered cognitive loss as a result of their disease and its treatment. This loss is evident from the reliable discrepancy between the patients' FSIQ and that of their siblings (28,41). Nevertheless, their FSIQs remain in the normal range, i.e., between 90 and 110. On CT brain scan no clear signs of gross brain abnormalities are noted; most of these patients have normal scans, although some may have evidence of minimal cortical atrophy. Furthermore, the neurological examination is unremarkable in most cases. On neuropsychological testing, the performance of these patients is often in the low normal range, particularly on tests of attention and memory and when using nonverbal, visuospatial material. There is, however, no evidence to relate this pattern of functioning to specific cerebral dysfunctioning. In addition, on longitudinal psychometric testing no deterioration is observed. However, because of the discrepancy in social and school performance between the patients and their healthy siblings, several patients may develop a negative self-image and experience adjustment problems. These patients may also have become overly test-anxious.

More Affected Patient

The more affected patients are not only impaired compared to their healthy siblings but also compared to the "normal" population. That is, their intelligence quotients are mostly in the dull normal range or lower (below 90). Furthermore, over time they tend to fall further behind their normally developing peers, and therefore their FSIQs decrease over time. This observation has also been made by other researchers, who have shown negative correlations between time since treatment and IQ (18,41). In terms of their medical profile, most of these patients have evidence of brain abnormalities on CT scan, e.g., intracerebral calcifications or severe cortical atrophy. Furthermore, some may have had CNS relapses, the neurological examination may reveal soft neurological signs, and a number of patients may be receiving treatment for an epileptic disorder. On neuropsychological evaluation, they present an attentional deficit as well as a global memory and learning impairment. In contrast to the first group, their impairment is often more pronounced for verbal or linguistic rather than nonverbal, visuospatial material. Careful clinical testing often demonstrates the presence of a word-finding deficit (anomia) as well as verbal comprehension problems that may be suggestive of restricted semantic knowledge. In addition, we observed personality changes, such as flat affect, lack of initiative, and increased distractibility.

IMPLICATIONS FOR REHABILITATION

The intervention and guidance for both groups begins with establishing close communication and mutual understanding between members of the team, the patients, and their parents. Where indicated, teachers and school principals may also be included in an effort to further delineate areas of strength, as well as to exchange information and to promote future rehabilitative efforts (24).

Patients in the first, less severely disabled group are informed that although they have suffered from the disease and its treatment they are not defective in psychological functioning nor are they learning-disabled (2). That is, even though they probably will not reach the same academic goals of their siblings, they are perfectly capable of finding a satisfying vocation and of leading an independent life. In order to alleviate the negative self-image and the anxiety associated with academic difficulties, some form of psychotherapy in combination with relaxation techniques may be required for a number of these long-term survivors. Furthermore, some patients and parents, confronted by the intellectual and emotional limitations, may need assistance in adjusting their hopes and expectations (24).

In contrast, the second group poses greater management problems for several reasons. Because of their attentional, memory, and learning defects, as well as the observed changes in personality structure, they are often unable to maintain themselves in the regular school system or in a regular work situation. Depending on the nature and severity of their deficits they will require a more sheltered and structured environment where they can be constantly supervised. Furthermore, any form of instruction will probably require clear and simple language and may have to be repeated several times. It is likely that their ability to learn new information or skills will be limited. Moreover, generalizations or different applications from what is learned in a specific situation to other situations are unlikely to occur (2).

We have argued that the observed attentional deficit some patients display emerges as a primary defect and, in terms of neuropsychological functioning, is of major consequence (5). It remains to be investigated if an improvement in the attentional abilities, through remedial intervention, also leads to an improvement in immediate and long-term memory functioning. Attentional processes may lend themselves to both pharmacological and neuropsychological intervention. In addition, new developments in the use of computer-aided cognitive rehabilitation programs may prove to be beneficial (46). Moreover, it needs to be studied whether other psychopharmacological agents that have been reported to selectively improve memory (9) can provide supportive therapy in the rehabilitation of these patients.

SUMMARY AND CONCLUSIONS

Changes in the treatment of childhood leukemia have resulted in prolonged disease-free survival and even cure for most patients. This progress in treatment has been obtained by using aggressive therapy, which in a small number of children may have resulted in adverse sequelae. We have argued that most of the long-term behavioral sequelae reflect cerebral dysfunction and are a presumed consequence of CNS preventive therapy.

We believe that a multidisciplinary team approach may provide a comprehensive method of approaching the child with long-term sequelae. It not only presents a forum offering guidance and counseling to the affected patients and their families but also creates a clinical research setting in which we can learn more about these sequelae. We hope that through these efforts late effect syndromes will become better understood, more widely known, and therefore detected sooner. Early identification of such patients might permit alteration in treatment or, possibly, early behavioral and pharmacological intervention, which might minimize these functional psychological deficits, spare these patients pain and frustration, and therefore improve their quality of life. Ultimately, we hope that new directions in the administration of CNS preventive therapy will lead to lower neurotoxicity, thereby reducing the number of long-term sequelae.

ACKNOWLEDGMENTS

I wish to thank Drs. D. Poplack and H. Moss (National Cancer Institute) and Dr. R. Riccardi (Universita Cattolica, Rome) for their continued support and the opportunity to study their patients. I also wish to acknowledge the support of Drs. P. Fedio, C. Cox, and F. Lalonde (National Institute of Neurological and Communicative Disorders and Stroke) in the design and administration of some of the neuropsychological procedures, as well as the support and enthusiasm of the other members of the Late Effects Team of the Pediatric Branch, National Cancer Institute. The work reported here was conducted while the author was a Fogarty Visiting Scientist from The Netherlands at the National Institutes of Health, Bethesda, Maryland.

REFERENCES

1. Bode, U., Oliff, A., Bercu, B. B., et al. (1980): Absence of CT brain scan and endocrine abnormalities with less intensive CNS prophylaxis. *Am. J. Pediatr. Hematol. Oncol.*, 2:21–24.

2. Brouwers, P. (1984): Behavioral problems and brain dysfunction in childhood cancer survivors: A multidisciplinary approach. In: *Proceedings of the Fifth National Cancer Communications Conference,* Washington, D.C.
3. Brouwers, P., Cox, C., Martin, A., Chase, T., and Fedio, P. (1984): Differential perceptual-spatial impairment in Huntington's and Alzheimer's dementias. *Arch. Neurol.,* 41:1073–1076.
4. Brouwers, P., Riccardi, R., Fedio, P., and Poplack, D. G. (1985): Long-term neuropsychological sequelae of childhood leukemia: Correlation with CT brain scan abnormalities. *J. Pediatr.,* 106:723–730.
5. Brouwers, P., Riccardi, R., Poplack, D., and Fedio, P. (1984): Attentional deficits in long-term survivors of childhood acute lymphoblastic leukemia. *J. Clin. Neuropsychol.,* 6:325–336.
6. Ceppellini, C., Merendi, M., Auriti, L., Zanetto, F., Romeo, T., Pandolfi, M., De Grandi, C., Scotti, G., and Masera, G. (1982): Neuropsychological evaluation in 34 children with ALL after treatment suspension. Paper presented at the Third International Symposium on Therapy of Acute Leukemias, Rome.
7. Coff, J., Anderson, H., and Cooper, P. (1980): Distractability and memory deficits in long-term survivors of acute lymphoblastic leukemia. *Dev. Behav. Pediatr.,* 1:158–163.
8. Crosley, C. J., Ronke, L. B., Evans, A., and Nigro, M. (1978): Central nervous system lesions in childhood leukemia. *Neurology,* 28:678–685.
9. Dimond, S. J., and Brouwers, E. Y. M. (1976): Increase in the power of human memory in normal man through the use of drugs. *Psychopharmacology,* 49:307–309.
10. Einsiedel, E., Weigl, I., and Gutjahr, P. (1979): The psycho-social status of children surviving a long time with acute lymphoblastic leukemia. *Therapiewoche,* 29:8669–8673.
11. Eiser, C. (1978): Intellectual abilities among survivors of childhood leukemia as a function of CNS irradiation. *Arch. Dis. Child.,* 53:391–395.
12. Eiser, C. (1980): Effects of chronic illness on intellectual development: A comparison of normal children with those treated for childhood leukemia and solid tumors. *Arch. Dis. Child.,* 55:766–770.
13. Eiser, C., and Lansdown, R. (1977): Retrospective study of intellectual development in children treated for acute lymphoblastic leukemia. *Arch. Dis. Child.,* 52:525–529.
14. Flament-Durand, J., Ketelbant-Balasse, P., Maurus, R., Regnier, R., and Spehl, M. (1975): Intracerebral calcifications appearing during the course of acute lymphocytic leukemia treated with methotrexate and x rays. *Cancer,* 35:319–325.
15. Freeman, J. E., Johnston, P. G., and Voke, J. M. (1973): Somnolence after prophylactic cranial radiation in children with acute lymphoblastic leukemia. *Br. Med. J.,* 4:523–525.
16. Goldman, P. S., and Nauta, W. J. H. (1977): An intricately patterned prefronto-caudate projection in the rhesus monkey. *J. Comp. Neurol.,* 171:369–386.
17. Holmes, H. A., and Holmes, F. F. (1975): After ten years, what are the handicaps and lifestyles of children treated for cancer? *Clin. Pediatr.,* 14:819–823.
18. Jannoun, L. (1983): Are cognitive and educational development affected by age at which prophylactic therapy is given in acute lymphoblastic leukemia? *Arch. Dis. Child.,* 58:953–958.
19. Koocher, G. P., and O'Malley, J. E. (1981): *The Damocles Syndrome: Psychosocial Consequences of Surviving Childhood Cancer.* McGraw-Hill, New York.
20. Last, B. F., van Veldhuizen, A., and de Ridder-Sluiter, J. G. (1982): Intelligentie en concentratievermogen van kinderen met leukemie en hun aanpassing op school. *Tijdschr. Kindergeneesk.,* 50:76–82.
21. Li, F. P., and Stone, R. (1976): Survivors of cancer in childhood. *Ann. Intern. Med.,* 84:551–553.
22. Martin, A., and Fedio, P. (1983): Word production and comprehension in Alzheimer's disease: The breakdown of semantic knowledge. *Brain Lang.,* 19:124–141.
23. Masterangelo, R., Poplack, D. G., and Riccardi, R. (1983): *Central Nervous System Leukemia: Prevention and Treatment.* Martinus Nijhoff, Boston.
24. McCalla, J. L. (1985): A multidisciplinary approach to identification and remedial intervention for adverse late effects of cancer therapy. *Nurs. Clin. North Am.,* 20:117–130.
25. McIntosh, S., Fischer, D. B., Rothman, S. G., Rosenfield, N., Lobel, J. S., and O'Brien, R. T. (1977): Intracranial calcification in childhood leukemia. *J. Pediatr.,* 91:909–913.
26. McIntosh, S., Klatskin, E. H., O'Brien, R. T., Aspnes, G. T., Kammerer, B. L., Snead, C., Kalavsky, S. M., and Pearson, H. A. (1976): Chronic neurologic disturbance in childhood leukemia. *Cancer,* 37:853–857.

27. Meadows, A., Massari, D., Fergusson, J., Gordon, J., Littman, P., and Moss, K. (1981): Declines in IQ scores and cognitive dysfunctions in children with acute lymphocytic leukemia treated with cranial irradiation. *Lancet,* 1:1015–1018.
28. Moss, H., Nannis, E., and Poplack, D. G. (1981): The effect of prophylactic treatment of the central nervous system on the intellectual functioning of children with acute lymphoblastic leukemia. *Am. J. Med.,* 71:47–52.
29. Ochs, J. J., Parvey, L. S., Whitaker, J. N., Bowman, W. P., Ch'ien, L., Campbell, M., and Coburn, T. (1983): Serial cranial computed tomography scans in children with leukemia given two different forms of central nervous system therapy. *J. Clin. Oncol.,* 1:793–798.
30. Peylan-Ramu, N., Poplack, D. G., Blei, C. L., Herdt, J. R., Vermess, M., and Di Chiro, G. (1977): Computer assisted tomography in methotrexate encephalopathy. *J. Comput. Assist. Tomogr.,* 1:216–221.
31. Peylan-Ramu, N., Poplack, D. G., Pizzo, P. A., Adornato, B. T., and Di Chiro, G. (1978): Abnormal CT scans of the brain in asymptomatic children with acute lymphocytic leukemia after prophylactic treatment of the central nervous system with radiation and intrathecal chemotherapy. *N. Engl. J. Med.,* 298:815–819.
32. Poplack, D. G. (1982): Acute lymphoblastic leukemia and less frequently occurring leukemias in the young. In: *Cancer in the Young,* edited by A. S. Levine. Masson, New York.
33. Price, R., and Birdwell, D. A. (1978): The central nervous system in leukemia. III. Mineralizing microangiopathy and dystrophic calcification. *Cancer,* 42:717–728.
34. Price, R., and Jamieson, P. (1975): The central nervous system in childhood leukemia. II. Subacute leukoencephalopathy. *Cancer,* 35:306–318.
35. Riccardi, R., Brouwers, P., Di Chiro, G., and Poplack, D. G. (1985): Abnormal computed tomography brain scans in children with acute lymphoblastic leukemia: Serial long-term follow-up. *J. Clin. Oncol.,* 3:12–19.
36. Ross, J. W. (1982): The role of the social worker with long-term survivors of childhood cancer and their families. *Soc. Work Health Care,* 7:1–13.
37. Rubinstein, L. J., Herman, M. M., Long, T. F., and Wilburn, J. R. (1975): Disseminated necrotizing leukoencephalopathy: A complication of treated central nervous system leukemia and lymphoma. *Cancer,* 35:291–305.
38. Soni, S., Marten, G., Pitner, S., Duenas, D. A., and Powazek, M. (1975): Effects of central nervous system irradiation on neuropsychological functioning of children with acute lymphocytic leukemia. *N. Engl. J. Med.,* 293:113–118.
39. Stehbens, J., Ford, M., Kisker, C., Clarke, W. R., and Strayer, F. (1981): WISC-R Verbal/Performance discrepancies in pediatric cancer patients. *J. Pediatr. Psychol.,* 6:61–68.
40. Stuss, D. T., and Benson, D. F. (1984): Neuropsychological studies of the frontal lobes. *Psychol. Bull.,* 95:3–28.
41. Twaddle, V., Britton, P. G., Craft, A. C., Noble, T. C., and Kernahan, J. (1983): Intellectual function after treatment for leukemia or solid tumors. *Arch. Dis. Child.,* 58:949–952.
42. Verzosa, M., Aur, R., Simone, J., Hustu, H. D., and Pinkel, D. P. (1976): Five years after central nervous system irradiation of children with leukemia. *Int. J. Radiat. Oncol. Biol. Phys.,* 1:209–215.
43. Walther, B., Gutjahr, P., and Beron, G. (1981): Therapiebegleitende und -ueberdauernde neurologische und neuropsychologische Diagnostik bei akuter lymphoblastischer leukaemie im kindesalter. *Klin. Paediatr.,* 193:177–183.
44. Wechsler, D. (1955): *Manual for the Wechsler Adult Intelligence Scale.* Psychological Corporation, New York.
45. Wechsler, D. (1974): *Manual for the Wechsler Intelligence Scale for Children—Revised.* Psychological Corporation, New York.
46. Wood, R. L. (1984): Management of attention disorders following brain injury. In: *Clinical Management of Memory Problems,* edited by B. A. Wilson and N. Moffat. Aspen Publications, London.
47. Zwartjes, W. J. (1979): Education of the child with cancer. In: *Proceedings of the National Conference of the Care of the Child with Cancer.* American Cancer Society, New York.

The Quality of Life of Cancer Patients,
edited by N. K. Aaronson and J. Beckmann,
Raven Press, New York © 1987.

Quality of Life of Cancer Patients: Review of the Literature*

Johanna C. J. M. de Haes and *Ferdinand C. E. van Knippenberg

*Institute of Social Medicine, University of Leiden, 2333 AL Leiden, The Netherlands; and
*Department of Medical Psychology, Medical Faculty, Erasmus University, 3000 DR
Rotterdam, The Netherlands*

Following the Second World War government policies in Western society shifted from restoring welfare to goals linked with psychological and social needs. Some major surveys into the well-being of the population were undertaken during the 1960s and 1970s in the United States (3,8,12,14). Findings from these studies were to help public policy to promote a better quality of life. The concept quality of life (QOL) was introduced into the debate on the goals of medical treatment at a later stage. It is used to draw attention to the fact that not only the cure and survival of patients but also their well-being must be considered important in medical care. This argument is especially important in oncology.

Cancer treatment has been directed traditionally toward prolongation of the patient's survival. Despite improved treatment results, for some tumor types cancer is still a fatal disease. At the same time cancer treatment is intrusive into the patient's physical, emotional, and social life. Surgery, radiotherapy, and chemotherapy have serious short-term as well as longer-lasting side effects. Nurses and physicians used the concept QOL initially to clarify the distinction between the medical and technical aspects of care and the other aspects of patient care. Being directly confronted with the suffering of patients, they have advocated paying more attention to supportive care.

More recently it has been stressed that QOL must be introduced as an endpoint in cancer treatment research (10,29). QOL was measured as an endpoint in only 4% of the cancer trials in 1975 and 1976 (5), but during the last few years more attention has been given to its measurement.

Quality of life research can be meaningful in several ways. QOL studies may give insight into the reaction of patients to cancer and cancer treatment and into the relations between different reactions and the overall QOL. The findings may support the patient information process and can influence decisions about the effectiveness of therapy: Costs and benefits can be weighed by the patient and by the person responsible for the treatment (10). It may also enhance supportive care.

---

* A version of this chapter appeared in *Social Science and Medicine*, 20(8): 809–817, 1985.

The research on QOL of cancer patients is reviewed in this chapter. Based on the literature, conceptual and methodological difficulties are described. Finally, some possible theoretical explanations for the results reported are given and suggestions for further research formulated.

RESEARCH ON THE QUALITY OF LIFE OF CANCER PATIENTS

A MEDLARS search up to December 1983 and an examination of the *Index Medicus* were carried out to obtain the largest possible number of cancer-related QOL studies. Only studies referring explicitly to QOL or well-being were included. These concepts are, as is usually the case, considered interchangeable (61). Studies on the QOL of cancer patients cover a wide range of patient groups. These groups differ from each other along medical dimensions: the type of tumor, the stage of disease, the treatment received, and the differing points in the treatment. Very different meanings are given to the concept QOL. Provisionally, the formulation of the authors is followed here. The studies are categorized as follows: (a) studies describing the QOL of a specific group of cancer patients; (b) studies comparing different groups of cancer patients, the independent variable being the type of treatment; (c) studies comparing cancer patients to noncancer patients: either patients with other diseases or nonpatients ("normals").

Descriptive Studies

It is seen from descriptive studies that side effects of treatment are a disruptive factor in the life of patients (21,26,48). Sexual difficulties and coping with a stoma are considered important problems for cured gynecologic cancer patients (21,66) who nevertheless seem to have settled into everyday life without undue difficulty (21). During chemotherapy behavioral disruption was reported more frequently than emotional discomfort (48). A positive attitude toward life or a fairly good overall QOL is reported in four of five studies (26,27,48,66).

Comparison of Groups of Cancer Patients

In some QOL studies supportive/palliative treatment is compared to a condition of no such treatment. Most often, however, two or more treatment regimens are compared. Some intensive radiotherapy and chemotherapy regimens are expected to be more toxic than others. Likewise, mutilating surgery is expected to have a more severe impact than other treatment modalities on the QOL of the patient. The primary question is whether the QOL is better after one treatment than after the other.

Palliation using BCG (bacillus of Calmette and Guérin) improved the QOL (i.e., the general condition) of lung cancer patients (4). Other forms of supportive therapy improved the QOL (i.e., loss of hair, bone marrow depression, vomiting, loss of appetite, and depression) of patients undergoing chemotherapy compared to controls (24).

A more intensive radiotherapy scheme induced more anxiety throughout most of the treatment, but no influence was found with respect to 20 other variables connected with well-being (55). Radiotherapy for prostate carcinoma affected the sexual functioning of patients less than surgery and was therefore considered to lead to a better QOL (42).

The impact of chemotherapy on the QOL of patients has been studied by various authors. In one study of 25 variables, intensive chemotherapy, compared to endocrine treatment, influenced only nausea, vomiting, constipation, and well-being in three of seven measuring points (54). In another study complaints were more severe in patients undergoing chemotherapy than in those coming to the hospital without treatment and disease-free. The general sense of well-being was not different between these groups (64). The disease-free cancer patients were found to differ from "normals" with respect to psychological complaints and satisfaction with life as a whole, whereas patients being treated with chemotherapy did not (43). Combination chemotherapy has been found to have a more negative impact on the QOL (interference with life as a whole, nausea, vomiting, malaise, alopecia) than a single drug treatment (53). Comparing two chemotherapy regimens, Burge et al. concluded that one was preferable to the other because of superior QOL (performance status) (9).

Several surgical procedures seem to influence the QOL of patients in a positive way. Lung resection compared to no resection is followed by an improved functional status of lung cancer patients (50). Patients who had undergone debulking surgery for advanced ovarian carcinoma had a less impaired activity level and report greater enjoyment of life than those who did not undergo such treatment (7). After sphincter-saving resection for rectal carcinoma, patients had better bladder function, food intake, work rehabilitation, sexual function, and mood than after abdominal-perineal resection (67). However, the hypothesis that limb-sparing surgery plus irradiation would provide a better QOL than leg amputation plus chemotherapy for sarcoma patients could not be substantiated. There was a difference with respect to sexual functioning in the opposite direction to that which had been hypothesized but not with respect to behavioral functioning, psychological functioning, economic consequences, or clinical assessment in these groups (60).

Finally, Schottenfeld and Robbins compared breast cancer patients with different stages of disease. The QOL (i.e., performance status) of patients with regional disease compared to local disease was inferior after 5 years but not after 10 years (57).

From these studies it may be concluded that differences between groups of cancer patients are primarily limited to certain factors related to QOL, such as physical complaints and activity level. In some cases the QOL consequences of treatment which on an *a priori* basis appear to differ dramatically with regard to impact on the lives of patients could be only partly confirmed empirically. Differences with respect to the overall QOL were seldom found.

Comparison of Cancer Patients and Other Groups of Patients or Nonpatients ("Normals")

It is commonly assumed that cancer and cancer treatment have a severe, negative impact on the QOL of patients. To test this hypothesis and to gain insight into the relative QOL of cancer patients, studies have been performed comparing cancer patients to noncancer patients. Many of these studies have been conducted among cancer survivors (18,19,35,38,56). Others refer to patients being treated or who were treated some months before measurement (16,23,35,36).

Cancer survivors were found to differ from noncancer patients with respect to marital status, the number of children, and insurance coverage (18); satisfaction with costs of living, taxes, national government, and leisure activities (38); psychosocial complaints, malaise, satisfaction with sleep, physical condition, and life as a whole (43); health concerns and self-control (56); and physical disability (19). However, no differences were found with respect to most QOL indicators: satisfaction with family, friends, work, income, values, activities, community, local government, health, the overall quality of life (38); psychological functioning (19); anxiety, depression, positive well-being, general mental well-being (56); daily activities (43); and work rehabilitation (18). Interestingly, survived cancer patients have reported more satisfaction with care from their partner and others than have healthy controls (43).

In the studies of patients being treated recently, the results appear similar. Mastectomized patients did not differ from benign controls with respect to QOL (36). Neither do chemotherapy patients differ from patients visiting a general practitioner or "normals" with respect to the level of well-being (23). The emotional well-being of melanoma patients being treated was found to be equal to that of "normals" and even superior to the well-being of patients with other dermatological disorders (16). No difference was found between chemotherapy patients and "normals" with respect to psychological complaints, satisfaction with life as a whole, and care from partner and others (43). Some differences were found, however, with regard to physical complaints (23,43) and sexual problems (36).

It is remarkable that comparisons between cancer patients and others do not seem to support the assumption that the QOL of cancer patients is, in general, poorer than the QOL of other groups. Actually, only Combes et al. (18), using objective indicators as their reference, found a marked difference between these groups.

It has been generally accepted (29,47) that cancer and cancer treatment cause a major disruption of life emotionally, socially, and physically. This assumption is confirmed in descriptive and comparative studies to some extent. However, results often do not point in the expected direction. This finding may be due to the operationalization of the concept, methodological aspects of the reviewed studies, or psychological mechanisms that have influenced the QOL of cancer patients but have not been taken into account.

DEFINING AND OPERATIONALIZING THE CONCEPT QUALITY OF LIFE

As Campbell et al. stated (12), "Quality of life is a vague and ethereal entity, something that many people talk about, but which nobody very clearly knows what to do about." When reading the studies on the QOL of cancer patients, this conclusion seems accurate. Fayos and Beland (25) gave a definition when advocating the assessment of QOL of cancer treatment: "the ability of patients to manage their lives as they evaluate it." In the research reported it is striking that QOL is never explicitly defined. Authors in other fields of study have given definitions of QOL. QOL is defined as: the "degree of need satisfaction within the physical, psychological, social, activity, material and structural area" (34); "a product of patient's natural endowment (NE) and the efforts made on his behalf by his family (H) and by society (S) (QL = NE × [H + S]) (58); "the global evaluation of the good or satisfactory character of people's life" (61); "the totality of those goods, services, situations and state of affairs which are delineated as constituting the basic nature of human life which are articulated as being needed and wanted" (32); and "the output of two aggregate input factors: physical and spiritual" (45).

If one compares these definitions, it becomes evident that they differ from one another along two dimensions. First, some authors explicitly refer to the subjective nature of QOL (25,34,61). Others refer to an objective situation (45,58). Objectivity may refer to objective, easily documented circumstances of life or to the fact that the evaluation of the QOL is made by an observer and not by the person evaluating his experience and perception of the situation. In cancer research this point has turned out to be very relevant because QOL is most often judged by those treating or nursing the patient. If QOL has been measured in cancer trials, physician-scored Karnofsky and Zubrod indices (40,69) are the instruments most commonly used (5). A new instrument has been developed to measure the QOL in cancer research (28,59) in which patients as well as physicians are expected to judge the QOL. The advantages of using a subjective evaluation of the situation have been discussed by Najman and Levine (49). Objective indicators are insufficient to understand QOL: The individual patient must be considered the only person able to weigh dissatisfactions and satisfactions (22,65).

Second, some authors define QOL as a global measure, an overall evaluation (25,61). Others define components of life that are important for the QOL (32,34, 45,58). Some authors combine these approaches in population-based research (3,12) by weighting components (domains, indicators, areas) as to their relevance for the global well-being of people in general or specific groups (e.g., cancer patients). Thus a global measure can serve as a criterion when assessing the interrelations among different components of life and the overall sense of well-being of cancer patients.

TABLE 1. *Operationalization of QOL in instruments developed to measure the QOL of cancer patients*

Instrument	Physical	Psychological	Social	Activities	Material	Structural	Global
Ability index (39)	x	x	x	x	x		x
ACSA (68)							x
ECOG (69)	x						
EORTC (1)	x	x	x	x			x
KPS (40)	x			x			
LASA (54,55)	x	x		x			x
QOL index I (28,60)	x	x	x	x			x
QOL index II (52)	x	x		x	x		x
RSCL (23,62)	x	x		x			x
Symptom checklist (35,44)	x	x		x			x
Vitagram (50)	x			x			x

Many researchers assume certain areas of life to be the operationalization of QOL. As a clear definition of QOL is lacking, the choice of these areas is often based on intuition. An overview of the indicators used by various authors is given in Tables 1 and 2. Included in Table 1 are instruments especially developed to measure QOL in cancer patients. In Table 2 are listed the operationalization of QOL in the single studies previously referred to. The areas suggested by Hörnquist are taken as the starting point, as they seem to be exhaustive (34). Also, the overall evaluation of QOL is embodied in the tables. It should be noted that, within the areas mentioned, some marked differences exist. Physical functioning, for example, may refer to bone marrow depression (24), gastrointestinal complaints (54), or the ability to consume a regular diet (7). Physical condition and activities may be overlapping areas (50).

Most authors include the physical condition of the patient, psychological well-being, and the performance of activities in their operationalization of QOL. However, fewer than half of the authors included social functioning or social support in their operationalization of QOL despite the suggestion that the quality of social support may account for some of the unexplained variance in the indicators of well-being (11,58). The material area proposed by Hörnquist (34) was included in only a few studies, even though the impact of disease on the economic welfare of the patient might be important: loss of jobs, expenses in paying for treatment, traveling, and special food. The structural component of life (the need of political participation, justice in society, and contacts with authorities) is considered in only one study. Intuitively, the relation between illness and this area is not evident. Surprisingly, Irwin et al.'s data suggested that patients are more dissatisfied with national costs than are "normals." Patients also show significantly higher levels of satisfaction with the media (38). The global evaluation of QOL by the patient has been taken into account in some studies. Unfortunately, this variable has only rarely been used as a criterion to weigh the relevance of different components of QOL. Physical complaints have proved important predictors of global well-being for cancer patients (23,43). In "normal" populations personal functioning, family life, and financial position turned out to be the best predictors of global well-being (3,12).

From Tables 1 and 2 it is evident that the choice of areas composing the QOL of cancer patients and the operationalization of these areas is not consistent. Furthermore, the choice of areas and the operationalization or the definition of the concept QOL has not been justified theoretically. Based on the comments made with respect to the definition of QOL, we suggest, following Szalaï (61), that QOL be defined as a subjective evaluation of the overall character of life.

SUBJECTS AND METHODS

The unexpected results of QOL studies might be due to methodological aspects of the research designs employed. One evident problem is that of sample size.

TABLE 2. *Operationalization of the QOL in individual studies into the QOL of cancer patients*

Study	Physical	Psychological	Social	Activities	Material	Structural	Global
Anthony et al. (4)	X	X					X
Blythe & Wahl (7)	X	X					
Burge et al. (9)	X			X			
Cassileth et al. (16)		X		X			
Combes et al. (18)			X		X		X
Craig et al. (19)	X	X	X	X			
Da Rugna & Buchheim (21)	X	X	X	X			
Edelstyn et al. (24)	X	X		X			
Giel et al. (26)	X	X	X	X			X
Gilbert et al. (27)	X			X			
Hutchinson et al. (36)	X	X	X				
Irwin et al. (38)	X	X	X	X	X	X	X
Leibel et al. (42)	X						
Meyerowitz et al. (48)	X	X	X	X	X		X
Palmer et al. (53)	X						X
Schmale et al. (56)	X	X					X
Schottenfeld & Robbins (57)	X			X			
Sugerbaker et al. (60)	X		X	X	X		
Vera (66)		X	X	X	X		
Williams & Johnston (67)	X	X		X			X

Van Dam et al. (63) have described a difficulty encountered by investigators when organizing QOL research in a clinical context: the noncooperation of physicians. Unfortunately, one of the consequences may be that the sample sizes are small (4,7,24,26,42,54,55,60,66) ($n \leq 25$), which makes it more difficult to discern any real existing group differences. A second issue has to do with control of background variables. Medical parameters, e.g., treatment, type of tumor, stage of disease, are assumed to be the independent variables influencing the QOL of cancer patients. Only in some investigations have the groups studied been compared with respect to age and sex differences and the time elapsed since treatment. However, demographic variables may explain a substantial part of the variance of the dependent variable, QOL, as they do in the general population (8,17). This factor has not been analyzed in any of the reported studies. Other variables possibly intervening in the explanation of QOL were analyzed only by Schmale et al. (56): Marriage and no change of job were found to be related to the level of general well-being experienced.

Third, attention should be given to the reliability and validity of the instruments used to measure QOL. Three groups of studies are distinguished. First, some authors developed ad hoc questions to measure QOL (4,7,9,18,19,24,26,36,42, 48,53,57,66). These authors did not report any findings on the reliability and validity of the instruments used. A second group of investigators used measures developed in other fields of social science to study the QOL of cancer patients. These scales, which refer to psychological adjustment and functional status, are the Sickness Impact Profile (25,60), the Katz Activities of Daily Living Scale (60), Bartel's Functional Scale (60), Psycho-Social Adjustment to Illness Scale (60), Present State Examination (46), the Mental Health Index of General Well-Being (16,56), and the HIS General Well-Being Measure (56). The reliability and validity of these measures have been demonstrated for noncancer patients, the general population, and psychiatric patients. The use of these instruments is advantageous as the evidence of reliability and validity may be quite extensive and as data on other populations may be available, thus enabling comparisons to be drawn. On the other hand, the condition of having cancer may be different, and therefore the QOL of cancer patients may have to be measured differently. That is, there may be certain problems specific to cancer that are not covered by these instruments. In a third type of study specific instruments have been developed to measure the QOL of cancer patients.

Some reliability and validity testing has been performed for most of these instruments. In Table 3 an overview is given of the information available on the reliability and validity of these instruments. To test reliability several indices have been used. It should be noted that because QOL is not defined as being stable for a specific period of time but is supposed to fluctuate according to circumstances (e.g., treatment periods), a test–retest index does not seem adequate to determine reliability. Likewise, interrater reliability can be adequate only if QOL is defined as the evaluation made by someone other than the patient him/herself.

Content validity is established by showing that the items are a sample of a

TABLE 3. Reliability and validity indices of the instruments measuring the QOL of cancer patients

Instrument	Reliability	Validity
Ability index (39)	—	—
ACSA (6,41)	Interrater	Content
ECOG (69)	—	—
EORTC (1)	Internal consistency 0.69/0.82	Discriminant/construct
KPS (40)	Test–retest = 0.66/interrater = 0.69	Concurrent/convergent/predictive
LASA (54,55)	—	—
QOL index I (28,59)	Internal consistency = 0.78/interrater = 0.81/0.84	Content/convergent/discriminant
QOL index II (52)	Internal consistency = 0.88/test–retest = 0.80	Content/construct/concurrent/discriminant
RSCL (23,62)	Internal consistency = 0.89	Content/concurrent/discriminant
Symptom checklist (35,44)	Internal consistency = 0.80/test–retest = 0.88	Content/discriminant/predictive
Vitagram (50)		Predictive

universe in which the investigator is interested (20). The content validity of the QOL measures is most often established by incorporating advice from health professionals. The opinion of patients is included explicitly only in the investigations of Spitzer et al. (59). Most investigators also consider other types of validity. Most often the calculated indices refer to the criterion-oriented approach (15,51). In this tradition a high correlation between the instrument under study and some criterion is seen as an indicator of validity. Predictive and concurrent validity indices have been employed in the QOL studies. It should be noted that different authors (44,50,68) use survival time as a criterion when presenting predictive validity. However, as survival is expected to be different from and independent of QOL, this criterion does not seem to be adequate. In recent years more emphasis has been placed on construct validity and the process of systematic validation in relation to theory testing (13,51). Several relations between the construct and the instrument under study and other constructs and instruments may be seen as indicators of construct validity. Spitzer et al. (59) used the expected correlations between two instruments, both intending to measure the construct QOL, as an indicator of validity (convergent). The terms construct validity and related methods are not always used in an appropriate manner in that expectations are seldom made explicit (52). For construct validation the embedding of the construct (QOL) in a theory should be elaborated

Research methods do not seem altogether adequate in many of the reviewed studies. Some have small sample sizes, many do not consider intervening variables, and the instruments used have not always proved reliable and valid. The design of studies has not always been sufficiently thorough. Therefore the unexpected results in the reported studies may be due to methodological shortcomings.

THEORETICAL NOTES

It has been assumed that some cancer treatment modalities are more disruptive to the QOL than others and that the QOL of cancer patients is worse than the QOL of the "normal" population. The fact that many results from QOL studies do not point in the expected direction may have to be taken seriously. It is possible that cancer and cancer treatment influence QOL less than is generally expected. However, if we agree that the QOL is a subjective evaluation of the patient, theoretical arguments can be raised to explain why such a seemingly disruptive disease as cancer does not consistently lead to a lowered evaluation of the QOL.

One explanation for the relatively high QOL of cancer patients may be provided by reference to Helson and Bevan's adaptation level theory (33). They formulated the theory with concern for determining what stimulus conditions lead to a judgment of "neutral" with a verbal rating scale technique. In their view the adaptation level of a person at any given instant is a weighted geometric mean of all stimuli, past and present, and their effects on the attribute being judged. The adaptation level changes when new stimulus objects are experienced. The neutral judgment corresponds to this adaptation level, and all other judgments are made relative to this level. If cancer patients are asked to judge their QOL, their judgment may be based on an adaptation level influenced by the experience of disease. As cancer patients may have experienced more extreme negative stimuli, their neutral point may refer to a more negative objective situation. Thus similar circumstances may lead to a more positive judgment of cancer patients than of "normals." For example, having experienced extreme nausea cancer patients may judge nausea as mild, whereas healthy persons pass a more negative judgment on the situation. This mechanism creates methodological problems. The score on a given scale may have a different meaning for cancer patients. This theory might explain why, in the study of Cassileth et al., cancer patients judged their situation more positively and more like "normals" than patients with skin diseases whose adaptation level may not have changed substantially (16).

A second explanation may be that the aggregation of the domains constituting the overall QOL changes. The overall explanation is determined by the aggregation of the evaluation of different areas of life (3,12). The weighing of the evaluation of different domains leads to an overall evaluation of life. For cancer patients this aggregation may have changed in two ways. First, their experience in some domains may have improved. Positive and negative emotions can contribute independently to the sense of well-being of persons (8). Positive experiences of cancer patients may occur along with negative experiences, thus leaving the overall level of QOL unchanged. For example, Meyerowitz et al. reported an amelioration of family and marital relations in patients undergoing chemotherapy (48). In research on the QOL of cancer patients, however, most emphasis has been put on negative aspects of well-being. Second, the value associated with certain domains of life may change (48). For example, being dissatisfied with one's job may have a different impact on the overall QOL of cancer patients than on that of "normals." Studies investigating the impact of the evaluation of different life domains on the overall QOL of cancer patients would lead to greater insight into the conditions of these patients.

A third argument is presented by the work of Campbell et al., who suggested that QOL has a cognitive and an affective component (12). Cognition refers to perception, reasoning, thinking, and satisfaction. Affect covers emotions and happiness. Circumstances may affect these components differently: "An individual who has achieved an aspiration towards which he has been moving may be said to experience the satisfaction of success. Another person may have lowered his aspiration level to the point which he can achieve and he might be said to experience the satisfaction of resignation. The two individuals might be equally satisfied in the sense of fulfilled needs but the affective content associated with resignation and success may well differ" (12). The distinction between cognition and affect has been demonstrated empirically by Andrews and McKennell (2). In their view measures of perceived well-being are attitudes that include affective (positive affect, negative affect) and cognitive components. Measures of affect are considered more sensitive to external circumstances. In patients with cancer, circumstances may have changed dramatically. If resignation has taken place, the satisfaction level may be relatively high, although the affective component of life quality may have changed.

This idea might explain why in the study of Irwin et al. (38) cured cancer patients were largely equal to "normals" with respect to their satisfaction with life as a whole and with certain areas of life. Schmale et al. (56) found a difference between cancer patients and "normals" with respect to worries, and Andrews and McKennel (2) found worries to be heavily loaded with negative affect. Thus it appears to be worthwhile to distinguish between cognition and affect in the study of QOL of cancer patients.

SUMMARY AND CONCLUSIONS

Studies of the QOL of cancer patients have been reviewed in this chapter. Some investigators used a descriptive approach, some compared the effect of different treatment regimens on the QOL of patients, and still others compared cancer patients to patients with other diseases or to "normals." In general, the results from comparative studies do not support the assumption that cancer or cancer treatment lead to a significantly lower QOL. Looking at the research more carefully it becomes evident that:

1. An explicit definition of the concept QOL is often lacking and a wide range in operationalizations is used.

2. Little attention has been given to intervening variables, whereas demographic variables are associated with the QOL in the population at large.

3. The number of patients involved in these studies is often small.

4. The reliability and validity of the instruments used are not always demonstrated.

5. Practically no attention has been given to theories explaining the origins of the QOL of patients.

Therefore it is suggested that future research must be better integrated into the tradition of the social sciences.

Obviously, the methodological difficulties encountered in QOL research must be overcome. More interesting, however, are the questions raised with respect to conceptual and theoretical problems. It has been assumed in this chapter that QOL is a subjective evaluation of the overall character of a person's life. From this starting point it is necessary to determine which aspects of life are related to subjective evaluation of QOL. These aspects may be tied either to external circumstances or to internal personal characteristics or adaptation mechanisms. A more refined theoretical approach may broaden insight into QOL. Knowledge of the conditions and the mechanisms of the QOL of cancer patients may have a positive influence on the care offered and thus lead to an improved situation for such patients.

ACKNOWLEDGMENTS

This work was funded by the Dutch Cancer Foundation "Koningin Wilhelmina Fonds." The authors wish to thank: I. P. Spruit, A. van Knippenberg, W. J. A. van den Heuvel, and M. C. Cuisinier for their critical comments on an earlier version of this chapter.

REFERENCES

1. Aaronson, M. K., Bakker, W., Stewart, A. L., Van Dam, F. S. A. M., Van Zandwijk, M. D., Yarnold, M. D., and Kirkpatrick, A. (1984): A multiple-dimensional approach to the measurement of quality of life in lung cancer clinical trials. In: *Proceedings from the 6th Workshop EORTC Study Group on Quality of Life*, Zürich.
2. Andrews, F. M., and McKennel, A. C. (1980): Measures of self-reported well-being: Their affective, cognitive and other components. *Soc. Indicators Res.*, 8:127–155.
3. Andrews, F. M., and Withey, S. B. (1976): *Social Indicators of Well-Being*. Plenum Press, New York.
4. Anthony, H. M., Madsen, K. E., Mason, M. K., and Templeman, G. H. (1978): A stratified randomized study of the intradermal BCG in patients with carcinoma of the bronchus: Prolongation of quality but not length of life in inoperable patients. *Cancer*, 42:1784–1792.
5. Bardelli, D., and Saracci, R. (1978): Methods and impact of controlled therapeutic trials in cancer. *UICC Techn. Rep. Ser.*, 36:75–97.
6. Bernheim, J. C., and Buyse, M. (1983): Amnestic comparative self assessment, a method to measure the subjective quality of life of cancer patients. *J. Psychosoc. Oncol.*, 4:25–38.
7. Blythe, J. G., and Wahl, T. P. (1982): Debulking surgery: Does it increase the quality of survival? *Gynecol. Oncol.*, 14:396–408.
8. Bradburn, N. M. (1969): *The Structure of Psychological Well-Being*. Aldine, Chicago.
9. Burge, P. S., Richards, J. D. M., Thompson, D. S., Prankerd, T. A. J., Sare, M., and Wright, P. (1975): Quality and quantity of survival in acute myeloid leukemia. *Lancet*, 2:622–624.
10. Bush, R. S. (1979): *Malignancies of the Ovary, Uterus and Cervix*. Edward Arnold, London.
11. Campbell, A. (1976): Subjective measures of well-being. *Am. Psychol.*, 117–124.
12. Campbell, A., Converse, P. E., and Rodgers, W. L. (1976): *The Quality of American Life*. Sage, New York.
13. Campbell, D. T., and Fiske, D. W. (1959): Convergent and discriminant validation by the multitrait-multimethod matrix. *Psychol. Bull.*, 2:81–105.
14. Cantril, H. (1965): *The Pattern of Human Concerns*. Rutgers University Press, New Brunswick, New Jersey.
15. Carmines, E. G., and Zeller, R. A. (1979): *Reliability and Validity Assessment*. Sage, London.
16. Cassileth, B. R., Lusk, E. J., and Tenaglia, A. N. (1982): A psychological comparison of patients with malignant melanoma and other dermatological disorders. *Am. Acad. Dermatol.*, 7:742–746.
17. Centraal Bureau voor de Statistiek (1981): *De Leefsituatie van de Nederlandse Bevolking 1977*. Staatsuitgeverij, The Hague.
18. Combes, P. F., Desclaux, B., Malissard, L., and Pons, A. (1977): Poids du diagnostic de maladie de Hodgkin sur la qualité de la vie des sujets qui en sont guéries. *Bull. Cancer (Paris)*, 64:395–408.
19. Craig, T. J., Comstock, G. W., and Geiser, P. B. (1974): The quality of survival in breast cancer: A case control comparison. *Cancer*, 33:1451–1457.
20. Cronbach, L. J., and Meehl, P. E. (1955): Construct validity in psychological tests. *Psychol. Bull.*, 4:281–302.
21. Da Rugna, D., and Buchheim, F. (1979): Lebensqualität und Komplikationen nach der Behandlung gynäkologischer Karzinome. *Ther. Umsch.*, 36:559–567.
22. De Groot, A. D. (1978): Bevordering van welzijn. In: *Over Welzijn*, edited by G. P. Baerends, J. J. Groen, and A. D. de Groot. Van Lochum Slaterus, Deventer, The Netherlands.
23. J. C. J. M., De Haes, Pruyn, J. F. A., and van Knippenberg, F. C. E. (1983): Klachtenlijst voor kankerpatiënten, eerste ervaringen. *Ned. Tijdschr. Psychol.*, 38:403–422.

24. Edelstyn, G. A., MacRae, K. D., and MacDonald, F. M. (1979): Improvement of life quality in cancer patients undergoing chemotherapy. *Clin. Oncol.,* 5:43–49.
25. Fayos, J. V., and Beland, F. (1981): An inquiry on the quality of life after curative treatment. In: *Head and Neck Oncology: Controversies in Cancer Treatment,* edited by A. R. Kager, pp. 99–109. Boston Hall, Boston.
26. Giel, R., Frankenburg, W., Oldhoff, J., Otten, B., van der Ploeg, E., Schrafford Koops, H., and Vermey, A. (1977): De Chirurg-oncoloog en de Kwaliteit van het Leven van Zijn Patiënten. *Ned. Tijdschr. Gen.,* 34:1315–1320.
27. Gilbert, H. A., Kagan, A. R., Nussbaum, H., Rao, A. R., Satzman, J., Chan, P., Allen, B., and Forsythe, A. (1977): Evaluation of radiation therapy for bone metastases: Pain relief and quality of life. *AJR,* 129:1095–1096.
28. Gough, I. R., Furnival, C. M., Schilder, L., and Grove, W. (1983): Assessment of the quality of life of patients with advanced cancer. *Eur. J. Cancer Clin. Oncol.,* 8:1161–1165.
29. Greer, S. (1984): The psychological dimension in cancer treatment. *Soc. Sci. Med.,* 4:345–349.
30. Deleted on proof.
31. Deleted on proof.
32. Harwood, P. de L. (1976): Quality of life: Ascriptive and testimonial conceptualizations. *Soc. Indicators Res.,* 3:471–496.
33. Helson, H., and Bevan, W. (1967): *Contemporary Approaches to Psychology.* Van Nostrand, Princeton.
34. Hörnquist, J. O. (1982): The concept quality of life. *Scand. J. Soc. Med.,* 10:57–61.
35. Huisman, S. (1981): Het Meten van Positieve Aspecten bij Kankerpatiënten. Psychologicol Laboratory, University of Amsterdam.
36. Hutchinson, A., Farnoon, J. R., and Wilson, R. G. (1979): Quality of survival of patients following mastectomy. *Clin. Oncol.,* 5:391–392 (abstract).
37. Hutchinson, T. A., Boyd, N. F., and Feinstein, A. R. (1979): Scientific problems in clinical scales as demonstrated in the Karnofsky index of performance status. *J. Chronic Dis.,* 32:661–666.
38. Irwin, P. H., Gottlieb, A., Kramer, S., and Danoff, B. (1982): Quality of life after radiation therapy: A study of 309 cancer survivors. *Soc. Indicators Res.,* 10:187–210.
39. Iszak, F. C., and Medalie, J. H. (1971): Comprehensive follow-up of carcinoma patients. *J. Chronic Dis.,* 24:179–191.
40. Karnofsky, D. A., and Buchenal, J. H. (1949): The clinical evaluation of chemotherapeutic agents in cancer. In: *Evaluation of Chemotherapeutic Agents,* edited by C. M. Macleod, pp. 191–205. Columbia University Press, New York.
41. Ledure, G., Souris, M., and Bernheim, J. (1981): Control study of amnestic comparative self assessment (ACSA). In: *Proceedings of the First EORTC Workshop on Quality of Life,* Amsterdam.
42. Leibel, S. A., Pino Y Torres, J. L., and Order, S. E. (1980): Improved quality of life following radical radiation therapy for early stage carcinoma of the prostate. *Urol. Clin. North Am.,* 7:593–604.
43. Linssen, A. C. G., Hanewald, G. J. F. P., Huisman, S., and van Dam, F. S. A. M., (1982): The development of a well-being (quality of life) questionnaire at The Netherlands Cancer Institute. *Proceedings of the Third EORTC Workshop on Quality of Life,* Paris.
44. Linssen, A. C. G., Hanewald, G. J. F. P., van Dam, F. S. A. M., and van Beek-Couzijn, A. L. (1981): The development of the complaint questionnaire at The Netherlands Cancer Institute. In: *Proceedings of the First EORTC Quality of Life Workshop,* Amsterdam.
45. Liu, B. C. (1974): Quality of life indicators: A preliminary investigation. *Soc. Indicators Res.,* 1:187–208.
46. Maguire, G. P. (1980): Monitoring the quality of life in cancer patients and their relatives. In: *Cancer Assessment and Monitoring,* edited by P. Syminton. Churchill Livingstone, New York.
47. Meyerowitz, B. E. (1980): Psychological correlates of breast cancer and its treatments. *Psychol. Bull.,* 87:108–131.
48. Meyerowitz, B. E., Watkins, I. K., and Sparks, F. C. (1983): Quality of life for breast cancer patients receiving adjuvant chemotherapy. *Am. J. Nurs.,* 2:232–235.
49. Najman, J. M., and Levine, S. (1981): Evaluating the impact of medical care and technologies on the quality of life: A review and critique. *Soc. Sci. Med.,* 15F:107–115.
50. Nou, E., and Aberg, T. (1980): Quality of survival in patients with surgically treated bronchial carcinoma. *Thorax,* 35:255–263.

51. Nunnally, J. C. (1967): *Psychometric Theory.* McGraw-Hill, New York.
52. Padilla, G. V., Presant, C., Grant, M. M., Metter, G., Baer, C., and Finnie, P. (1983): Quality of life index for patients with cancer. *Res. Nurs. Health,* 6:117–126.
53. Palmer, B. V., Walsh, G. A., McKinnae, J. A., and Greening, W. P. (1980): Adjuvant chemotherapy for breast cancer, side effects and quality of life. *Br. Med. J.,* 281:1594–1597.
54. Priestman, T. J., and Baum, M. (1976): Evaluation of quality of life in patients receiving treatment for advanced breast cancer. *Lancet,* 1:899–900.
55. Priestman, T. J., Baum, M., and Priestman, S. (1981): The quality of life in breast cancer patients. In: *Proceedings of the First EORTC Workshop on Quality of Life,* Amsterdam.
56. Schmale, A. M., Morrow, G. R., Schmitt, M. H., Adler, L. M., Elenow, A., Murawski, B. J., and Gates, C. (1983): Well-being of cancer survivors. *Psychosom. Med.,* 45:163–169.
57. Schottenfeld, D., and Robbins, G. F. (1970): Quality of survival among patients who have had a radical mastectomy. *Cancer,* 26:650–655.
58. Shaw, A. (1977): Defining the quality of life. *Hastings Center Rep.,* October:11.
59. Spitzer, W. D., Dobson, A. J., Hall, J., Chesterman, E., Levi, J., Shepherd, R., Battista, R. N., and Catchlove, B. R. (1981): Measuring the quality of life of cancer patients: A concise QL-index for use by physicians. *J. Chronic Dis.,* 34:585–597.
60. Sugerbaker, P. H., Barofsky, I., Rosenberg, S. A., and Gianola, P. J. (1982): Quality of life assessment of patients in extremity sarcoma clinical trials. *Surgery,* 91:17–23.
61. Szalaï, A. (1980): The meaning of comparative research on the quality of life. In: *The Quality of Life, Comparative Studies,* edited by A. Szalaï and F. M. Andrews. Sage, London.
62. Trew, M., and Maguire, G. P. (1982): Further comparison of two instruments for measuring quality of life in cancer patients. In: *Proceedings of the Third EORTC Workshop on Quality of Life,* Paris.
63. Van Dam, F. S. A. M., Linssen, A. C. G., and Couzijn, A. L. (1984): Evaluating quality of life. In: *Practice of Clinical Trials in Cancer,* edited by M. Staquet, R. Sylvester, and M. Buyse. Oxford University Press, Oxford.
64. Van Dam, F. S. A. M., Linssen, A. C. G., Engelsman, E., van Benthem, J., and Hanewald, G. J. F. P. (1980): Life with cytostatic drugs. *Eur. J. Cancer,* 1(Suppl.):229–233.
65. Van Dam, F. S. A. M., Somers, R., and van Beek-Couzijn, A. L. (1981): Quality of life: Some theoretical issues. *J. Clin. Pharmacol.,* 21:1665–1685.
66. Vera, M. I. (1981): Quality of life following pelvic exenteration. *Gynecol. Oncol.,* 12:355–366.
67. Williams, N. S., and Johnston, D. (1983): The quality of life after rectal excision of low rectal cancer. *Br. J. Surg.,* 70:460–462.
68. Yates, J. W., Chalmer, B., and McKegny, F. P. (1980): Evaluation of patients with advanced cancer using the Karnofsky Performance Status. *Cancer,* 45:2220–2224.
69. Zubrod, C. G., Schneiderman, M., Frei, E., et al. (1960): Appraisal of methods for the study of chemotherapy of cancer in man. *J. Chronic Dis.,* 11:7–33.

Editors' Note: Subsequent to this literature review, several pertinent articles have appeared regarding approaches to the measurement of quality of life in cancer. Of particular interest are the following: H. Schipper et al. (1984): Measuring the quality of life of cancer patients: The Functional Living Index—Cancer: Development and validation. *J. Clin. Oncol.,* 2:472–483; P. J. Selby et al. (1984): The development of a method for assessing the quality of life of cancer patients. *Br. J. Cancer,* 50:13–22.

The Quality of Life of Cancer Patients,
edited by N. K. Aaronson and J. Beckmann.
Raven Press, New York © 1987.

Quality of Life in Adults with Acute Leukemia

Robert Zittoun

Department of Hematology, Hotel-Dieu de Paris, F-75181 Paris Cedex 04, France

Many psychosocial studies have been performed in childhood leukemia, focusing especially on side effects of cranial irradiation, parental implications, and psychological sequelae (19,20,24). By contrast, little attention has been given to quality of life issues in adult patients with acute leukemia (11), with the exception of a special interest in patients in germ-free environments (13). Interindividual differences regarding somatic and psychosocial factors contribute to the complexity and difficulty of designing effective methodologies to address this concern. A preliminary clinical description of the disease and its treatment modalities is necessary, including the quality of life of the patients from the viewpoint of the hematologist. Such a description can help to define concretely the possible alterations of quality of life throughout the disease course, to focus on the main parameters that should be assessed, and to identify the patients who may require psychosocial support.

The specificity of the problems raised derives from the illness characteristics themselves, the most important being the systemic nature of the disease. From the onset, the entire body is involved, with permanent danger of death. Recovering or maintaining normal blood counts is considered essential for life. Supportive care—especially blood products transfusions—is necessary but contributes to a reduction in the patient's autonomy. This situation, characterizing acute leukemia at first presentation and during relapses, is also observed during the late phase of chronic leukemias: Chronic myelocytic leukemia is compatible with normal life but transforms into acute leukemia after an average duration of 3 years; chronic lymphocytic leukemia is mainly observed in the elderly and is characterized by a long survival with a near-normal quality of life in most cases, but decreased blood cell counts are usually observed at an advanced stage.

Medical intervention for acute leukemia consists primarily in chemotherapy. Treatment modalities are increasingly aggressive and vary according to age and prognostic criteria. The various treatment regimens for induction of complete remission and for consolidation require prolonged and repeated hospitalizations. They carry a noticeable risk of toxic death, induce side effects with serious repercussions, and result in a spectrum of situations for the patient, ranging between a severely deteriorated and shortened life to a relatively normal one.

Two specific aspects related to the course of acute leukemia and its treatment have been noted in the literature. First, each acute phase is seen as a menacing sign of imminent death and each remission as an escape from death and a hope for cure (25). Second, intensive chemotherapy is commonly performed within a protected environment, especially in the case of bone marrow transplantation. This situation results in greater patient isolation and affects the patient-caregiver relationship (23).

FIRST PHASE: HOSPITALIZATION AND INDUCTION TREATMENT

Two types of medical situations may be envisioned when the patient enters the ward. In the first the patient appears to have a good general health status, with the disease being discovered through a systematic blood count performed after moderate weakness or a minor infection. In the second situation the patient appears febrile and seriously ill and needs prompt treatment. The prognosis for these two situations is different, not only with respect to immediate risks but also with respect to chances of complete remission and longer survival. Performance status has been identified as a major initial prognostic parameter (15).

Nevertheless, all these patients receive the same treatment: hospitalization with isolation in a protected environment; repeated blood assays and bone marrow aspirations; intravenous infusion, often through a central catheter for chemotherapy; blood transfusion; and antibiotics. The rationale for such aggressive treatment is to induce a complete remission (10). Other types of treatment more respectful of quality of life have rarely been tried and are restricted to older patients (3,4,14). Moreover, the only parameter usually employed to assess the overall quality of life is the time spent out of the hospital (6,14).

The induction treatment of acute lymphoblastic leukemia is usually less aggressive at the onset, consisting in corticosteroids and weekly intravenous injections for 4 to 6 weeks, along with repeated lumbar punctures, sometimes poorly tolerated. The treatment of acute myelogenous leukemia is shorter with respect to initial chemotherapy, lasting about 1 week, but is followed by an unavoidable phase of severe aplasia with decreased blood cell counts for 2 to 4 weeks. This aplasia may be marked by highly febrile infections. Hemorrhagic risk is also present, and therefore platelet transfusions are given prophylactically.

The patient's quality of life during this induction phase can be variable. It may be examined in three contexts: the social context, the hospital milieu, and the psychological context.

Social Context

Illness and hospitalization represent a severe and sudden disruption of the patient's social relationships. This disruption may have negative consequences at the very beginning of the illness or secondarily, depending on the previous social profile, the conditions offered in the ward, and the information given to the patient by the health providers and other patients. Particularly for patients from rural areas or Third World countries, the remoteness, the disruption of family and social ties, and the brutal transplantation into a sophisticated hospital milieu may cause confusion and anxiety.

The discontinuation of work is equally problematic. This problem exists for craftsmen, salesmen, managers of small businesses, and farmers alike, many of whom have insufficient health insurance. They may also experience difficulties depending on the current employment situation, as others in the community compete for their jobs. This professional concern is applicable as well for students who are in the midst of obtaining their degrees and professional training.

Here again the illness may appear as either a tolerable restriction or, conversely, a family and social catastrophe. It can be very difficult to support patients who are in a precarious emotional and social balance (e.g., in the case of patients who left at home a handicapped child or sick relative). The families themselves, whether during the induction phase or more advanced treatment stages, frequently solicit information and emotional support from the therapeutic team.

Hospital Milieu

The second context refers to the patient's quality of life during his stay in hospital. One must stress the seemingly contradictory objectives of providing optimal psychological support while inflicting intensive medical treatments (i.e., isolation, continuous intravenous infusions).

Those techniques that are being developed to improve the treatment outcome unavoidably affect negatively the patient during hospitalization. The development of an ambiance that promotes quality of life is thus particularly needed. The warmth and compassion displayed by the caregivers is not only an individual endeavor; it is a mileu created by collective staff efforts. The patient's tolerance of isolation depends to a large degree on the appropriate preparation given through interviews, consultations, and special staff meetings (25). Staff availability may not always be optimal, but some median solution might be found that is satisfactory to both the staff and the patient.

Psychological Factors

Quality of life during the induction treatment depends in large measure on the patient's personality and his intrapsychic resources. The tolerance of treatment is not easily predicted through a simple psychological profile at the time of hospital admission. Patients who appear depressed before treatment sometimes adapt very well, whereas others who appear to be emotionally stable manifest anxiety, denial, introversion, and regression.

A certain amount of introversion is seen in many of the patients. Depression is also frequently manifested, although suicidal behavior is exceptional.

Briefly, there appear to be two interdependent factors that particularly affect quality of life during such treatments: the level of patient anxiety and the information made available about the illness, its treatment, and its evolution (32). The diagnosis is more frequently kept unpronounced than really ignored by the patient (12). However, more and more patients know their diagnosis precisely. When they do not receive it from their doctors, they may become aware of it through other patients. They may also guess the diagnosis through medical information delivered by the media, especially television, about treatments of hematological malignancies, by making comparisons with their own therapy (12). The results of blood counts are generally communicated, enabling the patient to follow his own disease course.

Perceptions of impending danger affect the patient and likewise reduce his quality of life during hospitalization. This situation is often manifested by fatigue, insomnia, anorexia, obsessions or ruminations fixed on blood counts and treatment, preoccupations with family or professional life, and a disturbance in sexual life. The support from the therapeutic team consequently represents an essential ingredient in patient treatment. This support implies that a psychologist or a psychiatrist should be available to the patient. The actual function of this person may vary from brief consultation with the medical staff to intensive psychotherapeutic interventions.

COMPLETE REMISSION: STRUGGLE FOR CURE AND QUALITY OF SURVIVAL

Necessity of Consolidation and Maintenance Treatment

Complete remission, frequently obtained after 1 to 3 months of induction treatment, is of indeterminable duration. Most of the prognostic criteria derived from large statistical series are useful to predict the remission induction but not its duration. One of the rare criteria that may yield some information is the facility by which remission is obtained. That is, the more quickly remissions are induced, the longer are their duration (16). All of the therapeutic attempts aimed at prolonging the duration of remission and increasing the number of patients who remain in their first remission more than 4 years—therefore with strong chance to be definitively cured—are based on combined, intensive cytotoxic chemotherapy (5,31). Consolidation treatments, which begin shortly after the first remission is obtained, are administered for several months and often require repeated hospital admissions. The value of low dose maintenance treatment has been debated in regard to acute myelogenous leukemia (9). Some protocols are based on intensive induction and consolidation treatment without complementary maintenance treatment during remission (5,29).

Hence comes the first contradiction of obtaining complete remission: Most adults with leukemia have a low chance for cure. Thus one might prefer returning to a short-term, relatively normal life as a treatment objective. However, the balance between intensive consolidation and quality of life during remission must not be considered lightly. Although intensive chemotherapy may compromise the quality of life of some patients, it is balanced by the increased proportion of patients alive and free of disease up to 4 years later (10). No patient in complete remission perceives himself as cured. Hope is present, but the risk of relapse is always discerned. Therefore intensive consolidations are rarely refused, at least during the first remission.

Side Effects of Intensive Chemotherapy

The patient's acceptance of intensive consolidation depends largely on the experience of the induction treatment, particularly as related to its side effects. Sometimes the induction treatment is successful and apparently devoid of major toxicity yet poorly tolerated by patients who claim that they would not want to undergo such distressing treatment again.

Physical side effects may delay the return to a normal life. Sequelae include cutaneous, dental, or painful rectal abscesses, fatigue, and weight loss (3). Fortunately, other complications that could more severely affect quality of survival are rarer, e.g., blindness, transient or permanent, due to retinal bleeding; deafness caused by drug toxicity; hemiplegia caused by cerebral venous thrombosis. One might imagine as well that in some cases the physician himself renounces the use of consolidation treatment. This was the situation in our service when a patient, after intestinal necrosis during a period of septic aplasia, had to undergo surgery leaving a definite colostomy. Yet the decision to avoid consolidation and maintenance treatment, which was hoped to permit the best quality of life possible, could not prevent the patient's subsequent depression, tied to his knowledge about his diagnosis and his fear of his impending relapse and death.

Returning to "Normal" Life?

For each therapeutic protocol, the proportion of patients able, during their remission, to be rehabilitated back into their usual family, affective, and sexual life is unknown. We can cite single instances which indicate that patients can resume a relatively normal life including returning to work after a few weeks of convalescence. Vacationing is frequent, as is the reestablishment of certain athletic activities. When after some years of remission the hope of cure becomes a reality, some patients marry and have healthy children. The fear of relapse is softened progressively with the length of remission, even though it probably never disappears in the minds of the patient or the physician, even if both have tacitly agreed not to discuss it. Finally, the patient may return to a relatively normal life, being followed up less regularly and being subject to common illnesses that have no relation to his leukemia. One can be surprised by the shared patient/physician indifference to this existential adventure that has barely passed.

Bone Marrow Transplantation During Remission

Planning a bone marrow transplant at the beginning of complete remission requires acceptance of prolonged constraint and considerable risks associated with the treatment. This discomfort is balanced against the increased chance of definitive cure instead of transient remission (7,28). Accordingly, the additional difficulties introduced into the leukemic patient's quality of life are multiple. If the patient hears of this treatment before or during induction, he may develop false hope, often to an excessively optimistic degree, even before a bone marrow donor is located. In the circumstance where a histocompatible sibling is not found immediately or where reawakened family conflicts lead to potential donor refusal, the patient's disappointment is considerable.

Once this treatment becomes a reality, the scheduled time for the marrow graft becomes the D-day. However, the risks are multiple. Rigorous isolation for several weeks in a life island "bubble" or sterile unit creates patient and family psychological reactions such as fear of germs. Increased staff tension is also not uncommon (23). Other difficult problems arise, especially the permanent infertility induced by the conditioning regimen with high dose chemotherapy combined with total body irradiation. However, aside from this major side effect, quality of life of patients surviving after the first months of transplantation and who are free of graft-versus-host disease is generally considered good or excellent (17).

FAILURES

Sudden or Progressive Distress

Failure of induction treatment or relapse after one or more complete remissions represents for some patients a sudden, dramatic event; for others it is manifested as slow and progressive deterioration. Treatment failures are distressing to the patient and the staff. Active treatments often correspond to patient requests, except for late experimental trials following numerous failures. In any case, one must try to understand the patient's wishes and keep communication open, even in emergency cases that need intensive care.

Repeated Relapses: Lassitude

When duration of remission becomes progressively shorter—years to months, months to weeks—the patient perceives his unstable nature. Even if he is in good general condition, he lives as if having been only briefly reprieved.

Sometimes this reprieve helps him to organize his life around his own priorities. The remission/relapse sequence involves serious repercussions for the patient, his family, and the staff, however, and carries with it unexpected behavioral responses. The psychological preparation for death can leave the patient and his family at a loss. Conversely, after new treatment that causes another remission, the patient must prepare to live, not die (25). The stages toward death hypothesized by Kubler-Ross (18), regardless of their correspondence to patients' actual experiences, are disrupted. Conflicts between patients, family members, or staff are not unusual. In contrast, unexpected relationships can be established (e.g., that between a nurse and the patient, which could extend to include the family and reach beyond the hospital confines).

The progressive loss of physical faculties with successive hospitalizations brings about a desire to preserve autonomy and to maintain control of the social environment. Consequently it is increasingly important for the patient to be vigilant about treatment, ward, and family relationships. Loss of control adds to distress and may result in emotional lability, total fatigue, and loss of hope (25). On the one hand patients may request additional treatments (experimental or unorthodox), and on the other they may refuse further treatment attempts.

Approaching the End: Quality of Life or Quality of Dying?

A careful clinical approach is essential to define optimal dying conditions for leukemic patients in the terminal phase. The physician must make a decision the moment he sets forth as his objective the relief of suffering and not the hypothetical prolongation of life. This decision is not made in isolation but comes from an understanding of the patient, the illness course, family interviews, and staff consultation. Communication with the patient helps to determine if and how he suffers, if he is aware of his illness course, and what he wishes. The request for new treatments or, conversely, for euthanasia originates more often from those around the patient, not the patient himself. In apparently noncurable situations "comfort" chemotherapy might still be appropriate. The anthracyclines can, in particular, have an analgesic effect if the pain is due to leukemia proliferation. However, major analgesics must promptly replace the cytostatics for most of the terminal cases. Neuroleptic or anesthetic prescriptions may be separately considered, depending on the alertness of the patient, patient wishes, and the persistence of uncontrolled pain.

The permanently acute character of the disease renders difficult a serene approach to the terminal phase based exclusively on pain relief, help for physical discomfort, and psychotherapy. Supportive care, including platelet transfusions to prevent hemorrhages and high dose antibiotics for treatment of infections in the immunocompromised patient constitute, until the last moment, a means of keeping the patient alive. This unrelenting fight to gain a marginally longer survival can make quality of life a subsidiary concern.

DISCUSSION

The paucity of studies devoted to quality of life of adult leukemic patients relates not only to the methodological difficulties of such studies in oncology but also to the poor prognosis and acute course of this disease. Quality of life of acute leukemic patients is severely compromised from the onset and remains poor during each hospitalization, whether for first induction treatment, relapses, or the terminal phase. Assessment of quality of life could seem, therefore, superfluous in such a situation where, in addition to chemotherapy, the main concern consists in supportive care. Various medical methods, e.g., central venous access (21), appear to be the easiest way to improve the quality of life during the intensive care period.

However, assessment of psychosocial parameters involved in quality of life should be considered a goal of paramount importance, even during the acute phases. In acute leukemia, as well as other cancers, most psychiatric syndromes consist in adjustment disorders (8), with anxiety and depression as central symptoms. These disorders are both detectable and amenable to treatment. Moreover, if one considers the immediate and permanent danger of death in acute leukemia at first presentation and during relapses, such adjustment disorders are expected to be frequent, and their study should be looked on as a priority. Information delivered to the patient is a basic component of coping strategies but cannot be viewed as a simple communication and educational process (32). Rather, it involves the development of close relations between the patient and the caregivers, who must be aware of possible defense mechanisms to be preserved.

The tentative description of quality of life provided in this chapter from the viewpoint of the oncologist, along with descriptions of disease course and treatment, could help to define properly designed psychosocial studies in such specific situations.

Time is a major parametric component of acute leukemia. Cycles of chemotherapy for consecutive induction and consolidation treatments lead to cyclic deterioration and improvement of the quality of life, which can be grossly assessed by scoring physical side effects and by computing the number of days spent in the hospital, total hospital costs, or both (22,29,30).

The first complete remission, the duration of which averages 1 year, can be followed by consecutive relapses and remissions, resulting in a broken line model of the whole course (26), with adjustment problems for remissions as well as for relapses. Therefore such a model advocates prospective psychosocial studies, with data collected several times at different phases of the illness or treatment. Another possibility is to focus the assessment of quality of life at the two possible endpoints of the disease. In terminally ill patients only the hematological unit is able to provide the palliative care and to accompany such dying patients, taking into account the need for specialized treatment up to the end. On the other hand, in long-term remitters with a high chance of cure, assessment of quality of life should be considered a major concern when comparing various treatment modalities, such as intensive consolidation chemotherapy versus bone marrow transplantation. Such comparisons are made currently and can contribute to the decision-making process. However, they are actually limited to the assessment of somatic side effects, e.g., graft-versus-host disease and sterility after bone marrow transplantation, performance status, and economic costs (1,2).

Finally, the systemic nature of acute leukemia gives specific characteristics to this disease, which can be compared only to some other cancers with widespread metastasis, high degree of chemosensitivity, but high risk of relapse such as small-cell bronchial carcinoma and nonseminomatous testicular cancer (27). Accordingly, the methodology of psychosocial research in oncology must be adapted not only to cancer in general but also to the specificity of such situations.

REFERENCES

1. Appelbaum, F. R., Dahlberg, S., Thomas, E. D., et al. (1984): Bone marrow transplantation or chemotherapy after remission induction for adults with acute nonlymphoblastic leukemia: A prospective comparison. *Ann. Intern. Med.*, 101:581–588.
2. Armitage, J. O., Ray, T. L., Klassen, L. W., et al. (1984): A comparison of bone marrow transplantation with maintenance chemotherapy for patients with acute nonlymphoblastic leukemia in first complete remission. *Am. J. Clin. Oncol.*, 7:273–278.
3. Burge, P. S., Richards, J. D. M., Thompson, D. S., Prankerd, T. A. J., Sare, M., and Wright, P. (1975): Quality and quantity of survival in acute myeloid leukaemia. *Lancet*, 2:621–624.
4. Castaigne, S., Daniel, M. T., Tilly, H., Herait, P., and Degos, L. (1983): Does treatment with ara-C low dosage cause differentiation of leukemic cells? *Blood*, 62:85–86.
5. Champlin, R., Jacobs, A., Gale, R. P., et al. (1984): Prolonged survival in acute myelogenous leukaemia without maintenance chemotherapy. *Lancet*, 1:894–896.
6. Curtis, J. E., Till, J. E., Messner, H. A., Sousan, P., and McCulloch, E. A. (1979): Comparison of outcomes and prognostic factors for two groups of patients with acute myeloblastic leukemia. *Leuk. Res.*, 3:409–416.
7. Deeg, H. J., Storb, R., and Thomas, E. D. (1984): Bone marrow transplantation: A review of delayed complications. *Br. J. Haematol.*, 57:185–208.
8. Derogatis, L. R., Morrow, G. R., Fetting, J., et al. (1983): The prevalence of psychiatric disorders among cancer patients. *JAMA*, 249:751–757.
9. Foon, K. A., and Gale, R. P. (1982): Controversies in the therapy of acute myelogenous leukemia. *Am. J. Med.*, 72:963–979.
10. Gale, R. P. (1979): Advances in the treatment of acute myelogenous leukemia. *N. Engl. J. Med.*, 300:1189–1199.
11. Gill, W. M. (1984): Measuring a patient's quality of life. *N. Z. Med. J.*, 97:329–330.
12. Gould, H., and Toghill, P. J. (1981): How should we talk about acute leukemia to adult patients and their families? *Br. Med. J.*, 282:210–212.
13. Holland, J. M., Plumb, J., Yates, S., et al. (1977): Psychological response of patients with acute leukemia to germ-free environments. *Cancer*, 40:871–879.
14. Kahn, S. B., Begg, C. B., Mazza, J. J., Bennett, J. M., Bonner, H., and Glick, J. H. (1984): Full dose versus attenuated dose daunorubicin, cytosine arabinoside, and 6-thioguanine in the treatment of acute nonlymphocytic leukemia in the elderly. *J. Clin. Oncol.*, 2:865–870.
15. Kansal, V., Omura, G. A., and Soong, S. J. (1976): Prognosis in adult acute myelogenous leukemia related to performance status and other factors. *Cancer*, 38:329–334.
16. Keating, M. J., Smith, T. L., Gehan, E. A., et al. (1980): Factors related to length of complete remission in adult acute leukemia. *Cancer*, 45:2017–2029.
17. Kersey, J. H., Ramsay, N. K., and Kim, T. (1982): Allogeneic bone marrow transplantation in acute nonlymphocytic leukemia: A pilot study. *Blood*, 60:400–403.
18. Kubler-Ross, E. (1969): *On Death and Dying*. Macmillan, New York.

19. Kupst, M. J., Schulman, J. L., Maurer, H., Honig, G., Morgan, E., and Fochtman, D. (1984): Coping with pediatric leukemia: A two year follow up. *J. Pediatr. Psychol.*, 9:149–163.
20. Maguire, G. P. (1983): The psychological sequelae of childhood leukaemia. *Recent Results Cancer Res.*, 88:47–56.
21. Newman, K. A., Schnaper, N., Reed, W. P., De Jongh, C. A., and Schimpff, S. C. (1984): Effect of Hickman catheters on the self-esteem of patients with leukemia. *South. Med. J.*, 77:682–685.
22. Peterson, B. A., Bloomfield, C. D., Bosl, G. J., Gibbs, G., and Molloy, M. (1980): Intensive five-drug combination chemotherapy for adult acute non-lymphocytic leukemia. *Cancer*, 46:663–668.
23. Raimbault, E., and Cludy, L. (1983): A psychotherapeutic approach of patients (and family) treated for acute leukemia in germ-free environment by bone-marrow transplantation and long term stay in isolator. EORTC Study Group on Quality of Life, Birmingham pp. 207–214.
24. Rowland, J. H., Glidewell, O. J., Sibley, R. F., et al. (1984): Effects of different forms of central nervous system prophylaxis on neuropsychic function in childhood leukemia. *J. Clin. Oncol.*, 2:1327–1335.
25. Scott, D. W., Goode, W. L., and Arlin, Z. A. (1983): The psychodynamics of multiple remissions in a patient with acute nonlymphoblastic leukemia. *Cancer Nurs.*, 6:204–206.
26. Spinetta, J. J. (1984): Measurement of family function, communication, and cultural effects. *Cancer*, 53(Suppl.):2330–2337.
27. Taylor, H. G., Brown, A. W., Jr., Butler, W. M., et al. (1981): Treatment experience with nonseminomatous testicular cancer in patients with stage II and stage III disease. *Cancer*, 48:110–115.
28. Thomas, E. D., Buckner, C. D., Clift, R. A., et al. (1979): Marrow transplantation for acute nonlymphoblastic leukemia in first remission. *N. Engl. J. Med.*, 301:597–599.
29. Vaughan, W. P., Karp, J. E., and Burke, P. J. (1980): Long chemotherapy-free remissions after single-cycle timed-sequential chemotherapy for acute myelocytic leukemia. *Cancer*, 45:859–865.
30. Vogel, L. L., Thorup, O. A., Kaiser, D. L., Zirkle, J. W., Harlan, J. F., and Hess, H. E. (1984): Acute leukemia in adults: Cost effectiveness of treatment. *South. Med. J.*, 77:51–55.
31. Weinstein, H. J., Mayer, R. J., Rosenthal, D. S., Coral, F. S., Camitta, B. M., and Gelber, R. D. (1983): Chemotherapy for acute myelogenous leukemia in children and adults: VAPA update. *Blood*, 62:315–319.
32. Zittoun, R. (1982): L'information des malades en hématologie. *Bordeaux Med.*, 15:51–57.

The Quality of Life of Cancer Patients,
edited by N. K. Aaronson and J. Beckmann,
Raven Press, New York © 1987.

Evaluation of Quality of Life in Women with Breast Cancer

Terrence J. Priestman

Queen Elizabeth Hospital, Birmingham B15 2TH, England

Having been ignored for many years, a great deal of attention has recently been devoted to the concept of quality of life in cancer patients. Between 1956 and 1976 less than 5% of publications reporting the results of clinical trials in cancer made any reference to the impact of toxicity on the patients' quality of life (1). Since that time, an increasing awareness of the limitations of cytotoxic chemotherapy has led to a greater emphasis on the assessment of the cost/benefit ratios of treatment, particularly with respect to subjective toxicity, and during the period 1978 to 1980 more than 200 papers on quality of life were published (3). There is no doubt that concern over quality of life is currently fashionable, but there is a danger that imprecise definitions and the absence of widely accepted methods of measurement are likely to prejudice clinical oncologists against the concept as they are confronted by increasingly complex, time-consuming, and unproved techniques for measuring their patients' subjective status, which many clinicians believe they can easily assess purely on the basis of personal judgment and experience.

It can be argued, however, that for breast cancer a number of studies related to quality of life have already provided results that have both increased understanding of the problems patients might encounter and influenced the medical management of the disease. The purpose of this chapter is to summarize a number of these findings and to briefly review the methods used.

SOME METHODS OF MEASUREMENT

A broad spectrum of techniques have been employed, ranging from questionnaires designed to give a global assessment of the patients' quality of life to methods intended to quantify a single subjective symptom or side effect that might influence well-being. One of the earliest attempts at subjective evaluation was the Karnofsky index (6). This 10-point rating scale, shown in Table 1, has been widely used for the last 30 years but has been criticized on the one hand for being a purely physical assessment made by an observer rather than the patient and on the other

TABLE 1. *Karnofsky scale*

Criterion	Score
Normal	100
Minor signs or symptoms	90
Normal activity with effort	80
Unable to continue normal activity but cares for self	70
Requires occasional assistance with personal needs	60
Disabled	50
Requires considerable assistance and medical care	40
Severely disabled and in hospital	30
Very sick: active support treatment necessary	20
Moribund	10
Dead	0

hand for being too complex, with simplified 4- or 5-point scales, such as the ECOG and WHO gradings, finding favor with many investigators. Reservations about the simplistic and physically oriented basis of these indices have resulted in the emergence of the more complex and sophisticated techniques outlined below. It is worth noting, however, that two studies have suggested that the Karnofsky scale is a reliable and valid measure in this situation, provided it is applied in a uniform and careful fashion (20,21).

More complex methods of assessment fall into two main groups: structured interviews and self-rating scales. Structured interviews use recognized psychological instruments such as the Present State Examination and the Standardized Social Interview Schedule to gain an insight into the subjective feelings of the patient. These methods, although of proved reliability, are time-consuming, require specially trained staff for their administration, and need expert analysis. They are thus not suitable for routine clinical use. Self-rating scales are generally simpler and more convenient, and a number of techniques have been devised, including visual and verbal scales (8).

Visual scales have been based on the technique of linear analogue self-assessment, where the patient is asked to mark on a 10-cm line how he feels in relation to the two extremes marked at either end of the line (Fig. 1). The scales can be used repeatedly to measure a patient's progress or deterioration, and questionnaires with as many as 25 parameters have been used to assess the results of therapy in breast cancer (2). Major disadvantages of this approach are the absence of a recog-

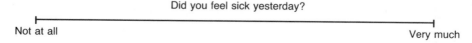

Did you feel sick yesterday?

Not at all   Very much

FIG. 1. Example of a linear analogue scale for self-assessment of subjective symptoms.

nized weighting for the variables that might be assessed and the fact that when patients are being compared sequentially equal changes in score with different patients may not signify equal degrees of improvement or deterioration. Verbal rating scales, although considered less flexible, overcome the latter difficulty to some extent by giving the patient a series of fixed options (usually four to seven) to choose from in response to a given question (Fig. 2). Once again a wide range of parameters may be explored, and the questionnaire may be repeated to obtain a dynamic view of patient response. A modification of the verbal rating scale is the diary card, on which a patient completes a daily questionnaire indicating the frequency and severity of certain specified symptoms or side effects. Global questions on overall well-being are also sometimes included (Fig. 3). A major problem with this technique is patient compliance. Very careful monitoring is necessary to ensure regular, and hence accurate, completion of the diary. As yet, none of these instruments has been sufficiently tested and refined to become a widely accepted measure, and work is still in progress comparing the various techniques. Nevertheless, some clinically relevant information has already been obtained with these as yet imperfect systems.

RESULTS IN BREAST CANCER

Although clinical observation, anecdotal reports, and uncontrolled series have for many years indicated significant psychological morbidity in patients undergoing mastectomy (13), it was not until the late 1970s that two controlled studies documented the scale of the problem; these studies used semistructured interviews and psychiatric rating scales to compare women undergoing mastectomy for cancer with those having surgery for benign breast disease. Levels of anxiety and depression were significantly higher in the mastectomy group, with 20% of patients suffering moderate or severe depression for 8 months or longer in Maguire et al.'s series (9) and 22% being depressed at 2 years after mastectomy in Morris et al.'s study (14). These two independent studies, with their careful methodology and similar findings, provided clear evidence of an extensive psychiatric morbidity, the extent and severity of which had almost certainly been previously unsuspected.

A logical progression from these initial findings was an assessment of whether expert counseling before and after mastectomy might serve to reduce the problems encountered. Maguire et al. reported the results of a controlled study in which

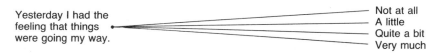

FIG. 2. Typical question from a verbal rating scale where the patient is asked to select the most appropriate response from a number of defined options.

Date . . . .

1. Did you have radiotherapy today?

   YES ☐   NO ☐

2. If YES, at about what time?

   . . . . .'a.m. OR . . . . p.m.

3. How severe has your nausea (sick feeling) been today?

   ☐ None

   ☐ Mild-did not interfere with normal daily life.

   ☐ Moderate-interfered with normal daily life.

   ☐ Severe-bedridden *due to nausea*.

4. How many times have you vomited (been sick) today.

   ☐ None

   ☐ 1 – 2 times

   ☐ 3 – 6 times

   ☐ More than 6 times.

5. How much have you eaten today?

   ☐ More than usual.

   ☐ Average amount for me.

   ☐ Less than usual.

   ☐ None at all.

6. Did you take any anti-sickness capsules today?

   YES ☐   NO ☐

7. If YES please record how many times on the chart below

Time	Number of white tablets (metoclopramide)	Number of white capsules (Nabilone)
Morning		
Afternoon		
Evening/Night		

8. Have the anti-sickness capsules upset you in anyway? Have you noticed any unusual effects? Explain below.

. . . .

. . . .

. . . .

. . . .

FIG. 3. Treatment diary card. This particular card was used in a study assessing two antiemetics in the control of radiation-induced nausea (17).

75 patients undergoing mastectomy who received counseling from a specialist nurse were compared with 77 women who received routine surgical care (11). Counseling failed to prevent psychiatric morbidity but did lead to early recognition of problems, with 76% of those who needed psychiatric help being recognized and referred for treatment by the nurse-counselor compared to only 15% in the control group. This referral resulted in significantly less psychiatric morbidity in the counseling group 12 months after mastectomy (12%) than in the control group (39%). A subsequent report confirmed that use of the nurse-counselor was not only of value in reducing the duration of psychiatric problems but was also cost-effective in terms of treatment saved by early diagnosis and referral (10).

Another obvious area for subjective evaluation in early breast cancer has been the impact of adjuvant cytotoxic therapy following mastectomy. In 1980 two reports appeared on this subject: One used self-rating questionnaires to compare low toxicity single agent adjuvant therapy with an aggressive cytotoxic regimen (15); the other employed Present State Examination interviews to compare women receiving CMF, melphalan, or no chemotherapy after mastectomy (12). In both studies the greater objective toxicity of the multidrug regimens was shown to adversely affect the patients' quality of life, and in Maguire et al.'s series (12) women receiving CMF had a significantly higher incidence of anxiety and depression, of sufficient severity to merit treatment, than those in the other two groups.

Although it is well documented that radiotherapy is frequently associated with anxiety and depression (4), little work has been done on assessing the effect of irradiation after either lumpectomy or mastectomy on the quality of life of breast cancer patients. One report did mention the use of linear analogue rating scales to compare the physical and psychiatric morbidity of two schedules for postmastectomy irradiation and indicated that daily fractionation appeared to be better tolerated than larger doses given two or three times each week (19), but the numbers involved were small.

Turning to recurrent or metastatic breast cancer, Priestman and Baum (16) reported on the use of visual analogue self-rating scales to assess response to systemic therapy and, having demonstrated the reliability and validity of the method, used a 25-point scale to monitor patients in a prospective trial comparing endocrine and cytotoxic therapy. The scale included 10 aspects related to symptoms of disease and side effects of treatment, five relating to psychological problems (e.g., anxiety and depression), five relating to physical state, and five covering personal relationships. Subsequent analysis (2) showed that patients receiving cytotoxic therapy experienced a far greater incidence of treatment-related side effects than those on hormonal treatment but, overall, scored significantly better for general well-being. It was thought that this apparent paradox was explained by the difference in objective response between the two groups—49% compared to 21% ($p < 0.02$) (18)—and that the toxicity of treatment experienced by the cytotoxic-treated patients was more than offset by the symptomatic relief they experienced as a result of objective tumor shrinkage. This view was reinforced by an analysis of the cytotoxic-treated patients comparing responders with nonresponders, where it was clear that if response was not apparent within 6 to 8 weeks of commencing therapy side effects rapidly became intolerable. It was concluded, therefore, that if tumor regression was seen even quite severe side effects, e.g., persistent vomiting and total alopecia, were well tolerated, but that if no response was apparent toxicity soon became unbearable.

Quality of life measures may also be used to assess new agents for advanced breast cancer. The initial version of an EORTC verbal self-rating scale (7) has been used as part of a phase II study evaluating high dose medroxyprogesterone acetate (MPA) therapy in advanced breast cancer. One reason for being particularly anxious to monitor the subjective response in this series was that previous reports had suggested that the increase in appetite, pain relief, and improved performance status, resulting in an improved quality of life, were sometimes seen in the absence of objective tumor shrinkage.

EORTC QUESTIONNAIRE

The EORTC questionnaire comprised some 35 questions: 12 related purely to physical performance, with simple yes or no responses; 10 related to mood (phrased positively, e.g., ''Yesterday I had the feeling things were going my way'') with the patient asked to answer from one of seven options ranging from ''very much so" to "not at all"; 11 questions again related to mood but phrased negatively (e.g., "Yesterday I felt depressed"), with the patient choosing from six answers; and finally two global questions relating to overall well-being with six and seven answers for reply, respectively.

Scores for subjective assessment were available for five patients who had an objective response and 12 with progressive disease. A repeated-measures analysis of variance for the responders and nonresponders who had completed data over the first 8 weeks of treatment showed that the mean difference in score between the two groups was statistically significant ($p = 0.05$). There were, however, marked fluctuations in scores for individuals, which suggested that the EORTC method may be an accurate measure of day-to-day quality of life. This does not, however, necessarily reflect the results of treatment alone but could be influenced by many other factors. Certainly there was no evidence from our survey to support the view that MPA has a euphoriant effect in those who fail to achieve an objective remission. Equally, however, there was no evidence that high MPA levels decreased the quality of life (5).

DISCUSSION

As yet, there is no universally accepted method for measuring quality of life in cancer patients. A number of approaches have been proposed, and some of these have been tested in clinical studies. The tasks of validating the various techniques, establishing acceptable methods of analysis, and comparing approaches in formal trials are at an early stage. Despite these limitations, it seems reasonable to suggest, on the basis of the results summarized in this chapter that, with breast cancer in particular, the close attention paid to the impact of the disease and its management has significantly influenced therapy policies. The clear delineation of the extent and severity of psychiatric morbidity associated with mastectomy has been one of a number of factors that have directed surgeons, whenever possible, toward lumpectomy and irradiation rather than more mutilating procedures. Similarly, the evidence of greatly increased levels of anxiety, depression, and other subjective problems associated with adjuvant cytotoxic therapy has been a major stimulus to oncologists, at least in Great Britain, to reconsider the place of such treatment and in many instances to abandon adjuvant therapy or to use less toxic endocrine approaches.

From studies in advanced disease it seems clear that objective regression of tumor is a major factor in improving the patient's quality of life and that if remission can be achieved even quite severe treatment-related toxicity is well tolerated. Conversely, to persist with unsuccessful therapy, especially if it gives rise to significant side effects, makes life intolerable for the patient.

Although there is no definitive measure for quality of life, the studies carried out so far in breast cancer have provided valuable information on the impact of treatment on the individual and allowed formal comparisons of the subjective benefits and side effects of various therapies. We now have accurate and sensitive instruments for evaluating subjective toxicity and, in a number of systems, a basis for relating such toxicity to the more global concept of quality of life. Although further refinement of the methodology is needed, it seems reasonable to suggest that some attempt to assess subjective toxicity should be now included in all evaluations of new agents and in all formal comparisons of therapeutic approaches to breast cancer.

REFERENCES

1. Bardelli, D., and Saracci, P. (1978): Measuring quality of life in cancer trials: A sample survey of published trials. *UICC Techn. Rep.*, 36:75–94.
2. Baum, M., Priestman, T. J., West, R. R., and Jones, E. M. (1980): A comparison of subjective responses in a trial comparing endocrine with cytotoxic treatment in advanced carcinoma of the breast. In: *Breast Cancer—Experimental and Clinical Aspects,* edited by H. T. Mouridsen and T. Palshof, pp. 223–226. Pergamon, Oxford.
3. Fayers, P. M., and Jones, D. R. (1983): Measuring quality of life in cancer clinical trials: A review. *Stat. Med.,* 2:429–446.
4. Forester, B. M., Kornfeld, D. S., and Fleiss, J. (1978): Psychiatric aspects of radiotherapy. *Am. J. Psychiatry,* 135:960–963.
5. Johnson, J. R., Priestman, T. J., Fotherby, K., Kelly, K. A., and Priestman, S. G. (1984): An evaluation of high-dose medroxyprogesterone acetate therapy in women with advanced breast cancer. *Br. J. Cancer (in press).*
6. Karnofsky, D. A., and Burchenal, J. H. (1949): The clinical evaluation of chemotherapeutic agents in cancer. In: *Evaluation of Chemotherapeutic Agents,* edited by C. M. MacLeod, pp. 199–205. Columbia University Press, New York.
7. Linssen, A. C. G., Hanewald, H., van Dam, F., and van Beek-Couzijn, A. L. (1981): The development of the complaint questionnaire at The Netherlands Cancer Institute. In: *Proceedings of the 3rd EORTC Quality of Life Workshop,* pp. 82–110.
8. Maguire, G. P. (1980): Monitoring the quality of life in cancer patients and their relatives. In: *Cancer—Assessment and Monitoring,* edited by T. Symington, A. E. Williams, and J. G. McVie, pp. 40–52. Churchill Livingstone, Edinburgh.
9. Maguire, G. P., Lee, E. G., Bevington, D. J., Kuchemann, C. S., Crabtree, P. J., and Cornell, C. E. (1978): Psychiatric problems in the first year after mastectomy. *Br. Med. J.,* 1:963–965.
10. Maguire, G. P., Pentol, A., Allen, D., Tait, A., Brooke, M., and Sellwood, P. (1982): Cost of counselling women who undergo mastectomy. *Br. Med. J.,* 284:1933–1935.
11. Maguire, G. P., Tait, A., Brooke, M., Thomas, C., and Sellwood, R. (1980): Effects of counselling on the psychiatric morbidity associated with mastectomy. *Br. Med. J.,* 281:1454–1456.
12. Maguire, G. P., Tait, A., Brooke, M., Thomas, C., Howat, J. M., Sellwood, R. A., and Bush, H. (1980): Psychiatric morbidity and physical toxicity associated with adjuvant chemotherapy after mastectomy. *Br. Med. J.,* 281:1179–1180.
13. Morris, T. (1979): Psychological adjustment to mastectomy. *Cancer Treat. Rev.,* 6:41–62.
14. Morris, T., Greer, H. S., and White, P. (1977): Psychological and social adjustment to mastectomy: A two year follow-up study. *Cancer,* 40:2381–2387.
15. Palmer, B. V., Walsh, G. A., McKinna, J. A., and Greening, W. P. (1980): Adjuvant chemotherapy for breast cancer: Side-effects and quality of life. *Br. Med. J.,* 281:1594–1597.
16. Priestman, T. J., and Baum, M. (1976): Evaluation of quality of life in patients receiving treatment for advanced breast cancer. *Lancet,* 1:899–901.
17. Priestman, T. J., and Priestman, S. G. (1984): An initial evaluation of nabilone in the control of radiotherapy induced nausea and vomiting. *Clin. Radiol. (in press).*
18. Priestman, T. J., Baum, M., Jones, V., and Forbes, J. J. (1978): Treatment and survival in advanced breast cancer. *Br. Med. J.,* 2:1673–1674.

19. Priestman, T. J., Baum, M., and Priestman, S. G. (1982): Die Lebensqualitat bei Brustkrebspatientin-nen. In: *Die Erkrankungen der Weiblichen Brustdruse,* edited by H. von H-J. Frischbier, pp. 248–251. Georg Thieme Verlag, Stuttgart.
20. Schag, C. C., Heinrich, R. L., and Ganz, P. A. (1984): Karnofsky Performance Status revisited: Reliability, validity and guidelines. *J. Clin. Oncol.,* 2:187–193.
21. Yates, J. W., Chalmers, B., and McKegney, F. P. (1980): Evaluation of patients with advanced cancer using the Karnofsky Performance Status. *Cancer,* 45:2220–2224.

The Quality of Life of Cancer Patients,
edited by N. K. Aaronson and J. Beckmann,
Raven Press, New York © 1987.

Silent Sadness of the "Cured" Breast Cancer Patient

Tina Morris

Faith Courtauld Unit, The Rayne Institute, London SE59NU, England

When she found she had cancer, Alice Trillin wrote (29):

> I felt immediately I had entered a special place, a place I came to call "The Land of the Sick People." The most disconcerting thing . . . was not that I found that place so terrifying but that I found it so ordinary . . . what had changed was *other people's* perception of me . . . everyone regarded me as someone who had been altered irrevocably.

The writer did not have breast cancer. Had she had breast cancer, she might have felt even more altered in the eyes of others. A fascinating study (21) of the perceptions of patients and nonpatients, men and women, about breast cancer found that whereas 59% of healthy men and 26% of healthy women think breast cancer is "the worst thing that can happen to a woman," only 6% of *patients* thought this. Thus even the patient with an excellent prognosis has a "guilty secret," for it is difficult to share the information that something *so terrible* in the eyes of the nonsufferer has happened to her.

This chapter has an emotive title because the feeling is an unseen, and largely unheard, sadness. Cancer is a taboo subject, and in the case of breast cancer the affliction is not visible to the outside world. Its psychological consequences are scarcely visible in psychiatric terms, although it is not because they do not exist.

This chapter covers (a) studies of the psychological morbidity of breast cancer; (b) studies of the characteristics of those who have difficulty adjusting to breast cancer; (c) studies of breast conservation; and (d) studies of ways to help breast cancer patients come to terms with, if not to adjust to, their illness.

WHAT PROPORTION OF PATIENTS CANNOT COME TO TERMS WITH MASTECTOMY?

There have been six studies (12,14,15,20,25,32) of mood disturbance and sexual problems following mastectomy, all involving relatively small numbers of patients. Their findings have been similar and suggest that 12 to 18 months after mastectomy

15 to 25% of patients have mood disturbance severe enough to warrant psychiatric intervention, and that about 30% of patients may have sexual difficulties. The study by Silberfarb et al. (25) found that sexual difficulties largely correlated with physical morbidity. A study (20) carried out in the Faith Courtauld Unit, using patients with benign breast disease as controls, found that sexual adjustment in patients with benign disease also deteriorated during the 2-year period of follow-up. Had controls been omitted from this study, we might erroneously have concluded that the deterioration in sexual relations in breast cancer patients was a consequence of breast cancer diagnosis.

In recent writings on coping with stress there has been serious criticism of the widely held belief in the "stage" model of adjustment to severe stress (26), i.e., the model proposed by Kubler-Ross (13) of a sequence of mood changes experienced by the individual as he or she reaches a "resolution" following a traumatic event. Silver and Wortman (26) found little experimental evidence to support such a cycle, and a great deal of evidence from studies of various traumatic events suggests that a large minority of victims have not "adjusted" even 5 to 6 years later.

WHAT ARE THE CHARACTERISTICS OF THOSE WHO HAVE DIFFICULTY ADJUSTING?

Studies of characteristics of those who find it difficult to adjust have been consistent in their findings. Several factors are associated with subsequent difficulties in adjustment: (a) a history of psychiatric treatment (31); (b) evidence of depression at the time of primary treatment (20,24,31); (c) general emotional lability (12,20,24); (d) anticipated or actual lack of support (2,5,10,31); and (d) lack of employment (2,5). Evidence of the value of these factors in predicting a sample of patients or subjects who will have difficulty adjusting is not confined to breast cancer but has been found in a wide variety of other stressful experiences, suggesting that subjects with these characteristics have difficulty adjusting to stress whatever its nature (3,4).

IS THERE EVIDENCE THAT SOME PATIENTS CANNOT ADJUST TO BREAST LOSS?

During the 1950s and 1960s, a series of illuminating reports on cancer patients were written by the psychologist Arthur Sutherland at the Memorial–Sloan Kettering Cancer Hospital in New York. Most were based on clinical observations, but all contained penetrating insights into the problems faced by cancer patients which have not been superseded by more sophisticated methods on the subject of breast loss. Sutherland wrote: "Mastectomy is an intolerable insult to women whose self-esteem and expectation of esteem from others is predicated to a large extent on their beauty and shapeliness" (27).

Three small studies (6,7,23) of the independent effect of breast loss in adjustment to breast cancer suggested that there are four factors particularly associated with an inability to accept the loss of the breast: (a) depression before surgery; (b) clearly and strongly expressed dread of mastectomy, e.g., "I'd rather be dead than lose my breast"; (c) poor sexual relationship; and (d) looking for a new partner. It is clear from this list that there is some interaction between the general background factors outlined earlier as predicting poor adjustment to the diagnosis of breast cancer and these more specific factors that influence adjustment to loss of the breast. For example, a history of depression, poor social relationships, a feeling of lack of support, *and either* the particular value the woman attaches to her breast *or* fears about the problem she will have adjusting in a new relationship where the woman's body has been part of the currency for beginning that relationship will be most likely to ensure a most difficult postoperative course for a woman "encouraged" to "go through with" mastectomy. In support of this probability, Dean et al.'s study (6) of immediate and delayed reconstruction found that women with poor marriages were both more likely to opt for and to benefit from breast reconstruction.

WOULD BREAST CONSERVATION SOLVE THE PROBLEM OF ADJUSTMENT TO BREAST CANCER?

There has so far been no controlled study of the psychological benefits and disadvantages of breast conservation. When women are routinely offered radiotherapy as a primary treatment, however, almost 100% prefer it (28).

In the Faith Courtauld Unit in London, we have interviewed 102 breast cancer patients as part of a larger study of psychological responses to cancer (18). All have early breast cancer ($T_{0,1,2}, N_{0,1}, M_0$) and have been treated by lumpectomy and radiotherapy, or simple or Halsted radical mastectomy with or without radiotherapy. Although data are currently available for only 3 months of follow-up (Table 1), scores on the Wakefield Depression Inventory, a self-rating scale of anxiety and depression used widely in the assessment of hospital patients, do not show any significant differences in the mean scores of the three main patient groups.

TABLE 1. *Wakefield Depression Inventory: comparison of means in breast cancer patients without and after radiotherapy*

Condition	No radiotherapy	Radiotherapy
All patients	9.24 (n = 38)	9.00 (n = 64)
Lumpectomy	7.60 (n = 5)	9.30 (n = 33)
Simple mastectomy	9.00 (n = 7)	8.48 (n = 29)
Halsted radical	9.37 (n = 27)	11.50 (n = 2)

This is not to suggest that differences may not emerge after a year or two of follow-up.

What the results do suggest, as so many writers have claimed, is that breast cancer is a severe stress, and that the operation itself is only one of a number of aspects of it to which the patient must adjust. There is a tendency to assume that cancer as a stress is *unique*. It is not. What is unique about breast cancer is *attitudes* to it. It is therefore naive to assume that less extensive surgery will eliminate the problem of adjustment for the "cured" patient because she has no visible sign of her disease. She still must live with continuing uncertainty about her prognosis (9).

This problem of the attitudes of others—the notion that for many healthy people, particularly men, breast cancer is "the worst thing that can happen to a woman"—may lead women to underreport the emotional distress they feel. We have a great deal of evidence (16,17,19,30) to that effect from studies carried out in our own Unit. Our latest study (18) demonstrated that, although there is a certain amount of psychiatric morbidity that is likely to result directly from a diagnosis of breast cancer and primary treatment, the scores of breast cancer patients on the Wakefield Depression Inventory are much closer to those of normal subjects than they are to those of psychiatric patients (Table 2). The symptoms on which the distressed breast cancer patient typically scores are not those that are likely to draw attention to her plight or to interfere with her "public" functioning—early morning waking, some weeping alone, lack of confidence, some loss of interest—and not enough usually to be labeled psychiatric illness. This mild morbidity may reflect underreporting for fear of being labeled "mad" as well as "bad." The psychiatric service is thus unlikely to be the most appropriate one to offer the well but psychologically distressed patient help. The service is unaccustomed to dealing with morbidity at this level.

WHICH PATIENTS NEED HELP? WHAT HELP IS LIKELY TO BE EFFECTIVE?

All patients need help around the time of surgery. They need psychological as well as medical assessment so that they can be given the primary treatment that

TABLE 2. Wakefield Depression Inventory: distribution of scores of breast cancer and psychiatric patients and normal controls

Subjects	Percent of patients by score of 0 to 30+			
	0–14 (normal)	15–21 (mild)	22–30 (moderate)	30+ (severe)
Breast cancer patients	83	11	5	1
Normal controls	93	4	3	0
Psychiatric patients	3	28	58	11

best suits their medical and psychological needs; they need information about their disease and its treatment; and they need help with practical aspects of rehabilitation, prostheses, and clothing. This statement seems axiomatic, but it is likely that only a few women in Europe and the United States receive a service of this type.

Unfortunately, those setting up services for breast cancer patients have often failed to distinguish between these *general* needs, which all new patients have, and the need to help patients who have recovered from their primary treatment and its aftermath but continue to be psychologically distressed. General needs are probably well served by the short-term rehabilitation/information group with nurse-counselors, social workers, physiotherapists, and patient volunteers along the lines of that run at Memorial–Sloan Kettering (8,22) or by nurse-counselors (11) or patient self-help groups (1).

Once physical recovery from breast surgery is complete, breast cancer patients may have little in common except their inability to adjust to stress. Groups and counselors specifically formed for such patients serve only to emphasize their common affliction, which is but a symbol of their general feeling of depression. Those who do not adjust, as we have seen, are emotionally vulnerable individuals for whom a cancer diagnosis is but one more difficulty. Even when there have been attempts to evaluate help for these mildly depressed patients, the components of the help offered have not been distinguished. Thus when an effect has been demonstrated, it is impossible to know whether it results from better information, early referral to other agencies, the use of drugs, or the counseling itself. Extensive research into levels of morbidity in breast cancer patients is unnecessary, as the facts are well established. There is, however, too little change in treatment delivery for most patients. Our overkill in research on morbidity and underemphasis on research into services to help patients may be related to three aspects of the situation with which we are dealing: (a) public fear of cancer; (b) our sense of helplessness, whether rational or irrational, when dealing with cancer; and (c) the fact that it is still mostly men who treat women with breast cancer.

We have seen that men's attitudes to the disease differ from those of women. It seems likely that men treating women, thinking the disease "the worst thing that can happen to a woman," either find the woman's distress too painful to deal with and ignore it or they overcompensate, perhaps with overanxious concern. Research needs now to move toward an examination of the attitudes of those persons who treat patients, toward establishing which forms of care are effective, and toward searching for ways to implement care programs, rather than continuing to search for the morbidity in the woman herself. Her burden can be much reduced by a change in *our* attitudes.

ACKNOWLEDGMENT

This work was supported by the Cancer Research Campaign.

REFERENCES

1. Adams, J. (1979): *Cancer Nurs.*, 2:95–98.
2. Bloom, J. R. (1982): *Soc. Sci. Med.*, 16:1329–1338.
3. Brown, G. W., and Harris, T. (1978): *Social Origins of Depression.* Tavistock, London.
4. Cobb, S. (1976): *Psychosom. Med.*, 38:300–309.
5. Cobliner, W. G. (1977): *Hosp. Physician*, 10:38–40.
6. Dean, C., Chetty, U., and Forrest, A. P. M. (1983): *Lancet*, 1:459–462.
7. Denton, S., and Baum, M. (1981): *Clin. Oncol.*, 8:375.
8. Euster, S. (1979): *Soc. Work Health Care*, 4:251–263.
9. Folkman, S., Schaefer, C., and Lazarus, R. (1979): In: *Human Stress and Cognition*, edited by V. Hamilton and A. M. Warburton, pp. 265–298. Wiley, Chichester.
10. Funch, D. P., and Mettlin, C. (1982): *Soc. Sci. Med.*, 16:91–98.
11. Gordon, W. A., Friedenbergs, I., Diller, L. et al. (1980): *J. Consult. Clin. Psychol.*, 48:743–759.
12. Hughes, J. J. (1982): *Psychosom. Res.*, 26:277–283.
13. Kubler-Ross, E. (1969): *On Death and Dying.* Macmillan, New York.
14. Maguire, G. P., Lee, E. G., Berington, D. J., et al. (1978): *Br. Med. J.*, 1:963–965.
15. Maguire, P., Tait, A., Brooke, M., et al. (1980): *Br. Med. J.*, 2:1454–1456.
16. Morris, T. (1980): *Cancer Detect. Prevent.*, 3:1.
17. Morris, T., and Greer, H. S. (1982): *Clin. Oncol.*, 8:113–119.
18. Morris, T., Blake, S., and Buckley, M. (1985): *Soc. Sci. Med.* 20:795–802.
19. Morris, T., Greer, S., Pettingale, K. W., and Watson, W. (1981): *J. Psychosom. Res.*, 25:111–117.
20. Morris, T., Greer, S., and White, P. (1977): *Cancer*, 40:2381–2387.
21. Peters-Golden, H. (1982): *Soc. Sci. Med.*, 16:483–491.
22. Sachs, S. H., David, J. M., Reynolds, S. A., et al. (1981): *Cancer*, 48:1251–1255.
23. Sanger, C. K., and Reznikoff, M. (1981): *Cancer*, 48:2341–2346.
24. Schonfield, J. J. (1972): *Psychosom. Res.*, 16:41–46.
25. Silberfarb, P. M., Maurer, C. H., and Crouthamel, C. S. (1980): *Am. J. Psychiatry*, 137:450–455.
26. Silver, R., and Wortman, C. B. (1980): In: *Human Helplessness, Theory and Applications*, edited by J. Garber and M. E. P. Seligman, pp. 279–375. Academic Press, New York.
27. Sutherland, A. M. (1967): *Int. Psychiatr. Clin.*, 4:75–92.
28. Tobias, J. S. (1980): *Cancer Topics*, 2:5–7.
29. Trillin, A. S. (1981): *N. Engl. J. Med.*, 304:699–701.
30. Watson, M., Pettingale, K., and Greer, S. In: *Psychological Aspects of Cancer, Advances in the Biosciences*, edited by M. Watson and T. Morris. Pergamon Press, Oxford (*in press*).
31. Weisman, A. D. (1976): *Am. J. Med. Sci.*, 271:187–196.
32. Worden, J. W., and Weisman, A. D. (1977): *Am. J. Med. Sci.*, 273:169–175.

Editors' note: The results of two randomized clinical trials comparing the psychosocial impact of mastectomy versus breast-conserving treatment have been published subsequent to the preparation of this chapter: J. C. J. M. de Haes and K. Welvaart (1985): Quality of life after breast cancer surgery. *J. Surg. Oncol.*, 28:123–125; W. Schein et al. (1983): Psychosocial and physical outcomes of primary breast cancer therapy: Mastectomy versus excisional biopsy and irradiation. *Breast Cancer Res. Treat.*, 3:377–382.

The Quality of Life of Cancer Patients,
edited by N. K. Aaronson and J. Beckmann,
Raven Press, New York © 1987.

Sexuality of Gynecologic Cancer Patients: Influence of Traditional Role Patterns

Gerjanne Bos

Department of Obstetrics and Gynecology, University Hospital,
2333 AA Leiden, The Netherlands

Almost 20% of all malignancies in women originate from the genital organs (11). Treatment can take the form of surgery, radiotherapy, chemotherapy, or combinations of these methods. For most gynecologic cancers, especially in stage I, the 5-year cure rate is over 80%. In stage II the rate is about 45% (30).

Gynecologic cancers are unique in that they have a direct impact on essential components of a woman's identity (15,16). In our society women are made to believe that their bodies, and in particular their genital organs, determine their female role (39). Thus their value as a woman and as a sexual partner is, to a great extent, determined by anatomic organs and functions (7,32). On an internalized level, many men and women believe that anything that affects female genital organs threatens part of a woman's femininity and sexual attractiveness.

EFFECTS OF TREATMENT

A report of the American National Cancer Institute (41) stated that the physical, psychological, and social loss that results from cancer treatment is a major determinant of a cancer patient's quality of life after treatment. The physical effects of surgical treatment may mean loss of the uterus, ovaries, fallopian tubes, upper portion of the vagina, bladder, rectum, clitoris, vulva, or vagina. It almost always causes functional losses (e.g., in the case of the first three organs, the disappearance of menstruation, loss of fertility, and hormonal disequilibrium). These changes in turn may influence sexual functioning, resulting in loss of sensory perceptions, loss of uterine contractions, and loss of lubrication and orgasm capacity, as well as dyspareunia, vaginal atrophy, and stenosis (3). It need hardly be said that, on the psychological level, mutilating operations are experienced as a serious assault on the body image and are therefore damaging to a woman's self-esteem (23,42). After gynecologic surgery many patients feel devalued as a woman, incomplete, no longer "whole," which may also have consequences for their sexuality.

207

EFFECTS OF CULTURE AND SOCIETY

Cultural and social influences may complicate the effects on the patient's psychological equilibrium and coping process, especially if the woman is influenced by myths and misconceptions. Cancer localization in the genital organs may have a certain connotation leading to feelings of shame (37). Women may find it difficult or indecent to mention these organs. A frequently heard remark, made especially by older patients, is: "I not only have cancer, but I have it in such an awful place!" From young or single patients it is known that they also feel ashamed about their scars and may avoid the "risk" of getting involved in intimate situations (6).

In *Illness as Metaphor,* Susan Sontag (40) pointed out that serious illness of any kind can elicit guilt in patients who interpret the disease as punishment for having done something wrong. It goes without saying that this situation may occur particularly in patients with genital cancer. Many patients feel guilty about real or imagined sexual "sins" or "transgressions" (17) such as masturbation, partner changes, contraceptive practices, and abortion. Although these guilt feelings are not realistic, ideas about sexuality, in young as well as older people, are amazingly conservative (26), and patients may try to cope by abstaining from sex. A special source of problems is the speculation frequently expressed in magazines about links between cervical cancer and promiscuity or poor hygiene of men. Partners may therefore accuse each other of being the cause of the disease (8). Furthermore, many patients fear that coitus will lead to recurrence because if coitus could cause the disease resumption would bring it back again. It is obvious that this misconception can also become a source of tension between the patient and her partner and thus can lead to fear of sex, loss of sexual desire, and sexual abstinence (2).

Cultural ideas also influence the way in which the medical and nonmedical staff advise patients and their partners about their future sex life. Reviewing the literature, it seems that priority is given to male-determined sexual preferences. Information and advice are mainly concerned with resumption of coitus and return to the frequency of intercourse as before the operation (10,12,38), with maintenance of a "normal" sexual life (27) or return to "normal" sexual functioning (20). Moreover, coitus is seen as a way to keep the vagina open in order to prevent atrophy and stenosis (43), even if intercourse is painful (36). In a large number of studies published in leading gynecologic and other journals treatment of sexual problems in gynecologic cancer patients is oriented almost exclusively toward the restoration of coitus (1,10,12,17,20,21,27,36,38,43). Other noncoital possibilities, which constitute female sexuality par excellence, might be more in accordance with the actual needs of these patients.

TRADITIONAL APPROACH

Although gynecologic cancer may have a severe impact on the quality of life of treated and cured patients, it is remarkable that so little research has been carried out in this area. The report of Newton (35) is an exception to this rule. Compared with female breast cancer, relatively little is known about the psychological consequences of gynecologic cancer. There is not a real lack of research interest, but the interest is largely traditionally determined, as the main concern is directed toward the sexual life and not toward the quality of life of gynecologic cancer patients. Worden and Weisman (44), however, remarked that overemphasis of sexual implications following cancer surgery may lead to underemphasis of more significant psychosocial concerns. Furthermore, this general overemphasis is focused mainly on quantitative aspects of sexuality, i.e., on the frequency of coitus and orgasms, thereby neglecting the qualitative aspects of the sexual and partner relationship. In a review of psychoanalytic writings on women, Baker Miller (5) commented that the greatest amount of material is on womens' sexuality instead of their psychology. This traditional approach is rather regrettable and may contribute to low self-esteem, especially in women with gynecologic cancer.

SEXUAL DYSFUNCTION

An accurate estimation of the seriousness of sexual dysfunction is important when studying female sexual problems. However, serious methodological difficulties are encountered as to operationalization and definition, and most investigators have different opinions about adequate and inadequate sexual functioning. It might be more realistic to assess sexual problems of women in terms of their sexual relationship. For example, women who are unable to achieve orgasm are not necessarily dissatisfied, whereas orgasmic women are not necessarily satisfied sexually (29). This means that orgasm alone is not a satisfactory criterion for assessing female sexuality.

In order to be able to describe sexual dysfunctions of gynecologic cancer patients, its incidence rates should first be described in the general population, in gynecologic patients, and in patients with breast cancer.

General Population

A social-sexologic study among 600 married individuals in The Netherlands performed by Frenken (19) indicated that 43% of the women lack enjoyment in their sexual interactions. Masters and Johnson (33) reported sexual problems in 50% of American marriages. Several studies on female orgasm behavior indicated that most women do not experience orgasm by coitus only: according to Fisher 80% (18), and according to Hite 70% (22). In both studies only 5% of the women were anorgasmic via masturbation. Can women bridge the gap between masturbatory orgasm and coital orgasm? De Bruijn (14) concluded that only one-third (35%) transfer their masturbation experience to a coital orgasm. Her data further indicated that only one of five women (20%) finds coital orgasm really important. According to the author's interpretation, many women are not primarily interested in orgasm during sex. For many of them orgasm is not their main source of sexual satisfaction—only one of them. Other sources are feelings of love, intimacy, sensuality and physical closeness, warmth, trust, and friendship. Kaplan (25), a sex therapist and psychoanalyst, stressed that a sexual encounter with orgasmic release is in fact not satisfying if other feelings are missing. From these data it is obvious that, for most women, coitus is one of the least effective techniques of reaching orgasm and a less preferred way of lovemaking.

Gynecologic Patients

Levine and Yost (29) investigated the presence of sexual problems in women attending a general gynecologic clinic for complaints not related to sex. Of these women, 34% were sexually dissatisfied. Dennerstein et al. (15) reported that, after hysterectomy for nonmalignant processes, 37% of the patients experienced deterioration in sexual relations.

Breast Cancer Patients

Two British groups investigated psychological and sexual functioning in breast cancer patients. Both studies used women with benign breast disease as control subjects. Morris et al. (34) reported that 2 years after treatment 32% of the breast cancer patients experienced sexual problems compared with 27% of the controls, and 22% developed psychological morbidity compared with only 8% of the controls. Maguire et al. (31) found that 1 year after mastectomy 33% of the patients had moderate to severe sexual problems compared with 8% of the controls, and 25% showed psychiatric morbidity compared with 10% of the controls. The incidence rates of sexual problems and psychological morbidity in both studies were nearly the same for the breast cancer patients, and there was also no difference between 1 or 2 years after mastectomy. However, it seems peculiar that in the Maguire study the frequency of sexual problems in the benign sample is much lower than in the general population.

Gynecologic Cancer Patients

Carenza et al. (13) investigated the prevalence of sexual problems in patients with cervical cancer. Of these patients, 60% were sexually active less than once a month or not at all. Many patients had little interest in sex but continued to have sexual activity in order to prove to themselves that they were the same as before or out of fear of losing their partner (also common in the general population).

A study of the American National Cancer Institute on the sexual behavior of patients with newly diagnosed gynecologic cancer at various sites (21) indicated that after the onset of symptoms and treatment 50% of these women are dissatisfied with their sex life. Coitus was avoided by 50% of them, and for an additional 30% the frequency had declined. The most often mentioned reasons for the reduction of coitus were bleeding or fear of bleeding, pain or fear of pain, and general anxiety. However, it was not mentioned in this study that cancer can also serve as an alibi to abstain from sex. Furthermore, patients were not asked if they had sexual activity other than intercourse.

Andersen and Hacker (3) excellently reviewed the literature on the psychosexual adjustment of gynecologic cancer patients. The incidence of diminished desire for coitus ranged from 20 to 33%. Interpretation of the results from various studies, however, was difficult owing to differences in research methodology. In their own study Andersen and Hacker (4) examined psychosexual adjustment following pelvic exenteration, an extremely mutilating operation. In this study, 80% of the patients reported having no sexual interest after treatment. All patients who underwent reconstructive surgery reported having been given inadequate information, leading to unrealistic ideas of what to expect from their neovagina. The authors commented that there seemed to be no basis to state before the operation: "Sexual intercourse will feel the same" or "You should be able to have intercourse just as you do now." Quite rightly, the authors further pointed out that sexual functioning should be assessed only as part of a general psychological evaluation. Feelings of anxiety and depression and changes in body image and self-esteem, which are often experienced by cancer patients, can significantly influence sexual behavior.

According to Bransfield et al.'s review of the literature (9), the reported incidence of sexual dysfunction differs greatly. It ranges between 12 and 73% for diminished sexual desire, between 19 and 90% for diminished frequency of sexual intercourse, and between 11 and 90% for diminished frequency of orgasm. As pointed out before, in most of these studies the frequency of vaginal intercourse and the frequency of orgasm have been used as major indices of sexual functioning.

INTIMACY

A study reflecting a more female-oriented view was conducted by Leiber et al. (28). They investigated the communication of affection between patients and their spouses. Male and female patients with various types of cancer were included in the study. The authors found a 60% decrease in sexual intercourse among female patients and a 27% decrease among male patients. On the other hand, they found an increase in physical closeness and intimacy among 60% of the female and among 40% of the male patients. They further remarked that physiological capacity did not seem to be a major factor in reduced sexual desire. It may be concluded that after a traumatic illness such as cancer there is a shift in the manner of expressing affectionate feelings. The observed decline in coitus frequency should by no means be interpreted as having a negative influence on the relationship; on the contrary, it may result in the development of a more conscious exploration of the partner relationship.

DISCUSSION

As early as 1937 Horney (24) commented that much of what seems to be sexuality has nothing to do with it in reality. The incidence of sexual problems is rather high in both women without cancer and those with gynecologic cancer. It is therefore not justified to attribute the sexual problems in women with gynecologic cancer mainly to this malignancy. After a gynecologic cancer experience, the development of a shift from coital to intimate behavior should be stimulated and seems to be possible. For that purpose, unconsummated possibilities in the patient should be explored. Sexuality of gynecologic cancer patients can be better understood by being aware of sexual preferences of women in general. These include a need for intimacy, physical closeness and stroking, trust, and warmth. Further research is necessary on psychotherapeutic interventions aimed at achieving a better quality of life and a more intimate relationship. A shift in this direction can be the start of a more emancipated way of living and loving for surviving gynecologic cancer patients.

REFERENCES

1. Abitbol, M. M., and Davenport, J. H. (1974): Sexual dysfunction after therapy for cervical carcinoma. *Am. J. Obstet. Gynecol.*, 119:181–189.
2. Amias, A. G. (1975): Sexual life after gynaecological operations. *Br. Med. J.*, 2:608.
3. Andersen, B. L., and Hacker, N. F. (1983): Psychosexual adjustment of gynecologic oncology patients: A proposed model for future investigation. *Gynecol. Oncol.*, 15:214–223.
4. Andersen, B. L., and Hacker, N. F. (1983): Psychosexual adjustment following pelvic exenteration. *Obstet. Gynecol.*, 61:331–338.
5. Baker Miller, J. (1973): Introduction. In: *Psychoanalysis and Women*, edited by J. Baker Miller. Penguin, London.
6. Bos, G. (1982): Gynecological cancer in the young woman. *J. Psychosom. Obstet. Gynecol.*, 2:176.
7. Bos, G. (1982): The influence of traditional sex-role patterns on the interpretation of psychosomatic complaints. In: *Advances in Psychosomatic Obstetrics and Gynecology*, edited by H. J. Prill and M. Stauber. Springer-Verlag, Berlin.
8. Bos, G. (1984): Psychological aspects of gynaecologic oncology surgery. In: *Surgery in Gynecological Oncology*, edited by A. P. M. Heintz, C. Th. Griffiths, and J. B. Trimbos. Martinus Nijhoff, The Hague.
9. Bransfield, D. D., Horiot, J. C., and Nabid, A. (1984): Development of a scale for assessing sexual function after treatment for gynecologic cancer. *J. Psychosoc. Oncol.*, 2:3–19.
10. Cain, E. N., Kohorn, E. I., Quinlan, D. M., Schwartz, P. E., Latimer, K., and Rogers, L. (1983): Psychosocial reactions to the diagnosis of gynecologic cancer. *Obstet. Gynecol.*, 62:635–641.
11. *1982 Cancer Facts and Figures* (1981): American Cancer Society, New York.
12. Capone, M. A., Good, R. S., Westie, K. S., and Jacobson, A. F. (1980): Psychosocial rehabilitation of gynecologic oncology patients. *Arch. Phys. Med. Rehabil.*, 61:128–132.
13. Carenza, L., Stentella, P., Albanese, M. G., and Etiope, S. (1982): Psychological and psychosomatic aspects in the sexual life of women following radical hysterectomy for carcinoma of the cervix. In: *Advances in Psychosomatic Obstetrics and Gynecology*, edited by H. J. Prill and M. Stauber. Springer-Verlag, Berlin.
14. De Bruijn, G. (1982): From masturbation to orgasm with a partner: How some women bridge the gap and why others don't. *J. Sex Marital Ther.*, 8:151–167.

15. Dennerstein, L., Wood, C., and Burrows, G. D. (1977): Sexual response following hysterectomy and oophorectomy. *Obstet. Gynecol.*, 49:92–96.
16. Derogatis, L. R. (1980): Breast and gynecologic cancers. *Front. Radiat. Ther. Oncol.*, 14:1–11.
17. Donahue, V. C., and Knapp, R. C. (1977): Sexual rehabilitation of gynecologic cancer patients. *Obstet. Gynecol.*, 49:118–121.
18. Fisher, S. (1973): *Understanding the Female Orgasm.* Basic Books, New York.
19. Frenken, J. (1976): *Sexual Aversion: A Social-Sexological Investigation Among 600 Married Individuals.* Van Loghum Slaterus, Deventer, The Netherlands.
20. Good, R. S., and Capone, M. A. (1980): Emotional considerations in the care of the gynecologic cancer patient. In: *Psychosomatic Obstetrics and Gynecology,* edited by D. D. Youngs and A. A. Ehrhardt. Appleton-Century-Crofts, New York.
21. Harris, R., Good, R. S., and Pollack, L. (1982): Sexual behavior of gynecologic cancer patients. *Arch. Sex. Behav.*, 11:503–510.
22. Hite, S. (1976): *The Hite Report.* Macmillan, New York.
23. Holland, C. B. J. (1976): Coping with cancer: A challenge to the behavioral sciences. In: *Cancer: The Behavioral Dimensions,* edited by J. W. Cullen, B. H. Fox, and R. N. Isom. Raven Press, New York.
24. Horney, K. (1975): The neurotic personality of our time. In: *Intimacy,* edited by J. van Ussel. Leven en Welzijn, Antwerp.
25. Kaplan, H. S. (1979): *Disorders of Sexual Desire.* Brunner-Mazel, New York.
26. Krop, M. F. (1983): Sexuality of the young woman. In: *Psychosomatic Aspects of Obstetrics and Gynaecology,* edited by L. Dennerstein and M. de Senarclens. Excerpta Medica, Amsterdam.
27. Lamberti, J. (1979): Sexual adjustment after radiation therapy for cervical carcinoma. *Med. Aspects Hum. Sex.,* March:87–88.
28. Leiber, L., Plumb, M. M., Gerstenzang, M. L., and Holland, J. (1976): The communication of affection between cancer patients and their spouses. *Psychosom. Med.,* 38:379–389.
29. Levine, S. B., and Yost, M. A. (1976): Frequency of sexual dysfunction in a general gynecological clinic: An epidemiological approach. *Arch. Sex. Behav.,* 5:229–237.
30. Mackay, E. V., Beischer, N. A., Cox, L. W., and Wood, C. (1983): *Illustrated Textbook of Gynecology.* Saunders, Philadelphia.
31. Maguire, G. P., Lee, E. G., Bevington, D. J., Kuchemann, C., Crabtree, R. J., and Cornell, C. E. (1978): Psychiatric problems in the first year after mastectomy. *Br. Med. J.,* 1:963–965.
32. Mantell, J. E. (1982): Sexuality and cancer. In: *Psychosocial Aspects of Cancer,* edited by J. W. Cullen and L. R. Martin. Raven Press, New York.
33. Masters, W. H., and Johnson, V. E. (1970): *Human Sexual Inadequacy.* Little, Brown, Boston.
34. Morris, T., Greer, H. S., and White, P. (1977): Psychological and social adjustment to mastectomy: A two-year follow-up study. *Cancer,* 40:2381.
35. Newton, M. (1979): Quality of life for the gynecologic oncology patient. *Am. J. Obstet. Gynecol.,* 134:866–869.
36. Rosenbaum, E. H., and Rosenbaum, I. R. (1980): *A Comprehensive Guide for Cancer Patients and Their Families.* Bull Publishing, Palo Alto.
37. Schain, W. S. (1981): Role of the sex therapist in the care of the cancer patient. *Front. Radiat. Ther. Oncol.,* 15:168–183.
38. Seibel, M. M., Freeman, M. G., and Graves, W. L. (1980): Carcinoma of the cervix and sexual function. *Obstet. Gynecol.,* 55:484–487.
39. Sloan, D. (1978): The emotional and psychosexual aspects of hysterectomy. *Am. J. Obstet. Gynecol.,* 131:598–605.
40. Sontag, S. (1977): *Illness as Metaphor.* Vintage Books, New York.
41. Sugarbaker, P. H., Barofsky, I., Rosenberg, S. A., and Gianola, F. J. (1982): Quality of life assessment of patients in extremity sarcoma clinical trials. *Surgery,* 91:17–23.
42. Vettese, J. M. (1976): Problems of the patients confronting the diagnosis of cancer. In: *Cancer: The Behavioral Dimensions,* edited by J. W. Cullen, B. H. Fox, and R. N. Isom. Raven Press, New York.
43. Weinberg, P. C. (1974): Psychosexual impact of treatment in female genital cancer. *J. Sex. Marital Ther.,* 1:155–157.
44. Worden, J. W., and Weisman, A. D. (1977): The fallacy in postmastectomy depression. *Am. J. Med. Sci.,* 273:175.

The Quality of Life of Cancer Patients,
edited by N. K. Aaronson and J. Beckmann,
Raven Press, New York © 1987.

Evaluation of the Quality of Life of Patients with Advanced Ovarian Cancer Treated with Combination Chemotherapy

Johanna, C. J. M. de Haes, *J. W. Raatgever,
**M. E. L. van der Burg, †Els Hamersma, and ‡J. P. Neijt

*Institute of Social Medicine, University of Leiden, 2333 AL Leiden; *Institute of Biostatistics,
Erasmus University, Rotterdam; **Rotterdam Radiotherapy Institute, Rotterdam; †The
Netherlands Cancer Institute, 1066 CX Amsterdam; and ‡Department of Internal Medicine,
University Hospital, Utrecht, The Netherlands*

It has been suggested that quality of life (QOL) must be introduced as an endpoint when evaluating cancer treatment: "The treatment of patients with cancer has two principal objectives: to reduce the threat to life posed by the disease and to increase the patient's level of ease and comfort" (2). These two objectives may well be at odds with one another. Therefore in the final analysis, to measure the value of treatment these endpoints have to be given relative weights in order to enable physicians, nurses, and patients to compare the benefits of each treatment. The need for establishing the impact of treatment on the well-being of patients becomes more urgent when an experimental therapy regimen is expected to have a considerable influence on the daily lives of patients on the one hand and an uncertain influence on survival on the other.

In earlier research the treatment of advanced ovarian carcinoma with a combination of cytostatic drugs proved to cause severe toxicity (12). For this reason, QOL has been measured in ovarian cancer patients who took part in a randomized multicenter trial comparing two combination chemotherapy regimens. All patients in this trial had advanced epithelial ovarian carcinoma and received either the standard therapy: hexamethylmelamine, cyclophosphamide, 5-fluorouracil, and methotrexate (Hexa-CAF); or the experimental therapy: cisplatin, adriamycin, hexamethylmelamine, and cyclophosphamide (CHAP-5). The results of this study as to medical parameters and toxicity have been reported extensively elsewhere (10,11). The overall response rate of patients assigned to the Hexa-CAF regimen was 50%. In the CHAP-5 group the overall response rate was 79%. Median overall survival of the Hexa-CAF group was 19.6 months compared to 26.1 months for those receiving CHAP-5. The toxicity of both regimens was considerable. However, it was apparent that the CHAP-5 schedule was more toxic than the Hexa-CAF regimen. Patients being treated with CHAP-5 experienced more moderate or severe myelosuppression, vomiting, hair loss, neurotoxicity, and renal toxicity. Consequently, it was expected that the QOL would be more significantly impaired by the CHAP-5 chemotherapy schedule.

In randomized trials the QOL has been largely ignored (6). In a review of cancer trials reported in the literature during 1975 and 1976, it was found that only 4% included some QOL measure (1). The Karnofsky index was most frequently used as a measuring instrument for QOL in these trials. However, this scale was proved to be poorly reproducible (7,15); moreover, as it covers only functional status, it operationalizes the concept of QOL in a limited way. Therefore a new instrument was developed for the current study. In this study QOL is assumed to be composed of physical and psychological symptoms, functional status, and the sense of well-being as evaluated by the patient (4).

PATIENTS AND METHODS

Patient Population and Chemotherapy Regimens

Patients with a histologically verified epithelial ovarian carcinoma in stage III or IV (FIGO classification) and a Karnofsky index of $\geq$ 70 were randomly assigned to one of two treatment arms in the Hexa-CAF/CHAP-5 trial. Patients were excluded if they had been previously treated with radiotherapy or chemotherapy. Furthermore, continuous patient follow-up had to be guaranteed.

TABLE 1. *Patients completing the questionnaire at different moments and number of questionnaires completed*

Parameter	Hexa-CAF	CHAP-5
Patients entered in the QOL study (No.)	28	34
No. of questionnaires completed	148	255[a]
Mean	5.3	7.5
Median	6	5.5
Range	1–10	1–42[a]
Median follow-up time	3.75 months	4
Range follow-up time	0–9 months	0–15.5
No. of evaluable patients completing the questionnaire during		
Entire course of chemotherapy	25	31
Treatment weeks	22	16
Rest periods	15	31
First period	17	26
Second period	15	22
Third period	12	12

[a] Two patients, receiving CHAP-5, filled in an excessive number of questionnaires (*n* = 35, 42). They account for the difference between Hexa-CAF and CHAP-5 with respect to the number of questionnaires completed.

If patients were assigned to the Hexa-CAF regimen, methotrexate 40 mg/m^2 and 5-fluorouracil 600 mg/m^2 were both given intravenously on days 1 and 8 in the outpatient clinic. Cyclophosphamide 100 mg/m^2 and hexamethylmelamine 150 mg/m^2 were each given orally on days 1 through 14. From day 15 to 28 no drugs were given. The cycle was repeated from day 29. Patients assigned to the CHAP-5 regimen received adriamycin 35 mg/m^2 on day 1 as an intravenous bolus injection prior to the administration of cisplatin. Cisplatin 20 mg/m^2 was given intravenously on days 1 through 5 in the hospital. Pre- and posthydration were administered. Starting on day 15, hexamethylmelamine 150 mg/m^2 and cyclophosphamide 100 mg/m^2 were both taken orally for 14 consecutive days. Thereafter the regimen was repeated starting on day 36 with adriamycin and cisplatin.

In three hospitals the oncologists involved in the Hexa-CAF/CHAP-5 trial asked the patients included in the trial to participate in the QOL study. If they agreed (90%), the oncologist or the responsible nurse handed out the questionnaire, to be completed either in the outpatient clinic or in the hospital. The patient filled in the questionnaire and returned it to the physician. The date of completion was filled in so as to make comparison of medical data and QOL data possible. This procedure was repeated on various visits. Thus each patient completed several questionnaires. Sixty-two patients took part in the QOL study. These patients received either Hexa-CAF ($n = 28$) or CHAP-5 ($n = 34$) therapy. Six patients completed the questionnaire only before therapy had started or after it had finished. As this number was too low, they were not considered evaluable. Table 1 shows the number of patients who completed the questionnaires and were analyzed for different treatment periods. The subjects' ages ranged from 28 to 67, with a mean of 56 years for patients treated with Hexa-CAF and 53 years for those treated with CHAP-5.

Measuring Instrument and Psychometric Analysis

To measure the QOL in this study, a questionnaire was designed that was short so as to be easily handled in a clinical context (2), easily completed by the patient (12), and included relevant domains of experience (10). Included in the questionnaire was, first, a list of 34 physical and psychological symptoms: the Rotterdam Symptom Checklist (RSCL) (Table 2). The patient was asked to report the extent to which she had been bothered by each symptom during the past 3 days. For every symptom a 4-point response scale (ranging from "not at all" to "very much") was used. The selection of symptoms was based on the Dutch version of the Hopkin's Symptom Checklist (9), the checklist developed by Linssen et al. (8), and the advice of oncologists and psychologists working with cancer patients.

Second, the patient was asked to rate the extent to which she could perform eight activities (Table 3). For every activity a 4-point response scale was used, ranging from "unable to perform" to "able to perform without help." An additive

TABLE 2. *Proportion of patients reporting the occurrence of individual symptoms at any moment during the course of treatment*

Symptom	Hexa-CAF ($n = 25$) (%)	CHAP-5 ($n = 31$) (%)
Lack of appetite	64	87.1[a]
Irritability	64	58.1
Tiredness	92	100
Worrying	76	87.1
Pain in muscles	76	61.3
Feeling depressed	68	87.1[b]
Lack of energy	84	87.1
Low back pain	60	54.8
Nervousness	84	90.3
Nausea	79.2	83.9
Desperate about future	56	67.7
Sleeplessness	76	87.1
Headache	56	64.5
Vomiting	52	74.2[b]
Dizziness	56	51.6
Loss of sexual interest	60	85.7[a]
Itching	20	19.4
Feeling lonely	56	58.1
Feeling tense	72	90.3[b]
Crying spells	60	38.7
Abdominal ache	72	67.7
Fear	60	61.3
Constipation	48	35.5
Diarrhea	32	48.4
Heartburn, belching	84	51.6[a]
Shivering	80	61.3
Tingling of hands/feet	56	54.8
Pain in mouth swallowing	40	41.9
Difficulty concentrating	68	77.4
Loss of hair	76	93.5[b]
Burning eyes	60	64.5
Deafness	28	38.7
Shortness of breath	52	35.5
Dry mouth	68	71.0

[a] $p \leq 0.05$, chi-square test.
[b] $p \leq 0.10$, chi-square test.

index of the item scores provided a measure of the functional status of the patient.

Third, the patients were asked to give a general impression of their physical sense of well-being during the past 3 days. The possible answers were "very well," "well," "not well/not ill," "ill," or "very ill." The reliability and validity of the three parts of the questionnaire have proved satisfactory (4,5,14). Questions regarding rest during daytime and medicine use were not answered reliably and were therefore omitted from the analysis (4).

In the current analysis the scores of the patients on the symptom checklist were used in two ways. First, the difference in experiencing individual symptoms was tested for both regimens. In addition, a factor analysis (13) was carried out

TABLE 3. *Daily activities*

Activity
Care for myself
Walk in the house
Housekeeping
Climb stairs
Odd jobs
Walk out of doors
Shopping
Go to work

on the 34 symptoms to construct scales based on the underlying patterns. As the number of questionnaires completed was not equal for all patients (Table 1), the mean scores on each symptom across questionnaire administrations were computed for every patient. These means served as the scores used in the factor analysis. As the number of patients was rather low ($n = 56$), symptoms with low mean scores for the total group of patients (mean ranging from 1 to 4 $\leq$ 1.50) and symptoms only weakly related to any other symptom (Pearson $r \leq 0.40$) were omitted. A principal components factor analysis with varimax rotation was conducted on the resulting 22 symptoms (Table 4) (13). Based on the explicability and the eigen-value curve, a four-factor solution was chosen. Included in the resulting factors were those items loading 0.40 or more (Table 4). Based on this factor analysis four multiitem scales (i.e., symptom indices) were constructed by adding the symptom scores included in each factor:

1. Psychological symptoms. The psychological factor included 10 symptoms and explained 42.2% of the variance. The reliability of this scale was found to be quite high (Cronbach's alpha of 0.94) (3).
2. Pain. The symptoms in the second factor refer to the experience of pain in different parts of the body. This factor explained 9.5% of the variance and exhibited satisfactory reliability (alpha of 0.81).
3. Gastrointestinal symptoms. The three symptoms included in the third factor— lack of appetite, nausea, and vomiting—clearly refer to gastrointestinal complaints. The factor explained 8.4% of the variance. The reliability of the scale is good (alpha of 0.88).
4. Fatigue. The fourth factor refers predominantly to fatigue (tiredness and lack of energy). It explained 6.4% of the variance. The reliability of this scale is satisfactory (alpha is 0.72).

It may be concluded that although the number of patients is rather low the results of the factor analysis are quite evident. A substantial proportion of the variance is explained by the extracted factors. Moreover, all of these factors clearly refer to a relevant domain of experience.

TABLE 4. *Factor loadings of 22 complaints on four factors extracted after varimax rotation (>0.40)*

Complaint	1	2	3	4
Irritability	0.53	—	—	—
Worrying	0.84	—	—	—
Feeling depressed	0.79	—	—	—
Nervousness	0.62	—	—	—
Desperate about the future	0.84	—	—	—
Sleeplessness	0.63	—	—	—
Feeling lonely	0.68	—	—	—
Feeling tense	0.77	—	—	—
Crying spells	0.43	—	—	—
Fear	0.88	—	—	—
Pain in muscles	—	0.66	—	—
Low back pain	—	0.65	—	—
Headache	—	0.66	—	—
Abdominal ache	—	0.64	—	—
Constipation	—	0.60	—	—
Lack of appetite	—	—	0.73	—
Nausea	—	—	0.81	—
Vomiting	—	—	0.95	—
Tiredness	—	—	—	0.60
Lack of energy	—	—	—	0.76
Shivering	—	—	—	0.46
Loss of sexual interest	—	—	—	—

It was expected that differences between treatment regimens with respect to the QOL might either reflect overall differences, differences related to treatment and rest periods, or differences related to the number of chemotherapy cycles received. First, to compare the overall differences between the Hexa-CAF and the CHAP-5 regimen, the proportion of patients reporting an individual symptom was computed. Additionally, the overall mean score for each question and each scale was computed for every patient (i.e., the scores of each patient across all occasions were averaged).

Second, Hexa-CAF and CHAP-5 were compared with respect to differences during the treatment weeks of the cycle and during the rest periods. Therefore for every patient a mean treatment score was computed by averaging the scores on the questionnaires completed during treatment weeks. A mean rest score was computed by averaging the scores from the rest periods of therapy courses for every patient.

Third, the two treatment regimens were compared at different time periods of the treatment as follows: first period, first and second therapy course; second period, third and fourth therapy course; third period, fifth and sixth therapy course. In the same way as described above, a mean score was computed for these three periods during the treatment. To evaluate the differences between the Hexa-CAF and the CHAP-5 schedule, chi-square tests and Student's *t*-tests were performed.

RESULTS

Overall Comparison

The proportion of patients suffering from an individual symptom is reported in Table 2. Of patients receiving Hexa-CAF, 80% or more reported tiredness, lack of energy, heartburn, and shivering. In the CHAP-5 schedule 80% or more reported tiredness, lack of appetite, worrying, feeling depressed, lack of energy, nervousness, nausea, sleeplessness, loss of sexual interest, feeling tense, and loss of hair. Patients undergoing CHAP-5 experienced greater lack of appetite, depression, vomiting, loss of sexual interest, tense feelings, and alopecia. Patients undergoing Hexa-CAF experienced more heartburn. The mean overall scores of patients receiving either Hexa-CAF or CHAP-5 were compared and the differences tested (Table 5). The findings indicated that patients receiving Hexa-CAF experienced more irritability and heartburn. Patients undergoing CHAP-5, however, experienced greater lack of appetite and loss of sexual interest. No differences were observed between the treatment regimens with respect to the indices constructed (psychological symptoms, pain, fatigue, and gastrointestinal symptoms), functional status, or sense of well-being.

Differences During Intensive Treatment Weeks and During Rest Periods

The results of the comparison of Hexa-CAF and CHAP-5 during intensive treatment weeks and during rest periods are given in Table 6. During the treatment weeks patients following the Hexa-CAF regimen reported more irritability, whereas

TABLE 5. *Overall comparison of Hexa-CAF and CHAP-5*

Condition	df	p Value[a] (≤ 0.05)	Outcome favored
Symptoms[b]			
Lack of appetite	54	0.05	Hexa-CAF
Irritability	54	0.04	CHAP-5
Loss of sexual interest	54	0.05	Hexa-CAF
Heartburn	54	0.02	CHAP-5
Psychological symptoms	54	—	—
Pain	54	—	—
Gastrointestinal symptoms	54	—	—
Fatigue	54	—	—
Functional status	51	—	—
Physical sense of well-being	53	—	—

[a] Student's *t*-test.
[b] Only those symptoms favoring one of the treatment regimens are reported.

TABLE 6. *Comparison of Hexa-CAF and CHAP-5 during intensive weeks and rest periods*

Condition	Intensive treatment weeks			Rest periods		
	df	p Value (≤0.05)	Outcome favored	df	p Value (≤0.05)	Outcome favored
Symptoms[a]						
Lack of appetite	36	0.001	Hexa-CAF	44	0.005	Hexa-CAF
Irritability	36	0.037	CHAP-5			
Nausea	36	0.001	Hexa-CAF			
Vomiting	36	<0.001	Hexa-CAF			
Loss of sexual interest	36			44	0.031	Hexa-CAF
Loss of hair				44	0.015	Hexa-CAF
Psychological symptoms	36	—	—	44	—	—
Pain	36	—	—	44	—	—
Gastrointestinal symptoms	36	<0.001	Hexa-CAF	44	—	—
Fatigue	36	—	—	44	—	—
Functional status	36	—	—	44	—	—
Physical sense of well-being	36	0.024	Hexa-CAF	44	—	—

[a] Only those symptoms favoring one of the treatment regimens are reported.

patients following the CHAP-5 schedule reported more lack of appetite, nausea, and vomiting; consequently, their gastrointestinal symptoms index score was higher. The sense of well-being was also worse for patients undergoing CHAP-5 than for patients receiving Hexa-CAF.

During the rest periods patients being treated with CHAP-5 were more distressed by lack of appetite, loss of sexual interest, and loss of hair. Neither the mean rest score for gastrointestinal symptoms nor the mean rest score for the sense of well-being differed significantly between groups. No difference between the two groups was evident on any of the other scales.

Differences During Successive Courses of Treatment

The differences between Hexa-CAF and CHAP-5 in different courses of treatment are given in Table 7. During the first period (first and second courses) patients being treated with Hexa-CAF suffered more from tiredness and shivering. They also reported higher distress on the fatigue scale. As to the other complaints and QOL indices, there were no differences between Hexa-CAF and CHAP-5.

During the second period (third and fourth treatment course), patients being treated with CHAP-5 reported more lack of appetite, depression, nausea, vomiting, difficulty concentrating, and diarrhea. The gastrointestinal symptoms of these patients were also more severe. As to the other indices, no differences were found during this period. During the third period (fifth and sixth treatment course), patients being treated with Hexa-CAF reported more abdominal aches, whereas patients being treated with CHAP-5 reported more lack of appetite and vomiting. The

TABLE 7. Comparison of Hexa-CAF and CHAP-5 during different periods in the course of theray

Condition	First period			Second period			Third period		
	df	p Value (≤0.05)	Outcome favored	df	p Value (≤0.05)	Outcome favored	df	p Value (≤0.05)	Outcome favored
Symptoms[a]									
Lack of appetite									
Tiredness	41	0.011	CHAP-5	35	0.006	Hexa-CAF	22	0.004	Hexa-CAF
Depressed				35	0.044	Hexa-CAF			—
Nausea				35	0.012	Hexa-CAF			
Vomiting	41	0.025	CHAP-5	35	0.036	Hexa-CAF	22	0.039	Hexa-CAF
Shivering									
Difficulty concentrating				35	0.047	Hexa-CAF			
Diarrhea				35	0.015	Hexa-CAF			
Abdominal ache							22	0.036	CHAP-5
Psychological symptoms	41	—	—	35	—	—	22	—	—
Pain	41	—	—	35	—	—	22	—	—
Gastrointestinal symptoms	41	0.008	CHAP-5	35	0.006	Hexa-CAF	22	0.037	Hexa-CAF
Fatigue	41	—	—	35	—	—	22	—	—
Functional status	30	—	—	32	—	—	19	—	—
Physical sense of well-being	39	—	—	35	—	—	22	0.033	Hexa-CAF

[a] Only those symptoms favoring one of the treatment regimens are reported.

latter suffered more from gastrointestinal symptoms, and their physical sense of well-being was inferior to that of patients receiving Hexa-CAF. There were no differences with respect to psychological complaints, fatigue, pain, and functional status.

DISCUSSION

When researching the value of cancer treatment, the impact of treatment on QOL must be considered. There have been no systematic studies on the effect of combination chemotherapy in ovarian cancer on the QOL. In this chapter, however, an investigation of the impact of the Hexa-CAF and CHAP-5 chemotherapy schedules is reported.

Although CHAP-5 is more toxic than Hexa-CAF, the overall comparison of the two regimens did not lead to a clear distinction. Only with respect to some individual complaints could a difference be found. As the cisplatin used in the CHAP-5 schedule produces many gastrointestinal symptoms, the reported difference in lack of appetite is quite understandable. Why patients undergoing Hexa-CAF reported more irritability and heartburn and patients receiving CHAP-5 more loss of sexual interest is not easily interpreted. The loss of sexual interest was especially apparent during the rest periods. Possibly loss of libido is less distressing during hospital stays, when other complaints are more dominant. During intensive treatment weeks, the number and intensity of gastrointestinal symptoms were clearly more prominent in patients receiving CHAP-5. Even the overall sense of well-being was worse in these patients. These findings are due to the severe effect of cisplatin on gastrointestinal functioning and are in accordance with medical expectations. It is not clear why irritability was more important in patients receiving Hexa-CAF. Like loss of sexual interest, loss of hair may be experienced as more distressing during rest periods because other symptoms are less distressing at that time.

The differences between Hexa-CAF and CHAP-5 during different periods in the course of treatment give another impression. During the first treatment cycles Hexa-CAF was evaluated as more burdensome because of fatigue. During subsequent cycles CHAP-5 therapy was assessed as more burdensome because of gastrointestinal symptoms, depression, difficulties in concentrating, and the physical sense of well-being. The reported abdominal ache in Hexa-CAF patients may be a consequence of recurrence of the disease.

It may be concluded that if one overall comparison is made between these two treatment modalities no clear-cut difference becomes evident. However, if a distinction is made for treatment weeks and rest periods and for successive cycles in the course of treatment, the CHAP-5 regimen seems more burdensome than the Hexa-CAF schedule. The most important symptoms reported by the patients were (a) for Hexa-CAF tiredness, lack of energy, and heartburn, and (b) for CHAP-5 tiredness, nervousness, feeling tense, and alopecia. Interestingly, in the registration of side effects by physicians (10) tiredness was never mentioned. Likewise, mood depression was recorded by physicians in less than 5% of patients, whereas psychological symptoms were mentioned frequently by patients. These differences may be due to a different evaluation of the situation: Patients reported their subjective judgment, whereas physicians were expected to judge the situation objectively. These perceptions may well be quite different.

CONCLUSION

It has been suggested that QOL must be included as an endpoint in cancer trials. A measuring instrument was developed for the study reported here. Using the single symptoms and the constructed scales, it has proved possible to discern differences between treatment modalities. The reliability of the measure has proved good. The differences in reported problems as a function of treatment received were, however, not as clear-cut as we had expected. This lack of specificity may be due to the fact that, in the present study, patients completed several questionnaires but not all at the same time and in the same number. Particularly because a number of treatment centers were involved in the study, it was difficult to organize the study systematically with respect to points of measurement. From the results of this study it becomes evident that the measurement of QOL has to take place at different moments during the treatment cycle and over the course of several cycles. Thus a longitudinal design is necessary. Future studies should be well organized, have clearly defined points of measurement, and have a systematic control of completion dates throughout the project, as is usual for medical parameters. Because QOL studies are still uncommon in cancer research, particular attention should be focused on problems of research implementation.

ACKNOWLEDGMENTS

This work was funded by the Dutch Cancer Foundation "Koningin Wilhelmina Fonds." We would like to thank The Netherlands Joint Study Group for Ovarian Cancer for their cooperation in the study, J. F. A. Pruyn for advice on the research design, and A. L. Stewart for her comments on an earlier draft of this chapter.

REFERENCES

1. Bardelli, P., and Saracci, R. (1978): Measuring the quality of life in cancer clinical trials. *UICC Techn. Rep. Ser.*, 36:75–79.
2. Bush, R. S. (1979): *Malignancies of the Ovary, Uterus and Cervix.* Edward Arnold, London.
3. Cronbach, L. J. (1951): Coefficient alpha and the internal structure of tests. *Psychometrika*, 16:297–334.
4. De Haes, J. C. J. M., Pruyn, J. F. A., and van Knippenberg, F. C. E. (1983): Klachtenlijst voor kankerpatiënten, eerste ervaringen. *Ned. Tijdschr. Psychol.*, 38:403–422.
5. De Haes, J. C. J. M., Raatgever, J. W., and Neijt, J. P. (1982): Measuring quality of life in cancer clinical trials. Paper presented at the International Society of Clinical Biostatistics, Rotterdam.
6. Greer, S. (1984): The psychological dimension in cancer treatment. *Soc. Sci. Med.*, 4:345–349.

7. Hutchinson, T. A., Boyd, N. F., and Feinstein, A. R. (1979): Scientific problems in clinical scales as demonstrated in the Karnofsky index of performance status. *J. Chronic Dis.*, 32:661–666.

8. Linssen, A. C. G., van Dam, F. S. A. M., Engelsman, E., van Benthem, J., and Hanewald, G. J. F. P. (1979): Leven met cytostatica. *Pharm. Weekbl. [Sci.]*, 114:501–515.

9. Luteijn, F., Kok, A. P., Hamel, L. F., and Poiesz, A. (1979): Enige ervaringen met een klachtenlijst. *Ned. Tijdschr. Psychol.*, 23:167–179.

10. Neijt, J. P. (1983): *Combination Chemotherapy in the Treatment of Advanced Ovarian Carcinoma.* ICG Printing, Dordrecht, The Netherlands.

11. Neijt, J. P., ten Bokkel Huinink, W. W., van der Burg, M. E. L., van Oosterom, A. T., Vriesendorp, R., Kooyman, C. D., van Lindert, A. C. M., Hamerlynck, J. V. T. H., van Lent, M., van Houwelingen, J. C., and Pinedo, H. M. (1984): Randomized trial comparing two combination chemotherapy regimens (Hexa-CAF vs. CHAP-5) in advanced ovarian carcinoma. *Lancet*, 2:594–600.

12. Neijt, J. P., van Lindert, A. C. M., Vendrik, C. P. J., Roozendaal, K. J., Struyvenberg, A., and Pinedo, H. M. (1980): Treatment of advanced ovarian carcinoma with a combination of hexamethylmelamine, cyclophosphamide, methotrexate and 5-fluorouracil (Hexa-CAF) in patients with and without previous treatment. *Cancer Treat. Rep.*, 64:232–326.

13. Thurstone, L. (1947): *Multiple-Factor Analysis.* University of Chicago Press, Chicago.

14. Trew, M., and Maguire, P. (1982): Further comparison of two instruments for measuring quality of life in cancer patients. In: *Proceedings of the Third EORTC Workshop on Quality of Life*, Paris.

15. Yates, J. W., Chalmer, B., and McKegney, F. P. (1980): Evaluation of patients with advanced cancer using Karnofsky performance status. *Cancer*, 45:2220–2224.

The Quality of Life of Cancer Patients,
edited by N. K. Aaronson and J. Beckmann,
Raven Press, New York © 1987.

Psychological Impact of Cancer: Its Assessment, Treatment, and Ensuing Effects on Quality of Life

Sidney Bindemann

Department of Clinical Oncology, Gartnavel General Hospital, University of Glasgow, GB 6B Glasgow G12 OYN, Scotland

Interest in the psychological component of a cancer diagnosis has grown considerably. Systematic studies are increasingly being undertaken and reported, and several relevant factors have been identified and commented on. The purpose of this chapter is to provide a brief review of such factors, together with an elaboration on key aspects that require measurement and assessment. Present trends and future possibilities for psychotherapeutic intervention with cancer patients are also reviewed and discussed.

The emotive connotations of the word "cancer" are universally recognized for their capacity to evoke psychologically disabling trauma and have been shown to occasion serious delay in the reporting of self-perceived symptoms (20,53,54). Once diagnosed, the extent of psychological dysfunction present is likely to be yet further modified by individual differences. However, evidence of cognitive and affective disorders may, together or separately, be symptomatic of an organic lesion or metabolic imbalance. Alternatively or concurrently they may be directly related to the noxious side effects of anticancer therapy as well as to the type of disease diagnosed (12,38). In most cases (apart from those affecting a few psychologically robust individuals) uncertainty, together with the degree of threat that is entailed in the diagnosis of malignant illness, is likely to induce yet further distress through fear and anxiety, disappointment, anger, guilt, and remorse (15,32). The effects of serious disruption to the cancer patient's domestic, social, and occupational functioning has also been observed and commented on (22).

Evidence of the presence of psychological dysfunction (rather than of a need for psychiatric intervention) more accurately describes the most commonly observed behavioral phenomenon in cancer patients. However, great care is required to ensure that anticipated and predictable mood and behavioral modification does not acquire a maladaptive component, thereby assuming psychopathological status. The need for such vigilance is evident in a growing literature describing the prevalence of psychiatric morbidity in cancer patients (26,29,30,36,50).

227

NEED FOR MEASUREMENT

Actual and precise measurement of the principal dimensions of psychological dysfunction is by no means easy to achieve. On the one hand, an acceptable degree of accuracy in the measurement of self-reported behavioral change, which can simultaneously be confirmed in the hospital ward by members of medical, nursing, and support staff (or in the home by members of the patient's own family), is feasible and often practicable. On the other hand, changes in the patient's mood and in his/her ability to maintain healthy adaptive balance in emotional functioning is notoriously more difficult to adequately and accurately assess, principally because of uncertainty about, and inaccessibility of, precipitating factors. Detailed knowledge, soundly based on systematically recorded data, about psychological and social premorbidity (a highly desirable prerequisite to satisfactory assessment) is rarely if ever available to the researcher. Adequate understanding about individual motivation and interest (as well as about opportunity afforded and inherent opportunity to fulfill them)—all of which are crucial to any valid and reliable statement about quality of life—is almost invariably equally difficult to achieve. Moreover, such instruments of measurement and assessment as are available for general usage in the attempt to accurately identify and describe behavioral, attitudinal, and mood modification are notoriously beset by methodological and procedural difficulties. Any self-report approach that greatly exceeds 40 items in overall length is likely to create problems due to fatigue and boredom of the patient. However, any significant reduction in such length may well raise serious doubts concerning the instrument's face and content validity. Finally, results from such ''pencil and paper'' tests, however robustly constructed in terms of item content and relevance, are unlikely to do anything like justice to the measurement of that vast, complexly interacting and competing array of variables that, when taken together, relate to individual well-being or quality of life.

Notwithstanding, and without prejudice to full recognition of the necessarily fragmentary nature of any attempt at measurement, several studies have been undertaken and their results documented in the search for important, relevant information about patient well-being in the face of life-threatening illness and its implications. These include the application of interviewing techniques and procedures (25,34), structured and otherwise; of nominal, ordinal, and interval-type scaling techniques (24,49), and of the Graphic Response Scale. The latter scale (which in the strict psychometric sense is really an item) is frequently referred to as the Visual Analogue Scale or the Linear Analogue Self-Assessment (LASA) scale (10,41). For the most part, this approach provides a range of fixed-choice responses, which, it is claimed, discriminates sensitively on variables relating to patient behavior, symptoms, and so on over a clearly defined period of time.

The need for accurate quantification has also involved the deployment of questionnaires and inventories that have been devised and constructed for purposes other than the measurement of well-being or quality of life in cancer patients. In some instances these have been used singly (18), at other times in combination (28), and most commonly for the purpose of assessing patient groups on the basis of well-known personality parameters or traits, e.g., reactive depression, or "state" as opposed to "trait" anxiety (48). Such means of measurement have in many cases been validated on large samples of the general population and therefore give immediate access to relevant normative data. This method has been shown to have real value in achieving a better understanding of the cancer patient and his needs. Several studies have been undertaken that have deployed questionnaires constructed for the precise purpose of measuring well-being or quality of life in the cancer patient (2,44,52). On the whole, the LASA method appears to have been most widely favored for attempted measurement of the quality of life of cancer patients.

An alternative method for patient self-assessment has been proposed by the author and his colleagues (4,6) that requires subjects to respond on a semantic-differential type scale. The scale deploys a well-researched distribution of items in the form of bipolar alternatives, e.g., "often feel tired—seldom feel tired," "apprehensive—confident," for response to the "actual self," i.e., "the kind of person I am," descriptive criterion and the "ideal self," "the kind of person I should like to be," descriptive criterion. Data obtained via patients' responses are subjected to factor analysis, a statistical procedure that facilitates the reduction of large amounts of data into smaller homogeneous clusters, or factors. Such factors may thereafter be treated as single variables, for which a factor score may be computed for any well-defined group response within the data. In the case of a factor, say, of "anxiety," such factor scores accurately indicate the self-perceived location for the "actual" and the "ideal" self-descriptive criteria. It is hypothesized that determination of the size of the discrepancy between self-perceived reality on the one hand and aspiration on the other, will prove to be informative about patient well-being or quality of life: When the discrepancy is large, subjective assessment of quality of life is unsatisfactory; conversely, when the discrepancy is small, subjective evaluation, as indicated by individual or group factor scores (whichever the case may be), indicates a self-perceived satisfactory and acceptable quality of life.

The advantages and disadvantages of this particular approach have been fully described and discussed elsewhere (4). However, it does appear to successfully negotiate notorious problems associated with attempted measurement of psychological premorbidity. Moreover, this approach has in fact been successfully applied to cancer patients and has demonstrated a facility for measurement that concurs powerfully with patient perceptions and "rater" perceptions of behavior modification in response to patient training in relaxation therapy (5).

TREATMENT POSSIBILITIES

Uncertainty as to the most effective means of treatment for psychological dysfunction in the cancer patient is clearly reflected in the wide (though not mutually exclusive) range of therapeutic strategies and procedures known to be currently available. Psychotropic drug therapy in the form of anxiolytic and antidepressant-type drugs appears to constitute the most widely applied "crisis," or short-term, approach. However, the cancer patient's need for continuing support is rarely short-term. Moreover, there is mounting evidence of an articulated need for an alternative approach, preferably in the form of self-management, that can avoid both the short- and the long-term adverse effects of chemically induced mood and behavioral modification, e.g., disorientation, isolation, and threat to supportive bonds through isolation and possible dependence on the drug.

Two broad strategies of management that require patient compliance and involvement are:

1. A supportive facility whereby the patient is encouraged to overcome or to reduce to manageable proportions anxiety related to his illness and the intense personal problems it so frequently engenders

2. A directive facility through which the patient may avail himself of instruction and training in simple, self-applied procedures that are directed toward the recovery of confidence and hope for the future

Role of Supportive Therapy

Some form of patient support is likely to be routinely available to all hospital patients. However, it presumably differs widely, in the source from which it emanates as well as in the specialty with which it deals. Personal contact with patients by members of the hospital's medical and nursing staffs, both informally and on the ubiquitous ward round, certainly seem to constitute the most commonly available supportive service. However, a relatively new concept of supportive care is emerging in the form of the "team" approach (1). This approach has effectively widened the concept of patient service to embrace an impressive diversity of formally structured disciplines, e.g., psychological, social, psychotherapeutic, dietary. Additionally, group as well as individually administered counseling services in all such specialties are increasingly being reported (14,47). Support for the families of cancer patients demarks yet another important area of need that is increasingly being acknowledged and understood (35). The hypothesis that shared experiences outweigh potential difficulties nevertheless requires scientifically controlled evaluation.

Although it seems reasonable to assume that the area of need for supportive therapy, as is apparent from the foregoing, is always fairly diffuse, the first line of defence against that degree of anxiety and fear engendered by uncertainty is confidence, which in the case of the cancer patient finds its central focus in the consulting physician or surgeon. Indeed, reports indicate that patients who manifest difficulty in handling such dependency are themselves likely to display anger and paranoid symptoms (37). Some patients are known to almost compulsively scrutinize their every bodily function between hospital and clinic appointments. Consequently, each follow-up attendance is likely to raise apprehension that is best resolved by friendly explanation, suggestion, and reassurance. Evidence has also cogently demonstrated and illustrated the value of continuing sound relationships between the patient and the consulting physician or surgeon. In just one such example, Twycross (51) indicated how improved relationships between terminal care patients and their attending physicians facilitated a reduction in the need for pain-relieving drugs.

It seems unlikely and indeed undesirable that there should emerge some future "blanket" form of psychological support that aims to provide an equal measure of benefit to every patient suffering from malignant disease. Indeed, it can be persuasively argued that the most effective and satisfactory deployment of supportive resources is that which succeeds in early identification of those patients who experience difficulty coping with the implications of their illness and its treatment. The quantifiable consequences of individual differences, e.g., level of intelligence, current beliefs and opinions, and psychosocial functioning, all of which are complexly related to coping ability levels, requires a supportive approach that is tailored to meet individual needs. Moreover, what is likely to appeal to a patient who, for example, has an acute awareness of spiritual need, may convey little if any meaning to the patient who manifests no such awareness of need. Similarly, any given trial or study of supportive techniques may evoke a positive response in only a few potential subjects eligible for such a study.

It is, above all, absolutely essential that the emergence of obstacles and difficulties in measurement and assessment of quality of life should not deter from the attempt to evaluate what is evaluable and thereby to improve what is being offered by way of support. There is no doubt that the demands of "necessity" and "sufficiency" criteria are met most frequently via a protocol design that facilitates adequate preliminary investigation, selection, and stratification. Such a design is often required well before the application of such familiar terms as "experimental" and "control" to mutually exclusive patient groups in research trials.

Role of Directive Therapy and Autogenic Training

The principal aim of directive therapy and autogenic training is to facilitate the patient's potential for adaptability in the direction of insightful awareness and, when feasible, resolution of those psychological and personal problems known to be associated with a malignant illness. Directive therapy involves regular, periodic repetition of an exercise such as is entailed in, for example, Progressive Muscle Relaxation (PMR). Such systematic behavioral regulation, achieved by means of coping skills training, is swiftly developing into one of the most extensively investigated areas of inquiry in applied psychology with the cancer patient. PMR was first proposed and formalized into a systematically applied program for relaxation by Jacobson (23). The lengthy and cumbersome procedure he originally outlined has been successively refined and modified, principally by Wolpe (55) and more recently by Bernstein and Borkovek (3), into a more wieldy and viable format for its successful application. Where applied, attention is repeatedly focused on the "common to all" somatic component of relaxation experienced in particular muscle groups. Patients are encouraged similarly to attend to physical tension, noting both gross and subtle differences entailed in these two contrasting states of awareness. In a series of publications, PMR has been shown to possess a capacity for adaptability to the point where it might reasonably be perceived as facilitating an active coping skill (8,27). Thus PMR constitutes an acceptable training format whereby individual patients may readily learn progressively to relax gross muscle groups by the "tense–relax" method. Commitment to a belief in the individual patient's reactive potential for self-control is also evident in the development of physiological monitoring and feedback facilities. In broad terms, relaxation is perceived as a psychophysiological state that is achieved via parasympathetic dominance over multiple visceral and somatic symptoms. Psychophysiological feedback (biofeedback), in fact, refers to a set of procedures whereby the individual may develop learned control over a wide range of physiological processes. By this means it becomes at least theoretically possible to modify smooth muscle and autonomic nervous system activity, e.g., heart rate, blood pressure, and electrodermal activity, and thereby consciously induce the desired state of parasympathetic dominance with its attendant sense of relaxation and well-being.

Its use with cancer patients as an adjunctive form of relaxation therapy has been proposed (40), and actual studies have been reported (9). Systematic evaluation of the potential worth of this relatively new therapeutic approach is urgently required if its potential reinforcement for coping skills training is to be fully realized. However, to date, relatively few adequately controlled studies involving cancer patients in biofeedback-assisted relaxation have been reported.

Hypnosis has also been proposed for the management of emotional distress in the cancer patient (11,13). The present-day perception and interpretation of what in the past was frequently regarded as an aberration, and hence a therapeutic tool of dubious worth, has changed dramatically. Indeed, the historically derived association of hypnosis with mysticism and patient gullibility has weakened considerably, mainly because of well-documented evidence of its status and role as an altered state of consciousness, possessing profound and exciting therapeutic implications (16,17,42). A particularly valuable characteristic of the hypnosis-assisted relaxation response resides in its proved ability to eliminate sensory distraction while simultaneously facilitating and heightening an ability to attend selectively. The well-documented "ego-strengthening" routine (21) adapted to encompass the individual patient's psychological needs and goals is most commonly employed in the application of such treatment with cancer patients. Hypnosis and relaxation training schedules have also been effectively used in the management of psychogenic vomiting after administration of cytotoxic chemotherapy (8,33,42) and in the control of chronic pain in cancer patients (43,56).

In a study carried out by the author and his colleagues (7), relaxation training (ReT) was applied to 68 cancer patients (27 men and 41 women) who were undergoing treatment for their physical illness in a clinical oncology treatment unit. The patients concerned had developed psychological problems that were unrelieved by anxiolytic or antidepressant drugs. In the particular instance of this study, compliant patients were introduced to ReT that comprised simple breathing exercises, PMR, and lightly induced hypnosis. Following their initial training, patients continued to themselves induce profound relaxation by means of an audio tape recording of ReT. Progress was reviewed at prescribed intervals, i.e., 48 hr, 1 week, and 4 weeks, and qualitative changes in "psychological," "social," and "other behavioral" criteria were observed and recorded by the patients themselves, their immediate relatives, and members of the oncology, medical, and nursing staff. Concordance in such levels of assessment was impressively high. Reported and observed benefits of ReT indicated marked improvement in quality of life, including improved psychological and social functioning, with an accompanying reduction of the need for analgesic and psychotropic drug intake. Some patients clearly indicated an enhanced ability to tolerate further chemotherapy. Moreover, ReT appeared to make a valuable contribution during the period of terminal care. In general, its principal advantages over other methods of treatment appear to reside in its apparent capacity to mobilize a resource for self-control and thereby reduce the sense of loneliness and isolation that some patients are known to feel and which is not infrequently exacerbated by the administration of psychotropic drugs. This mobilization of personal resources is especially valuable for patients attending a chemotherapy unit where the rather formal and technological atmosphere might very well generate loneliness, fear, and feelings of passivity and loss of control. A more detailed account of the method, together with a full discussion of results obtained, is reported elsewhere (7). A randomized study has also been completed (5) and will be reported on in the near future.

Other Claims for Supportive and Directive Therapies

A considerably more controversial component of directive therapy and autogenic training is that which aims not merely at enhancing quality of life through self-regulation and control but which proposes a dynamic force of faith as the basis for actual recovery from physical disease. For some time now, clinicians and researchers have focused on the psychological differences of cancer patients who do well (survive longer) as distinct from those who do poorly (rapidly succumb) (19). Several reports and indeed volumes have indicated support for the thesis that hope is a significant factor in survival from cancer and that, conversely, psychological dysfunction and the impact of unfavorable social factors may heighten patients' susceptibility to disease and impede recovery (31,45,46). Such observations as these appear *prima facie* to be directly related to the association between emotional decomposition and depression and elevation of adrenal cortical steroid hormones and the awareness that cortisol may be immunosuppressive. The experimental data undeniably support the hypothesis that experimentally induced tumor growth and metastases may be modified by neuroendocrinological reactions to stress (39). However, this work has been achieved in animal models almost at the other pole to man on the phylogenetic scale, and it is indeed hazardous, to say the least, to draw similar conclusions concerning tumor growth in humans.

Whatever the effect of stress hormones on endocrine and immunological defences, it seems unlikely that the relation is as simple and straightforward as the more enthusiastic devotees of this persuasion would have us believe. Moreover, it is a well established fact that tumors do proceed through periods of acceleration, deceleration, and stasis and have occasionally been known to regress spontaneously. At the present time, therefore, there simply is no known body of entirely favorable and incontrovertible evidence that corroborates the thesis that psychological factors do influence cancer prognosis. Of course, this state of affairs, so needful of accurate assessment, by no means invalidates the worth of its contribution any more than it reduces the attractiveness of its allure. However, science is about method, entailing empirical observation, control, and due consideration of other "necessity" and "sufficiency" criteria such as are required to satisfy the rigorous demands prediction entails. Good science is the only science there is. It would be a matter for regret if any who are concerned with the treatment of cancer patients are on the one hand prepared to make claims for the treatments they offer (but which remain unsubstantiated by evidence in the form of data) while on the other hand remaining unprepared to expose such treatments to properly constituted clinical trials. Sadly, it is the case that unsupported claims of this sort are not only unhelpful and misleading to cancer patients but serve frequently to inflict unnecessary pressures on the more vulnerable (among whom are of course relatives and loved ones) by encouraging false rather than appropriate hope and by undermining essential belief, faith, and confidence in available oncology services.

FUTURE NEEDS AND POSSIBILITIES

The purpose of this chapter is, first, to identify the notable and well-documented aspects of psychological dysfunction that are known to be associated with a cancer diagnosis; second, to briefly review known and applied methods of measurement and assessment of their impact on patient well-being or quality of life; and third, briefly to consider the possibilities for current studies of psychotherapeutic intervention and its potential for behavioral and attitudinal modification in favor of enhanced quality of life.

One effect of such a review and discussion as has here been attempted is to reflect the fragmentary nature of work that has been achieved in the past, as well as that which is currently known to be in progress. Although there is a certain inevitability about such a state of affairs, a plea for the pooling of ideas and resources so far as future studies are concerned seems wholly appropriate. Happily, there are now emerging accounts, albeit isolated, of interdepartmental, multidepartmental, and even multinational research projects that greatly enhance the flow of ideas and exciting possibilities for comparative analysis and evaluation. Such joint and corporate undertakings are, after all, commonplace in clinical medicine—to the considerable advantage of all who are prepared to explore possibilities and motivations for the sharing and pooling of resources, training facilities, and so on.

At the present time, there is little by the way of "hard" data to indicate relative benefits obtained from supportive and directive therapies. This problem is difficult to resolve, as it is not infrequently the case that cancer patients who are receiving directive therapy in the form of PMR or in accordance with an alternative model for relaxation training are also the recipients of supportive therapy in that they are simultaneously being counseled, receiving ongoing support from others who are actively concerned with their care, or both. Unless information about the total psychotherapeutic input (whether of a formal or informal nature) is available, and this is rarely if ever likely to be the case, it is hazardous to attribute results to one particular approach when such benefits may well relate to the influence of an undefined factor or group of factors. There does therefore exist a pressing need for a systematic attempt, difficult though it may be to achieve, to adequately screen patient groups whenever possible and practicable in order to determine the nature of confounding variables.

Finally, it seems highly appropriate to enter the plea for fuller appraisal of the inherent possibilities for greater involvement (where appropriate) of relatives in the direction and indeed in the application of easily administered supportive measures. It is of interest to note in Meares' anecdotal account of a "spontaneous regression" previously referred to (31) that the patient's girlfriend (later to become his wife) was credited with a major role and contribution in the application of therapy from which considerable benefit was obviously derived. It makes good sense at least to explore this potential resource for the following reasons.

1. Relatives are almost invariably highly motivated in the direction of a search for opportunities to be of real assistance.

2. The nature of the relationship between patient and relative is frequently one that is characterized by mutual fidelity and trust.

3. Relatives are most likely to be on the spot almost all the time, and possibilities are further enhanced by the uninterrupted flow of their attendance and attention.

The author is in the process of exploring very simple possibilities for greater involvement of selected relatives, subject to the assurance of the provision of ongoing interest, advice, and support. It is his experience that relatives are not only willing to be so involved but are also ready to attempt to keep careful records in accordance with a simple format that has previously been explained to both patient and relative. Although this approach may involve only a few patients, much greater attention might profitably be directed toward any possibilities inherent in this potential resource. There are also good grounds for postulating and testing the hypothesis that, in the event of death of the patient, relatives who have been so involved more satisfactorily manage the bereavement period and process and are more likely ultimately to seek an outlet for their learned and developed sensitivities and skills through patient and relative support groups.

The understandable fascination with and interest in quality of life that is currently reflected in the literature concerning the treatment of malignant illnesses demands much more than its mere definition and evaluation as a concept. There is urgent need for greater evidence of the pursuit and search for valid means leading to its enhancement as a factor that shares at least an equal status with the aim for survival.

ACKNOWLEDGMENT

The author is supported by a grant from the Cancer Research Campaign (CRC) Education Panel.

REFERENCES

1. Belis, L., Weiss, R. B., and Thrush, D. (1980): The oncology clinic: A primary care facility. *Cancer Nurs.*, 3:47–52.
2. Bernheim, J. (1980): Anamnestic comparative self-appraisal: A measure of quality of life in cancer patients. *Proc. ASCO*, 21:357.
3. Bernstein, D. A., and Borkovek, T. D. (1973): *Progressive Relaxation Training: A Manual for the Helping Professions*. Research Press, Champaign, Illinois.
4. Bindemann, S., Kaye, S. B., Welsh, J., Habeshaw, T., and Calman, K. C. (1985): A method for measurement of the quality of life in cancer patients: Determination and evaluation comparatively, of their actual- and ideal-self perception of placement on derived factors. Submitted for publication.
5. Bindemann, S., Kaye, S. B., Welsh, J., Habeshaw, T., and Calman, K. C. (1986): Relaxation training in cancer patients; a randomised study of effect. Unpublished to date.
6. Bindemann, S., Milsted, R. A. V., Kaye, S. B., and Calman, K. C. (19xx): The assessment of quality of life in cancer patients; a fresh approach. *Br. J. Cancer*, 48:1, 387.
7. Bindemann, S., Milsted, R. A. V., Kaye, S. B., Welsh, J., Habeshaw, T., and Calman, K. C. (1985): Enhancement of quality of life with relaxation training in cancer patients attending a chemotherapy unit. In: *Proceedings of 1st Annual Conference of the British Psychosocial Oncology Group*. Pergamon, Oxford (*in press*).
8. Burish, T. G., and Lyles, J. N. (1981): Effectiveness of relaxation training in reducing adverse reactions in cancer chemotherapy. *J. Behav. Med.*, 4:65–78.
9. Burish, T. G., Shartner, C. D., and Lyles, J. N. (1981): Effectiveness of multiple muscle-site EMG biofeedback and relaxation training in reducing the aversiveness of cancer chemotherapy. *Biofeedback Self Regul.*, 6:523–535.
10. Coates, A., Dillenbeck, C. F., McNeil, D. R., et al. (1983): On the receiving end. II. Linear Analogue Self-Assessment (LASA) in evaluation of aspects of the quality of life in cancer patients receiving therapy. *Eur. J. Cancer Clin. Oncol.*, 19:1633–1637.
11. Crasilneck, H. H., and Hall, J. A. (1976): Hypnosis: Its use with cancer patients. In: *Clinical Hypnosis: Principles and Application*, pp. 109–116. Grune & Stratton, New York.
12. Devlin, B. H., Plant, J. A., and Griffin, M. (1971): Aftermath of surgery for anorectal cancer. *Br. Med. J.*, 3:413–418.
13. Ellenburg, L., Kellerman, J., Dash, J., Higgins, G., and Zelter, L. (1980): Use of hypnosis for multiple symptoms in an adolescent girl with leukaemia. *J. Adolesc. Health Care*, 1:132–136.
14. Ferlic, M., Goldman, A., and Kennedy, B. J. (1979): Group counselling in adult patients with advanced cancer. *Cancer*, 43:760–766.
15. Frank-Stromberg, M., Wright, P. S., Segalla, M., and Diekmann, J. (1984): Psychological impact of the "cancer" diagnosis. *Oncol. Nurs. Forum*, 11:16–22.
16. Fromm, E. (1979): Quo vadis hypnosis: Predictions of future trends in hypnosis research. In:

Hypnosis: Developments in Research and New Perspectives, new and revised 2nd ed., edited by E. Fromm and R. E. Shor, pp. 687–704. Aldine, New York.

17. Fromm, E. (1979): The nature of hypnosis and other altered states of consciousness: An ego psychological theory. In: *Hypnosis: Developments in Research and New Perspectives,* new and revised 2nd ed., edited by E. Fromm and R. E. Shor, pp. 81–104. Aldine, New York.

18. Graham, C., Bond, S. S., Gerkovich, M. M., and Cook, M. R. (1980): Use of the McGill Pain Questionnaire in the assessment of cancer pain: Replicability and consistency. *Pain,* 8:77–87.

19. Greer, S., Morris, T., and Pettingale, K. W. (1979): Psychological response to breast cancer: Effect on outcome. *Lancet,* 2:785–787.

20. Hackett, T. P., Cassem, N. H., and Raker, J. W. (1973): Patient delay in cancer. *N. Engl. J. Med.,* 289:14–20.

21. Hartland, J. (1971): *Medical and Dental Hypnosis and Its Clinical Applications,* pp. 196–204. Baillière-Tindall, London.

22. Holland, J. (1980): Understanding the cancer patient. *CA,* 30:103–112.

23. Jacobson, E. (1938): *Progressive Relaxation.* University of Chicago Press, Chicago.

24. Karnofsky, D. A., and Burchenal, J. H. (1948): Clinical evaluation of chemotherapeutic agent in cancer. In: *Evaluation of Chemotherapeutic Agents,* edited by C. M. McLeod. Columbia University Press, New York.

25. Knopf, A. (1974): Changes in women's opinions about cancer. *Soc. Sci. Med.,* 10:191–195.

26. Levine, P. M., Silberfarb, P. M., and Lipowski, Z. J. (1978): Mental disorders in cancer patients— a study of 100 psychiatric referrals. *Cancer,* 42:1385–1391.

27. Lyles, J. N., Burish, T. G., Krosely, M. G., and Oldham, R. K. (1982): Efficacy of relaxation training and guided imagery in reducing the aversiveness of cancer chemotherapy. *J. Consult. Clin. Psychol.,* 50:509–524.

28. Lyon, J. S. (1977): Management of psychological problems in breast cancer. In: *Breast Cancer Management—Early and Late,* edited by B. A. Stoll.

29. Maguire, G. P., Lee, E. G., Bevington, D. J., et al. (1978): Psychiatric problems in the first year after mastectomy. *Br. Med. J.,* 1:963–965.

30. Maguire, G. P., Tait, A., Brooke, M., et al. (1980): Psychiatric morbidity and physical toxicity associated with adjuvant chemotherapy after mastectomy. *Br. Med. J.,* 281:1179–1180.

31. Meares, A. (1979): Mediation: A psychological approach to cancer treatment. *Practitioner,* 222:119–122.

32. Miller, T. R. (1977): Psychological aspects of cancer. *Cancer,* 39:413–418.

33. Morrow, G. R., and Morrell, C. (1982): Behavioural treatment for the anticipatory nausea and vomiting induced by cancer chemotherapy. *N. Engl. J. Med.,* 307:1476–1480.

34. Morrow, G. R., Chiarello, R. J., and Derogatis, L. R. (1978): A new scale for assessing patients' psychosocial adjustment to medical illness. *Psychol. Med.,* 8:605–610.

35. Naysmith, A., Hinton, J. M., Meredith, R., et al. (1983): Surviving malignant disease—psychological and family aspects. *Br. J. Hosp. Med.,* 30:22, 26–27.

36. O'Malley, J. E., Koocher, G., Foster, D., and Slavin, L. (1979): Psychiatric sequelae of surviving childhood cancer. *Am. J. Orthopsychiatry,* 19:608–616.

37. Peck, A. (1972): Emotional reactions to having cancer. *AJR,* 114:591–592.

38. Peck, A., and Boland, J. (1977): Emotional reactions to radiation treatment. *Cancer,* 40:180–184.

39. Peters, L. J., and Mason, K. A. (1979): Influence of stress on experimental cancer. In: *Mind and Cancer Prognosis,* edited by B. A. Stoll, pp. 103–123. Wiley, Chichester.

40. Phillips, K. C. (1979): Biofeedback as an aid to autogenic training. In: *Mind and Cancer Prognosis,* edited by B. A. Stoll, pp. 154–167. Wiley, Chichester.

41. Priestman, T. J., and Baum, M. (1976): Evaluation of quality of life in patients receiving treatment for advanced breast cancer. *Lancet,* 1:899–900.

42. Redd, W. H., Andresen, G. V., and Minagawa, R. Y. (1982): Hypnotic control of anticipatory emesis in patients receiving cancer chemotherapy. *J. Consult. Clin. Psychol.,* 50:14–19.

43. Savitz, S. A. (1983): Hypnosis in the treatment of chronic pain. *South. Med. J.,* 76:319–321.

44. Schipper, H., Clinch, A., Murray, A., and Levitt, M. (1984): Measuring the quality of life of cancer patients; The Functional Living Index—Cancer: Development and validation. *J. Clin. Oncol.,* 2:472–480.

45. Simonton, O. C., and Simonton, S. M. (1981): Cancer and stress: Counselling the cancer patient. *Med. J. Aust.,* 679–683.

46. Simonton, O. C., Simonton, S. M., and Creighton, J. (1978): *Getting Well Again.* Tarcher, Los Angeles.

47. Spiegel, D., Bloom, J., and Yallom, I. (1981): Group support for patients with metastatic cancer. *Arch. Gen. Psychiatry,* 38:527–533.
48. Spielberger, C. D., Gorsuch, R. L., and Lushene, L. E. (1970): *STAI Manual for the State-Trait Anxiety Inventory.* Consulting Psychologist's Press.
49. Spitzer, W. O., Dobson, A. J., Hall, J., et al. (1981): Measuring the quality of life of cancer patients—concise QL-index for use by physicians. *J. Chronic Dis.,* 34:584–597.
50. Streltzer, J. (1983): Psychiatric aspects of oncology: A review of recent research. *Hosp. Community Psychiatry,* 34:716–724.
51. Twycross, R. G. (1975): Relief of terminal pain. *Br. Med. J.,* 4:212–214.
52. Van Dam, F. S. A. M., Linssen, A. C. G., Engelsman, E., et al. (1980): Life with cytostatic drugs. *Eur. J. Cancer Clin. Oncol. (Suppl. 1).*
53. Watson, M., Greer, S., Blake, S., and Shrapnell, K. (1984): Reaction to a diagnosis of breast cancer: Relationship between denial, delay and rates of psychological morbidity. *Cancer,* 53:2008–2012.
54. Welch, D. A. (1981): Waiting, worry and the cancer experience. *Oncol. Nurs. Forum,* 8:14–18.
55. Wolpe, J. (1969): *The Practice of Behaviour Therapy.* Pergamon, New York.
56. Zeltzer, L., and Lebaron, S. (1982): Hypnosis and non-hypnotic techniques for reduction of pain and anxiety during painful procedures in children and adolescents with cancer. *J. Pediatr.,* 101:1032–1035.

The Quality of Life of Cancer Patients,
edited by N. K. Aaronson and J. Beckmann,
Raven Press, New York © 1987.

Terminally Ill Patient: Medical and Nursing Care

Richard Hillier

Countess Mountbatten House, Southhampton University Hospitals, Southampton SO3 3JB, England

The two major problems for patients with far advanced cancer and their families have been inadequate understanding of their psychosocial problems and poor symptom control. Physical symptoms, particularly pain, frequently dominate the clinical scene and prevent appropriate management of the psychosocial issues. Because most clinicians deal with both aspects of quality of life, it is essential that the patient be rendered physically comfortable before his emotional, psychological, and spiritual problems can be successfully addressed. In short, anxiety, depression, fear, isolation, and hopelessness are not only masked but aggravated by physical symptoms (7).

This chapter is unashamedly about some of the physical aspects of terminal care. Some, such as pain, vomiting, and dyspnea, are controlled by doctors, but the nurse is preeminent in the management of mouth and bowel care, fungating wounds, pressure sores, and incontinence. Unless both disciplines work closely together, the patient with complex problems—and there are many—is managed badly. Competence, cooperation, and good communication are the keys to setting and attaining clear objectives rapidly.

Fortunately, symptom control is usually synonymous with disease control, so that curative therapy also alleviates symptoms. When end-stage disease occurs, there may be a conflict between these two aims, and the judgment of the clinician and nurse may be sorely tested when attempting to alleviate symptoms and to do no harm.

Successful control of symptoms depends on what the clinician does and how he or she does it. The inexperienced doctor or nurse may fail by adopting one of the following inappropriate tactics.

1. Because the patient is dying of cancer, he requires no treatment at all.

2. Because he has cancer, intensive investigation is required that may be prolonged and distressing. Symptoms are not treated unless or until a cause is found, which may delay appropriate treatment for days or weeks.

3. Symptoms are treated, but no effort is made to diagnose their cause.

Effective management precludes all three. An accurate history, appropriate examination, and relevant, simple investigations should be performed. After weighing

239

the evidence, which may be incomplete, a presumptive diagnosis is made and treatment commenced. If treatment fails, the diagnosis is reviewed and tactics are changed.

It may be argued that this protocol is merely good medical care. So it is, but in those with terminal cancer it is often forgotten in the turmoil of distress caused by incurable disease, emotional pressure from the patient and family, and, not least, the difficulty many nurses and doctors openly admit to when dealing with the dying.

MEDICAL CARE

Pain

The incidence of severe, unrelieved pain in cancer patients is approximately 9% (4). As death approaches, this figure rises to almost 60%. The sensation of pain is complex but, at its simplest, consists in two parts. First is nociception— the perception of the painful stimulus. Second is the emotional response to the pain that is perceived. For example, someone who has been overeating views his abdominal pain quite differently from a patient who knows that his pain is due to incurable abdominal cancer.

The nature of cancer pain differs from both acute and chronic pain (Table 1), so it follows that the management of cancer pain is also different (Table 2) (10). Before treatment the importance of making an adequate assessment of pain is essential. The history, severity, and cause of discomfort must be sought; the response to previous treatment is crucial when making a useful evaluation. In addition to the usual questions determining site, periodicity, character, and possible exciting causes of the pain, the effect of analgesics used previously must be examined. Do they have *any* effect on the pain? Do they relieve or only reduce it? How long are they effective? Do they have unpleasant side effects? Which is the *patient's* preferred analgesic, and which does he dislike?

These questions elicit surprising answers. Patients frequently prefer a mild, nonsedative analgesic to a powerful drug that causes drowsiness. The secret of good pain control is to learn to use powerful drugs (e.g., the opioids) without

TABLE 1. *Characteristics of cancer pain*

Prolonged acute pain (not chronic)
Becomes worse
Purposeless and demoralizing
Aggravated by nature of illness
    Past experience, e.g., close relative died of cancer
    Anxieties, e.g., pain inevitable and uncontrollable
    Ends in death
May become "total pain"
Iatrogenic variation common

TABLE 2. *Management differences between acute pain and cancer pain*

Therapy	Acute pain	Cancer pain
Aim	Pain relief	Pain relief
Sedation	Useful	Undesirable
Desired duration of effect	2–4 hr	As long as possible
Timing	On demand	In anticipation (regular)
Dose	Standard	Individually determined
Route	Parenteral	Oral
Adjuvant medication	Rare	Frequent

From Twycross (9), with permission.

side effects. Table 3 outlines the principles of good pain control, and Table 4 summarizes common sites of pain and their appropriate treatment.

Special Pains

Bone Metastases

With carcinoma of the lung and breast and some other tumors, prostaglandin E_2 and other prostaglandins in the E series cause increased bone destruction and sensitize free nerve endings to painful stimuli (3). Patients with bone metastases from these diseases may require an analgesic but may receive more benefit from prostaglandin synthetase inhibitors of which the nonsteroidal antiinflammatory drugs are the most useful. Unfortunately, some tumors (e.g., multiple myeloma, lymphomas, and some prostatic tumors) produce bone metastases which, although they secrete osteoclastic factor, do not produce prostaglandins in the same way, making the tumors less sensitive to nonsteroidal antiinflammatory drugs. In order of preference, the following drugs may be used: aspirin, flurbiprofen, or indomethacin in conventional doses. Sometimes, however, higher doses are required, and as much as 1,200 mg of aspirin every 4 hr may be necessary.

TABLE 3. *Principles of good pain control*

Diagnose cause.
Choose appropriate analgesic.
Anticipate pain; do not pursue it.
Use regular, not as-needed, dosage.
Use individually determined doses.
Maintain alertness.
Avoid depression or euphoria.
Avoid injections.
Dependence is not a problem.
Tolerance occurs but is seldom a problem.
Treat constipation and nausea early.
Increased pain complaints mean increased pain.
Inadequate pain control—seek advice.

TABLE 4. *Pain sites and their treatment*

Site/condition	Treatment
Visceral	Opioids alone
Bone Skin infiltration }	Opioids + nonsteroidal antiinflammatory drugs
Nerve compression Elevated intercranial pressure }	Opioids + corticosteroids
Lymphedema	Compression sleeve + opioids + ? antibiotics + ? corticosteroids
Pressure sores	Nursing techniques + special equipment + antibiotics
Muscle spasm	Muscle relaxants

Nerve Compression Pain

Nerve compression pain tends to be nonresponsive to opioids unless used in high doses. Glucocorticoids may reduce tumor mass in steroid-sensitive tumors (e.g., breast, lymphoma, small-cell carcinoma of the bronchus) or may relieve pain by reducing edema around tumors of the brain or spinal cord or those involving peripheral nerves (9). High dose analgesics remain the drug treatment of choice, and a course of dexamethasone 16 mg daily for 1 week will indicate if it is to be effective. If not, it is stopped. If the patient benefits, the dose is reduced to a level just above that which causes a return of symptoms.

Other physical measures may be useful, such as nerve blocking procedures, transcutaneous nerve stimulation, or occasionally neurosurgery. Frequently, whatever measure is employed, the pain is reduced but not relieved. It is then essential to help the patient cope with the pain residue. This aim is best achieved by physiotherapy, relaxation exercises, and remobilization even in the presence of motor weakness.

Secondary Infection

Secondary infection may occur in superficial ulcerating tumors and is best treated with systemic antibiotics, adding metronidazole if anaerobic infection is present.

Lymphedema

Lymphedema occurs commonly in the arms of patients who have had a radical mastectomy or radiotherapy to the axilla, or who have recurrent axillary disease. It also occurs in the legs of patients with pelvic tumors or disease in the inguinal, pelvic, and paraaortic glands. The so-called pain of lymphedema is due to pressure exerted by edema fluid and the weight of the arm pulling on the neck, brachial plexus, or, in the case of the legs, the hips. The discomfort therefore is not a pain that readily responds to analgesics. Thus treatment is aimed at reducing the edema by a compression cuff, diuretics, or occasionally antibiotics in the infected patient. Placing the arm in a position to avoid tugging at the brachial plexus is obligatory, and the value of a course of exercises prescribed by someone familiar with the problem cannot be overstressed.

Bowel Obstruction

Acute obstruction of the bowel produces three difficult symptoms: colicky abdominal pain, vomiting, and constipation with spurious diarrhea. Surgery is appropriate in some patients; but if not, several treatment measures are required (2).

The bowel contents may be softened with dioctyl sodium sulfosuccinate, allowing easy passage of a soft stool past the obstruction. High roughage diets must be avoided, as must peristaltic laxatives. Pain may be alleviated by using antispasmodics such as loperamide or diphenoxylate with atropine. Some patients may respond to sublingual hyoscine. Contrary to popular opinion, morphine does not increase the pain in these patients and should be prescribed. Whatever measures are used, these symptoms are difficult to treat. If the above methods fail, the patient may need to be taught to live with his symptom and to accept occasional intermittent pain and occasional vomiting. If explained to them properly, most patients do this well, provided every effort is made to first alleviate the symptoms.

Headaches

The common causes of headaches are muscle tension, elevated intracranial pressure, head and neck tumors, and bone metastases in the cervical spine or occiput causing referred pain. Tension headaches must be diagnosed by exclusion because, on the whole, they are uncommon in cancer patients. Elevated intracranial pressure responds to a small dose of analgesic and dexamethasone up to 16 mg daily. With this regimen elevated intracranial pressure is rarely a problem.

Head and neck tumors grow in a particularly sensitive area with many free nerve endings. A small reduction in tumor size or peritumor edema is of disproportionate help, so corticosteroids may be useful. However, many patients complain of throbbing discomfort or pressure pain that frequently can be only partially relieved. These patients benefit from sensitive and imaginative nursing care.

Finally, cervical spine disease can be treated with radiotherapy, but occasionally patients find a soft collar useful. Hard collars are rarely helpful, even when the cervical spine is unstable, although they are frequently prescribed because of anxiety of the caregivers.

DRUGS FOR PAIN

Table 5 lists a few simple drugs, the use of which controls most pain (5). Long lists of drugs are unhelpful. The clinician must choose a few effective agents and become familiar with them.

As there is no standard dose, an appropriate regimen for each patient is required. If drugs of one strength are ineffective, a stronger analgesic (not one of similar strength) should be substituted. Once the pain is controlled, it must not be allowed to return. Thus regular dosage is essential; *pro raise nata* (prn) doses should never be used in a patient with continuous pain. For severe pain, morphine and diamorphine are still the drugs of choice for those with a limited life expectancy. Once a patient is known to be terminal, whether this means weeks, months, or years, opioid analgesics are entirely appropriate and, if properly used, do not cause problems of dependence or tolerance.

Morphine and Diamorphine

Morphine and diamorphine are well absorbed when taken by mouth, reaching peak blood levels rapidly. The dose should be individually adjusted in order to relieve pain for approximately 4 hr (6). More frequent dosage is difficult to maintain either in hospital or at home and should be avoided. The potency ratio of morphine to diamorphine is 1.5:1.0, and although the literature indicates that these drugs are interchangeable experience suggests that diamorphine causes less sedation and less nausea at high doses. Also 70% of patients require less than 30 mg morphine every 4 hr, and patients needing more should be carefully reviewed. For example, is the pain nonopioid-responsive? Is there superimposed anxiety or depression? If so, the patient requires coanalgesics, anxiolytics, or antidepressants. A coanalgesic is any drug (or device) which, though not intrinsically analgesic itself, contributes to pain relief when used with conventional analgesics.

Morphine is best given by mouth and prescribed as follows: morphine 5 mg in chloroform water to 10 ml. The initial dose is 5 mg every 4 hr day and night and is gradually titrated against the pain by raising the dose at 5-mg intervals to 20 mg, 10-mg intervals to 60 mg, and 20-mg intervals thereafter. These last high doses are rarely necessary. In the frail elderly, an initial dose of morphine 2.5 mg t.i.d. may be required, again gradually titrating the dose upward until pain relief is achieved.

The only indications for parenteral morphine in those with terminal cancer are uncontrolled vomiting, an inability to swallow, and very rarely overwhelming pain or failure to absorb the drug because of upper gastrointestinal disease. Once the pain is controlled by injection, an oral regimen can usually be resumed.

TABLE 5. *Drugs for pain*

Drug	Dose	Comments
Mild pain: nonnarcotic analgesics		
Aspirin	300–900 mg 4 hourly	Bone pain. Gastric irritation common.
Paracetamol	0.5–1.0 g 4 hourly	Bone pain and breakthrough pain.
Moderate pain: weak narcotics		
Codeine	30–60 mg 4 hourly	Constipating.
Dextropropoxyphene	32.5–65 mg 4–8 hourly	Longer duration of action causes drowsiness.
Severe pain: intermediate strength narcotics		
Dipipanone	10 mg 4–8 hourly	Dizziness common. Combined with antiemetic in Diconal.
Nepenthe	1–2 ml 4 hourly	Precipitates out in concentrated solution. Measured dose of morphine + other opium alkaloids.
More severe pain: potent narcotics		
Diamorphine	2.5–100 mg 4 hourly ⎫	Drugs of choice. Treat constipation and nausea caused by higher doses. Warn patient of initial drowsiness.
Morphine	2.5–150 mg 4 hourly ⎬	
Morphine sulfate, continuous	10–100 mg 12 hourly	New slow release narcotic useful for continuous pain. Probably causes more sedation and nausea than the above.
Very severe pain: above + adjuvants		
? Coanalgesics		Analgesics of different groups potentiate one another. Other groups indicate the complexity of pain control.
? Steroids		
? Antiemetics		
? Anxiolytics		
? Antidepressants		
? Sedative		
? Anticonvulsant		
? Muscle relaxants		

Narcotic Side Effects

Strong opioids cause drowsiness, constipation, and nausea; they do *not* cause tolerance, dependence, or destruction of the personality. All patients prescribed strong analgesics require a laxative, and those receiving more than morphine 20 mg every 4 hr require a nonsedative antiemetic (haloperidol 0.5 mg t.i.d.). If anxious, a slightly sedative antiemetic may be indicated (prochlorperazine 5 mg every 4 hr). If grossly agitated and distressed, chlorpromazine 10 to 25 mg every 4 hr is the drug of choice. Chlorpromazine is usually overprescribed to patients who do not need it.

There is no place for adding these agents to an analgesic mixture. Polypharmacy (several drugs) may be necessary, but polypharmaceuticals (several drugs in the same preparation) are not. Tolerance to drowsiness occurs within a few days of commencing treatment. Tolerance to analgesia is not a clinical problem. If the patient complains of increased pain, the pain is almost certainly due to the extending tumor.

As with many other drugs, physical dependence occurs; but should alternative treatments, e.g., radiotherapy, hypnosis, or acupuncture, render the use of analgesics unnecessary, morphine can be reduced gradually over a period of 2 weeks without fear of withdrawal symptoms.

NAUSEA AND VOMITING

The common causes of nausea and vomiting (8) in cancer patients are shown in Table 6. Those most amenable to treatment are as follows.

Hypercalcemia

Hypercalcemia is common in patients with bone metastases from breast, lung, or kidney cancers but less so with other solid tumors. Mild hypercalcemia may be treated with rehydration, prednisolone 30 mg daily, and oral phosphate unless it causes diarrhea. Salmon calcitonin may be used in an emergency but is expensive and does not control serum calcium levels unless used continuously. Mithramycin, a cytotoxic agent, in a single dose of 25 μg/kg is useful, but side effects occur if used repeatedly.

TABLE 6. *Causes of nausea and vomiting*

Drugs
  Digoxin
  Estrogens
  Opiates
Biochemical causes
  Uremia
  Hypercalcemia
  Infection
  Steroid responsive vomiting (cause unknown)
Gastric irritation
  Drugs
  Tumor
  Ulceration
Intestinal obstruction
Elevated intracranial pressure
Constipation

Elevated Intracranial Pressure

In addition to headaches, elevated intracranial pressure causes vomiting, usually in the morning; it is often projectile and frequently severe. Dexamethasone 16 mg daily with cyclizine 50 mg t.i.d. (an antiemetic that acts specifically on the vomiting center) controls most patients. If it fails, the addition of a phenothiazine is helpful.

Drugs

Apart from chemotherapeutic agents, a number of drugs and toxic substances cause vomiting in advanced cancer. Digoxin, opioids, other analgesics, and estrogens may be implicated. Uremia, hypercalcemia, and nonspecific toxemia from necrotic tumors may also induce vomiting. The use of dialysis in the uremic terminally ill patient is inappropriate. Unfortunately, this cause of vomiting is difficult to control, and chlorpromazine in sedative doses, which may also eliminate troublesome hiccups in these patients, may be necessary. Other drugs mentioned cause vomiting by their action on the chemoreceptor trigger zone. Phenothiazines or occasionally a dopamine antagonist such as metoclopramide or domperidone should eliminate the problem.

Bowel Obstruction

Bowel obstruction is common with abdominal malignancies, particularly recurrent bowel disease, ovarian tumors, or pelvic obstruction. High obstruction due to a massive tumor at the gastric outlet is often difficult to manage surgically or by any other method including drugs.

In addition to the measures described, steroids may be useful in a few patients whose tumors infiltrate the bowel wall. Because of vomiting oral medication may be difficult, and suppositories, intramuscular injections, or continuous subcutaneous infusion may be useful. The latter can maintain a patient's independence as the apparatus requires charging only once every 1 to 3 days. This method enables patients, despite bowel obstruction, to remain at home and be maintained by their family doctor or community nurses. Antiemetics may act on the vomiting center, the chemoreceptor trigger zone (adjacent to the respiratory center), and at peripheral sites in the esophagus and stomach. When vomiting is difficult to control, drugs acting on one or all of these centers may be used together.

1. Phenothiazines. Prochlorperazine may be given as 5 mg orally every 4 to 8 hr, by suppository 25 mg every 8 hr, or by injection 6.25 mg every 4 to 8 hr. More sedative is chlorpromazine 12.5 to 25 mg orally every 4 hr, by suppository 100 mg every 8 hr, or by injection 12.5 to 25 mg every 4 to 8 hr.

2. Antihistamines. Cyclizine 50 mg t.i.d. may be useful as an additive antiemetic when phenothiazines alone fail. It can be given by mouth or by injection and is the drug of choice for vomiting caused by elevated intracranial pressure.

3. Dopamine blockers. Metoclopramide 10 mg t.i.d. before meals may alleviate vomiting due to delayed gastric emptying. Domperidone 20 mg t.i.d. has a similar action but does not cross the blood-brain barrier. Thus extrapyramidal side effects are uncommon and enable the drug to be used in much higher doses if required.

If all else fails, most vomiting can be reduced by drugs to one or two episodes per day. Most patients tolerate this frequency if the doctor explains what is happening and offers continued support and advice.

DYSPNEA

The causes of dyspnea (1) are shown in Table 7 and may be treated with one or more of the following drugs.

Glucocorticoids

Prior to radiotherapy, dexamethasone 16 mg daily may control dyspnea caused by glands or tumor compressing the superior vena cava. Lymphangitis carcinomatosa

TABLE 7. *Causes of dyspnea*

Increased demand
  Fever
  Exercise
  Metabolic, e.g., uremia, diabetes mellitus
  Anemia

Decreased capacity
  Obstruction of air passages
    Extrinsic compression
    Intrinsic obstruction
    Bronchospasm
  Reduced lung elasticity
    Bronchitis and emphysema
    Lung fibrosis
  Diminished lung tissue
    Tumor
    Infection
    Pleural effusion
    Pulmonary edema
    Lymphangitis carcinomatosa
    "Muscle weakness"

Psychological causes
  Inappropriate activity
  Fear

may respond dramatically to corticosteroids, and patients with bronchospasm resistant to bronchodilators benefit. Corticosteroids reduce peritumor edema and have an antitumor effect that may reduce the dyspnea of bronchial obstruction, especially if the patient has received maximum irradiation and has a tumor insensitive to chemotherapy. There is some evidence that patients with rapidly developing pleural effusions benefit from glucocorticoids when continuous aspiration becomes unhelpful or distressing.

Antibiotics

Whether to treat a chest infection in a terminally ill cancer patient often presents a dilemma. Fortunately, the decision to treat or not to treat is usually obvious. A relatively strong patient often survives an untreated pneumonia, whereas a much weaker patient succumbs to pneumonia despite the antibiotics. Failure to treat the first group considerably reduces the quality of life; therefore when in doubt, treatment is obligatory.

Opioids

The well-known side effect of opioids—respiratory depression—is actually beneficial to the breathless cancer patient. By reducing the ventilatory drive the overwhelming desire to breathe is diminished and anxiety is reduced. Patients with dyspnea from intrathoracic disease or pleural effusions benefit from this "side effect." Morphine or morphine sulfate continuously may reduce dyspnea from a terrifying life-threatening symptom to a mere nuisance. Agitated patients may require a tranquilizer such as chlorpromazine or diazepam. Only trial and error can dictate which patient does best on which drug.

In severe terminal dyspnea morphine 5 to 20 mg i.m. with diazepam 10 mg i.m. may be necessary to sedate the patient. It is unethical to allow patients within a day or two of death to suffocate in terror because of inadequate sedation. Yet old habits die hard, and the fear of sedation, even when the patient is in extremis, often prevents them from having adequate therapy. Families and nurses never forget the badly managed respiratory death.

Hyoscine

Hyoscine 0.4 to 0.8 mg subcutaneously dries up bronchial secretions and prevents the so-called "death rattle." Normally a central nervous system (CNS) depressant, it occasionally causes agitation and should always be given with morphine 5 mg to prevent these effects. The "death rattle" in a ward or home causes considerable anxiety to relatives, and hyoscine is a useful but underused drug that can transform a ghastly, bubbling death into a gentle and peaceful one.

Oxygen

Benefits conferred by oxygen are usually psychological, based in the belief that oxygen helps all breathlessness. Unfortunately, few patients with terminal cancer benefit from its physiological properties, but once a breathless patient uses oxygen, he does not easily give it up. It should be offered only to patients who need it.

NURSING CARE

Nursing care of the terminally ill patient was discussed fully by Twycross and Lack (11).

Dry Mouth

The commonest cause of dry mouth are drugs, especially antidepressants, phenothiazines, analgesics, and other anticholinergic drugs. Dehydration, anorexia, and mouth breathing make further contributions. Patients benefit more from good mouth care than from intravenous fluids. The following aids to mouth care are essential.

The mouth is washed routinely after all food intake with a soft toothbrush. Glycerine and citric acid mouth washes are popular and may be a local stimulant to saliva production. Ice cold washes and carbonated soda are particularly refreshing, but sweet drinks should be avoided. Effervescent ascorbic acid tablets counteract a tendency to oral thrush and are well tolerated. If thrush does develop, nystatin suspension 2 ml every 2 to 4 hr for 24 hr and every 4 hr thereafter are usually effective. Amphotericin B lozenges placed under the tongue at night may help in severe cases, but they dry the mouth. Oral ketoconazole may eradicate systemic candidiasis but is less effective locally than is nystatin. Although it causes liver damage, this complication is not a serious consideration in the terminally ill.

Sialorrhea (Drooling)

Excessive salivation in patients with tumors of the mouth is distressing. Atropine drops (2%) may temporarily reduce the production of saliva, but longer effects are achieved with atropine tablets 0.6 mg b.i.d., at the cost of side effects of dry mouth and occasionally agitation. Some patients respond to amitriptyline 25 mg at night for 3 weeks, after which dribbling may take several weeks to return. Excessive salivation is difficult to treat, however, and radiotherapy is occasionally necessary to destroy the salivary glands. However, even this measure is usually disappointing. Thus constant mopping by the patient or nurse may be all that can be done. Most patients with severe sialorrhea are usually sufficiently ill to survive only a short time.

Constipation

To be constipated is to pass a hard stool infrequently and with difficulty. The causes are shown in Table 8. Most dying patients become constipated. Thus treatment should be anticipated and vigorous to avoid fecal impaction. The bowel habits of patients must be carefully assessed. Ask about constipation, but if in doubt perform a rectal examination. Even then, no stool may be found and, in the patient who is eating but not having his bowels open, an enema often produces good results. Constant attention to the bowels with regular rectal examination avoids many unnecessary hospital admissions.

Patients must be encouraged to exercise whenever possible, maintain fluid intake, and consume bulk purgatives in the diet. Bran is unacceptable to many ill patients, causing discomfort, belching, and flatus. Fybogel and isogel are preferable. If a commode is placed next to the bed, patients are encouraged to answer the call to stool instead of waiting until someone is available to help them. Depression aggravates constipation and should be treated. When constipating drugs are used with dying patients, a laxative should be prescribed routinely.

Peristaltic agents are best, so Dorbanex (danthron and poloxamer) 5 to 10 ml b.i.d. is useful. Many similar agents are available and also contain stool softeners. If the feces becomes impacted, the following may be necessary: (a) manual removal of rock-hard feces; (b) glycerine or stimulant suppository; (c) softening of a hard stool with arachis oil followed by a normal saline enema or a Fletcher's phosphate enema (the latter is disposable and ideal for home use); and (d) regular laxatives prescribed thereafter.

Unfortunately, despite adequate oral laxatives, some patients still require routine suppositories or an occasional enema. Thus constant vigilance is necessary.

TABLE 8. *Causes of constipation in cancer patients*

Diminished food consumption
Inadequate roughage
Poor fluid intake
Reduced exercise
Specific bowel problem
Failure to answer call to stool
Depression
Drugs
Analgesics
Anxiolytics
Antiemetics
Antidepressants

Patients with spinal cord compression caused by local bone metastases may become paraplegic and lose control of their bowels. Laxatives should be avoided and manual evacuation performed regularly, twice a week 1 hr after a small dose of diazepam to relieve the patient's distress. Patients usually tolerate this procedure well and between evacuations remain continent and comfortable.

Urinary Incontinence

Urinary incontinence occurs with some pelvic tumors, bladder neck problems, and paraplegia and in the confused or weak elderly patient. Urinary tract infection should be sought and in patients with bladder spasm an antispasmodic prescribed.

If these measures fail, a wet bed ensues; pressure sores are more likely, constant changing of bed linen exhausts elderly relatives, and the persistent smell of urine distresses families and staff. In such patients the long-term risks of catheterization are far outweighed by the current problem, and a catheter should be inserted with appropriate antibiotic cover. This measure improves the general situation and condition of the patient and enables many relatives to nurse a patient at home when previously it would have been impossible.

Fungating Tumors

The commonest fungating tumor is carcinoma of the breast, but occasionally carcinoma of the vulva or more rarely carcinoma of the rectum fungate externally. Satellite lesions may form, break down, become infected, and produce painful, ulcerated, stinking lesions. They are always distressing and a constant reminder, day and night, of spreading disease. Treatment should be as follows.

1. Local radiotherapy and chemotherapy may be effective initially, but even then regression is usually temporary.

2. Aserbine (Bencard) may be used for desloughing the area.

3. Infected lesions are cleaned with half-strength eusol or hydrogen peroxide, after which the lesion is cleaned with normal saline.

4. If the lesion needs to be packed, gauze soaked in half-strength eusol and liquid paraffin is applied twice daily.

5. Gentian violet is a useful antiseptic, and some patients benefit from it and oral metronidazole 200 mg every 8 hr.

Topical antibiotics are contraindicated because sensitivity reactions are common. Neomycin may be absorbed by the lesion and causes deafness. Regular, frequent attention to these lesions with clean dressings to soak the often profuse discharge is mandatory. Temporary hospital admission gives the family or nursing staff a break from what is undoubtedly an onerous and unpleasant task.

Occasionally, persistent capillary or small arterial bleeding occurs. Pads soaked in epinephrine 1:1,000 may be useful for capillary bleeding, but single fraction radiotherapy is most effective when the bleeding is more profuse and does not cease spontaneously as it often does. Severe bleeding is a radiotherapeutic emergency.

Smell can be prevented by the use of charcoal-containing Denidor pads. Mechanical deodorizers are now so effective smell need no longer be a major problem.

CONCLUSION

Issues in this chapter are rather different from those found in other sections of this volume. However, patients usually approach doctors and nurses because of physical symptoms, and so it is essential to understand them if the physical aspects of quality of life are to improve.

There is a more important issue than this, however. By paying sufficient attention to the details of symptom control, the staff can always return to the patient with something more to offer, and they need never say or believe that there is nothing more to be done. This measure increases the caregiver's confidence, improves communication with the patient, and enables compassion—that virtue so highly rated by patients—to be imparted without embarrassment or shame.

REFERENCES

1. Baines, M. (1985): Control of other symptoms. In: *The Management of Terminal Diseases*, edited by C. M. Saunders. Edward Arnold, London.
2. Baines, M. J. (1984): The medical management of malignant bowel obstruction. In: *Cancer Chemotherapy and Selective Drug Development*, edited by K. R. Harrup, W. Davis, and A. H. Calvert. Martinus Nijhoff, Boston.
3. Ferreira, S. H. (1972): Prostaglandins, aspirin-like drugs and analgesia. *Nature*, 240:200–203.
4. Foley, K. M. (1979): Pain syndromes in patients with cancer. In: *Advances in Pain Research and Therapy*, Vol. 2, edited by J. J. Bonica and V. Ventafridda. Raven Press, New York.
5. Hanks, G. (1985): Pain control in cancer patients. *Cancer Top.*, 5:54–56.
6. Hillier, E. R. (1983): Oral narcotic mixtures. *Br. Med. J.*, 287:701.
7. Hinton, J. (1972): *Dying*. Penguin, London.
8. Saunders, C., and Baines, M. (1983): *Living with Dying: The Management of Terminal Disease*. Oxford University Press, Oxford.
9. Twycross, R. G. (1979): Non-narcotic, corticosteroid and psychotropic drugs. In: *The Continuing Care of Terminal Cancer Patients*, edited by R. G. Twycross and V. Ventafridda. Penguin, Oxford.
10. Twycross, R. G., and Lack, S. A. (1983): *Symptom Control in Far Advanced Cancer: Pain Relief*. Pitman, London.
11. Twycross, R. G., and Lack, S. A. (1984): *Therapeutics in Terminal Cancer*. Pitman, London.

The Quality of Life of Cancer Patients,
edited by N. K. Aaronson and J. Beckmann,
Raven Press, New York © 1987.

Care of the Dying*

Loma Feigenberg

Karolinska Sjukhuset, S-10401 Stockholm, Sweden

Dying is painful, alarming, and fraught with questions. Even so, people have always tried to succor a person whose life is drawing to a close.

Thanatology, as it is now called, started from this care of dying persons, but in its professional form thanatology has come to include many other aspects of life and death. The literature on clinical thanatology is not easily translated into the daily language of hospital care. An attempt is made here to communicate the content of psychological care of the dying without requiring that the reader is acquainted with abstruse psychological theory. The approach described here is applicable wherever dying persons are cared for, whether at hospitals or homes for the aged, hospices, or highly specialized departments for intensive care. It applies, moreover, to doctors as much as to nurses, to persons of religion as much as to social workers, and so on.

DYING: WHAT IS IT?

Dying is the process a person goes through from his or her first inkling, suspicion, or awareness of dying on up to the time when death occurs. It may take seconds, as when death results from a well-aimed bullet or a fatal accident, or it may last weeks or months if the agent is a stroke or cancer. In this chapter we concentrate on dying due to cancer; in principle it does not differ from other dying, though it may be easier to study because the course tends to be more protracted.

There is a biological dimension to dying that cannot be averted or altered. Far more important is the psychological dimension, with its fluctuations, upheavals, and transformations. It is a process wherein the dying person goes through a great deal and another person can be of great assistance, making a contribution that is meaningful for both.

REQUIREMENTS FOR CARE OF THE DYING

Three things are required of those who want to provide good psychological care in health and sickness, not least when caring for persons who are dying. They are knowledge, empathy, and self-awareness.

---

* A version of this chapter appeared in *Terminal Care: Friendship Contracts with Dying Cancer Patients.* Brunner/Mazel, New York, 1980.

Knowledge and Skills

General knowledge concerning thanatology is best acquired from anthologies (1,2,5,7). There is also the author's survey of the literature on psychological care of dying persons (3).

Basic insight into the psychology of dying can be acquired from a textbook by Kastenbaum and Aisenberg (6). Some prior knowledge of psychology and psychiatry is often needed when reading in this field. There are many articles and books to choose from, depending on one's knowledge and experience. Among the best are those of Weisman (9) and Shneidman (8).

Reading is by no means the only source of knowledge and skills. Contacts and talks with dying persons are at least as important, as is the exchange of experience with friends and associates in group meetings, discussions, role play, and so on. Fiction is a never-ending source of knowledge and understanding in these matters.

Empathy

Empathy concerns our ability to feel our way into and share another person's situation, what that person is feeling and going through. It involves trying to identify with and join in the other's reality so far as one possibly can. It is conceivable that the talent for empathy varies, but it is clear that empathy is also an ability that can be improved by practice. One way is to think of the dying person as someone who is close to you (a parent, son or daughter, husband or wife) and then try to imagine how that person would feel and react in the dying person's situation.

Self-Awareness

In all work there is a psychological motivation for—and perhaps also against— what one is doing. Coping with the task, which is unquestionably onerous, of keeping close to a person who is dying presupposes that many aspects of one's personality are harnessed to the work. Some persons are afraid and unwilling to care for the dying, just as others are overeager. Some degree of self-knowledge about one's motives is necessary.

Persons whose work—as a doctor, nurse, social worker, church representative— brings them into touch with many people have opportunities for introspection. From one's reactions to different personalities and situations one can soon learn that one has no trouble talking with some people but cannot abide others, just as one is excessively protective in some instances and aggressive in others. Such observations are the first step toward studying and understanding how one interreacts with other people.

IS CARE OF THE DYING PSYCHOTHERAPY?

Caring for dying persons is liable to arouse one's own anxiety and elicit depression and bereavement. Many consider that the work is unsuitable or even harmful for the practitioner. Although it is unduly demanding for some, the work is also truly rewarding, which tends to be overlooked. It widens one's horizon, granting meaningful and moving experiences of the realities of life.

It is argued by some, either from professional pride by some psychotherapists or from a contemptuous somatic viewpoint, that this work is in fact tantamount to psychotherapy. According to Feigenberg and Shneidman (4), care of the dying cannot be equated with psychotherapy. In our view, psychotherapeutic knowledge is part of the foundation for psychological care of the dying; but although such care is related to psychotherapy, there are essential differences. In simple terms, psychotherapy invariably aims at ultimately leaving the patient feeling better, feeling more healthy, and functioning better. This is not the case in care of the dying. The person is dying and knows it, as does the therapist, and both are aware that their relationship is to be terminated by death. This fact is the crux of all work with dying persons.

This is not to say that knowledge of psychotherapy is irrelevant to such work. Indeed, many clinical thanatologists have psychotherapeutic training. The danger lies in being tied down by psychotherapy's strict rules, so that one makes the mistake of "digging too deep," interpreting too much, and raising anxiety-provoking subjects and problems that the dying person no longer has the strength to tackle. When working with dying persons it is essential to be as flexible as possible.

CARING FOR DYING PERSONS

Many hesitate to undertake psychological care of the dying because they are afraid of causing harm. This risk is, in fact, slight. Others are simply afraid of being alone with a dying person. Such fears are groundless if one can display respect and warmth. What matters is that one manages to establish a natural relationship, listens in an interested, involved way, and initiates and maintains a meaningful dialogue.

A dialogue involves one person saying something and the other reacting in an adequate, understandable way, whereupon the first person reacts in a manner that, for him, is reasonable and logical and expresses his feelings. The dialogue between the two then continues and in this case ceases only when the dying person is no longer able to communicate.

If the contact is to be satisfactory for the therapist and meaningful for the dying person, it presupposes the three requirements mentioned earlier: knowledge, empathy, and self-knowledge. One cannot say that any one of these is more important than the other two. What is called for is a good mixture. Some people with empathy and self-knowledge manage to do excellent work with only a modicum of knowledge. Others have extensive knowledge and a fair amount of empathy but do more harm than good for want of self-knowledge. It may be one's own needs rather than concern for dying persons that prompts one to undertake this work. A typical example is a need to make amends for an unprocessed bereavement. Generally speaking, these three requirements are adequately met by a great many people who really do want and are able to care for dying persons in an atmosphere of solidarity and companionship and who consequently help many persons to die ''better'' than is usually the case at present.

The person who is best suited in the individual case is preferably chosen by the person who is dying. Personal contacts are formed without heeding organizational rules. Thus when one has been initiated with a doctor, nurse, social worker, or anyone else and the dying person so wishes, the relationship should be developed and strengthened in such time as remains.

FRAME FOR THE WORK

No two persons are exactly alike, and neither are their deaths. Consequently, the work of caring for dying persons cannot be specified in detail. Its nature requires that arrangements vary.

A person who wishes to work with psychological care of the dying must in the first place convey to the subject that he or she is prepared to do so. This message should be communicated explicitly, or not, as the case may be. A regular introductory talk may be called for in some situations, whereas in others a contact with, say, a doctor or nurse may gradually turn into psychological terminal care.

What is imperative is that once a terminal contact has been offered and accepted, the promise must be kept. To fail such a contact is a serious breach of another person's confidence. One should indicate early on how often one intends to come and then be sure to stick to the schedule. At first it may be a question of meeting once a month or perhaps once a week. It is always beneficial and particularly so during this phase to consult the doctors and nurses in charge concerning the medical situation.

More frequent visits are necessary as the patient gets worse and death approaches. By changing spontaneously to visits twice a week and ultimately every day, one confirms—without having to say so explicitly—one's knowledge that the patient's condition has deteriorated.

The interval between meetings should be shortened in accordance with the circumstances. There is seldom any need to call more than once or twice a day and at this stage one should not tax the patient with long sessions. It would be wrong to sit with the dying person all day. Relatives may pay a visit at certain times, and the daily routines are handled by the regular staff. Even if it happens to be, for example, the duty nurse who is providing psychological terminal care in addition to her professional functions, it is sufficient to come for a limited time each day and make it clear that the visit is for the special purpose of continuing with the dialogue that is in progress.

It should also be stressed—though it ought to be self-evident—that whatever is said in the course of the contact is personal and private. It must not be revealed to others. If the contact is to be meaningful, the dying person must come to understand that it is safe to bring up difficult matters, e.g., relations with close relatives or a husband or wife. The dying person must feel certain that, even when the subject of the difficulty is present, the partner in the contact has the tact and good judgment not to divulge what has passed between them.

The possibility of privacy varies with the circumstances. In a large institution where the beds are close together, a confidential exchange may be difficult to achieve. At the same time, there have been cases where I found reason to carry through the contact so that the relatives were completely excluded from it; in such cases I conclude a specific contract both with the dying person and with the relatives. This method (3), which is appropriate in certain rather special situations, calls for particular thanatological experience. In most cases of psychological terminal care, such strict confidentiality is not required; but the recurrent meetings should be arranged with reasonable privacy.

CONTENT OF THE MEETINGS

The subjects that arise in the course of contacts with dying persons are infinite. It should be emphasized that *nothing* the person talks about is uninteresting, unimportant, or indifferent. On the contrary, whether the imminent death is being talked about openly, all the dying person's internal perceptions are stamped with the threat of death. Therefore he or she does not have the time, the possibility, or the strength to talk about anything except what is of central importance.

It follows that those who work with dying persons should be very attentive, even to what may seem irrelevant. One should try to remember everything that is said; moreover, the things that are not said should be registered too. As the contact proceeds, something is bound to come up that relates to, or perhaps contradicts, an earlier remark. Being able to refer back to it is then of great value as an indication that one remembers and has understood, that the listener attaches importance to everything the dying person has to say.

However widely the dying person may range in the course of the talks, the subject matter can generally be assigned to one of three areas: the past, the present, and what lies ahead. The dying person always wants to talk about his or her life, about *what lies in the past:* childhood, growing up, youth, and school; religious, political, and occupational ties; achievements and setbacks; loved ones and intimate relationships; children; all the dreams and fantasies, all the ideals and hopes that have been cherished in the past.

The second area is *the present.* Everything that is now happening to the dying person from day to day is of crucial importance to him. It influences his perception of past events, of what remains of life, and of what may follow after death. A state of flux and upheaval is thus at the heart of dying. Taking part in this process and sharing as far as possible in the dying person's experience is the kernel of psychological terminal care.

The third area is the dying person's thoughts and conceptions of what we usually refer to as *life after death*. The dying person must be given a chance of verbalizing anxiety about what may lie ahead, of talking about religious matters, about fear of punishment and hope of atonement. He must be able to express a belief in eternal life or a conviction that after death there is nothing, as the case may be. This area, in other words, concerns conceptions of life, matters to do with ethics, philosophy, and religion.

Although the dying person's philosophy or religious beliefs should be respected during these talks, it is also important that one is honest, if asked, about one's own ideas and beliefs. One is not there to influence, persuade, or convert. It is a question of showing that the listener appreciates the dying person's point of view even if it is not shared.

During the contact it is the dying person who decides the subjects to talk about. Whereas psychotherapy, for instance, sticks to certain subjects or takes up one problem at a time in accordance with a plan, talks with a dying person frequently shift from topic to topic. One needs to be flexible in order to follow such changes during the terminal process. It is also important that changes of opinion are accepted with understanding. A disparaging remark about a relative in the morning may be followed by a need later in the day to correct or modify it or look for mitigating circumstances.

DIMENSIONS OF DYING

Death comes to us all and is therefore in a sense banal and commonplace. However, just as each life is unique, so is its conclusion. In this section is described what takes place on the psychological or human plane and what one aims at when trying to participate in, understand, and even share another person's dying.

A number of dimensions, spectra, or polarities that have proved relevant when working in relationships with dying persons are formulated. These dimensions, which serve as the basis of *questions one should ask oneself* continuously during such a contact, are provisional. The intention is neither to include every conceivable dimension, which would be impossible, nor to erect distinct boundaries. On the contrary, these dimensions are interrelated and fuse more and more as death approaches. Applying as much empathy and flexibility as possible, one must try to feel one's way in the psychological sphere, understanding needs and finding means of meeting them.

Time: The Central Dimension in Dying

Time and death are inextricably combined. The regular passage of time is accompanied by great changes at many levels in the dying person. Death is made dramatic by the existence of time.

A distinction can be made between chronological, biological, and subjective time. Chronological time is time as measured by clocks. It is a strictly subdivided, linear account of a progression we have agreed to measure in a particular way.

Subjective time is our perception of time. Its rhythm is entirely different from that of chronological time. Happy experiences cause us to forget time, and we complain that time is too brief; painful experiences cause time to seem interminable.

Like biological time, which is not considered here, subjective time continuously undergoes convulsive changes during the process of dying. There is a constant struggle to reconcile the time that has passed with the time that remains. Present time becomes chaotic.

The perception of time becomes more diffuse as dying progresses, partly for psychological reasons and partly because of the medicines administered. Hospital routines follow their chronological schedule, and the patient is upset by the discordance between what is going on around him and what he is experiencing.

By calling at an agreed time, regularly at first and then more and more frequently, one can represent a kind of continuity for the dying person. This continuity can help him or her hold on to the perception of time, as it were, from outside. We must also learn to understand and accept that the dying person's subjective time fluctuates and changes. We may consider that he is wrong; but his perception of time is not right or wrong—it simply *is*.

Denial and Acceptance

Denial is a common defense mechanism, and medical personnel are learning more and more to recognize and accept it. When something that we have been aware of and able to talk about becomes too threatening—when anxiety exceeds a certain threshold—we may seek protection in denial, in "forgetting" reality. This attitude is often dismissed contemptuously as "weakness," as childish or inappropriate behavior. Yet we all practice denial to some extent in respect to some aspect of our life. We succeed to varying degrees in denying death and the threat of death that resides in each of us.

The important point about this dimension is that dying persons never deny everything fully and completely, neither do they accept everything fully and completely; instead they move to and fro between these two extremes. Many factors in the process of dying cause this fluctuation; they are mostly psychological, but there is also the physical consequence of the person's disease. Those who work with terminal patients need to recognize, tolerate, and respect the fact that we all, to some extent, deny the realities we encounter in the course of our lives.

Right to Know and to Not Want to Know

This chapter is not the place to discuss the complex problem of whether patients should or should not be told the truth about their disease, its course, and likely outcome. A vast amount has been written on the subject, and the number of opinions is legion. It seems that the aim should be to say at each meeting whatever is best for the dying person's physical and mental health at that time. The more psychological insight one acquires and the more discerning one becomes, the better will one know what to say and, at least as important, how to say it. This function, so essential in all medical care, calls for knowledge and skills, empathy, and self-knowledge, as emphasized earlier.

A patient who really wants to know about his condition has a right to be told, but the reverse applies too: One must accept that a patient, or in this case a person who is dying, may not want to acknowledge more than part of the truth. The dying person is entitled not to want to know and to decide for himself how much he wants to know. A further point to remember is that a dying person nearly always knows and understands more than we realize, just because he is dying, but it is by no means certain that he wishes to talk about his innermost knowledge with just anyone or in just any situation. A person who is able to accompany the patient's journeys to and fro along this dimension is increasingly equipped to provide support and understanding.

Losses and Gains

Dying always involves a series of losses. All one's dreams must be relinquished. Many bodily functions are lost. One is to leave all those he loves, all those who have been of significance; and finally comes the hardest blow of all—the loss of one's self.

To offset all these losses to some extent, we can try to give something of our own selves. Taking a dying person seriously, showing respect and warmth and sharing his experiences as far as is possible—these can be substantial gains for that person. This aspect is not always recognized in medical care.

Hope and Despair

Hope can be seen as an internal, deeply rooted sense of being welcome in the world and a feeling that one's existence is in some way good and desirable. The feeling of hope is often established during childhood and endures through life. In terminal patients it is not a matter of a naïve hope of survival. They know that they are going to die, and few expect a miracle.

The converse of hope is despair or total surrender. One can provide support and be of great assistance by constantly asking oneself where on this dimension the patient happens to be. One needs to recognize the factors in that particular person's life which underpin and increase his hope; one needs to appreciate why he despairs. It is a matter of trying to share what is happening and yet maintain sufficient distance to avoid despairing oneself.

Will to Live and Desire to Die

The will to live and the desire to die, opposites, are related to hope and despair. Our profound wish to live has not been studied much and is little understood. Clearly we may also entertain a wish to die, as manifested in suicidal wishes, ideas, and actions. It is understandable that a dying person's view of his situation may induce a wish to terminate it. Sharing a person's feelings between the two extremes of this painful dimension, allowing him to talk frankly, is a way of affording relief and comfort. Medical caregivers at present have difficulty allowing patients to express a longing to die. Such feelings usually arouse contempt or anxiety in the listener.

Revolt and Submission

Dying patients are obviously liable to revolt. Their protest may be directed against God, the medical service, a relative, fate, or much besides. However, it also happens that, for no apparent reason, a dying person submits and even says disparaging or contemptuous things about himself. Numerous factors are included in this dimension, which is closely related to the dimension of identity versus dissolution. Many people revolt when they sense that their identity is disintegrating; others succumb in submission and self-effacement. It is up to us to stay close, hold the dying person's hand, listen to what is said, and perhaps refer back to what was said some days or weeks ago when that person was stronger. Things the dying person has said about his life can be used to illuminate, explain, or perhaps refute, in a constructive way, what he now brings up.

Security and Insecurity

Many patients are aware that their behavior is trying, that they have cried or screamed, been aggressive, that in their present state they smell, look unpleasant, and so on. They fear that this is how they will be remembered; they are apprehensive about what people will say of them afterward. It is up to us to reassure them, to explain that one understands the way things are, and that one is going to stand by them.

By continuing to return, even though the dying person has changed and may appear frightening, one can create at least some security for him. Dying persons often ask if one has been present at a deathbed before. Such questions may imply a fear that one will stop coming when things get really bad. They may also indicate a need to know if a person has stayed on until the end and if it is bearable to watch the coming of death.

Dying persons usually ask if one will remember them after they have gone.

Assurance on this point provides a measure of security. Perhaps it should be added that anyone who has really managed to be with a dying person certainly remembers him.

Dignity and Humiliation

It is common nowadays to talk about people "dying with dignity," to say that we should contribute to a "dignified death." I am not so sure if this involves preconceptions about how people "ought" to die—that they should be "strong," or grateful to those around them, or friendly and courteous. This amounts to imposing some of our own ideas about what is and is not dignified. Only the person who is dying knows what is dignified for him. Our job is to help him in this respect. During the process of dying the dignified and the undignified, the ugly and the beautiful, move closer and closer together; their beings become increasingly interwoven.

Living and Dying

A dying person is evidently dying, with all that this implies. However, he is still alive and has a right to be treated and regarded as a living person. It means that he should be permitted to perform all the activities of which he is still capable. Nothing should be "taken over" by the staff or others that the patient can still manage. One must talk *to* the patient and not *about* him in his presence. All the respect we show to living persons, whoever they may be, is still due when they are dying. The time will come when the dying person is less able to cope and needs more and more assistance. Responding to this need in ways that are not humiliating can be difficult, but it is essential throughout the process of dying and not least during the final stage. Thus the primary aim of what we call clinical thanatology is to help the dying person to live until he dies.

REFERENCES

1. Feifel, H., ed. (1959): *The Meaning of Death*. McGraw-Hill, New York.
2. Feifel, H., ed. (1977): *New Meanings of Death*. McGraw-Hill, New York.
3. Feigenberg, L. (1980): *Terminal Care: Friendship Contracts with Dying Cancer Patients*. Brunner/Mazel, New York.
4. Feigenberg, L., and Shneidman, E. S. (1979): Clinical thanatology and psychotherapy: Some reflections on caring for the dying person. *Omega*, 10:1–8.
5. Fulton, R., ed., in collaboration with Bendiksen, R. (1976): *Death and Identity*. Charles Press, Bowie, Maryland.
6. Kastenbaum, R., and Aisenberg, R. (1972, 1976): *The Psychology of Death*. Springer, New York.
7. Shneidman, E. S. (1976): *Death: Current Perspectives*. Mayfield, Palo Alto.
8. Schneidman, E. S. (1978): Some aspects of psychotherapy with dying persons. In: *Psychosocial Care of the Dying Patient*, edited by C. A. Garfield, pp. 201–218. McGraw-Hill, New York.
9. Weisman, A. D. (1972): *On Dying and Denying: A Psychiatric Study of Terminality*. Behavioural Publications, New York.

The Quality of Life of Cancer Patients,
edited by N. K. Aaronson and J. Beckmann,
Raven Press, New York © 1987.

Self-Care of Cancer Patients

Jean F. A. Pruyn and H. W. van den Borne

IVA, Institute for Social Research, University of Tilburg, 5000 LE Tilburg, The Netherlands

With respect to self-help and mutual support groups in cancer, Holland and Rowland (4) ended their historical review with the following passage:

> Oncology has been cautious in accepting the "fellow" patient concept of employing contemporary patients in the cancer treatment process to help one another; the caution, however, is diminishing. This is particularly true as oncologists recognize the unique nature of fellow-patient support, which goes beyond that available in the medical setting and is of mutual benefit to those who receive and provide it. These social and mutual patient help efforts are being increasingly accepted by the medical community and reflect the current trend toward greater willingness to utilize psychological and social interventions.

As distinct from Holland and Rowland (4), who seemed to expect a rather positive attitude toward fellow-patient support in the medical setting, a study in which data were collected in 146 Dutch hospitals reported some negative reactions from professional caregivers (13). Until now there are few data available on the background, functioning, and effects of contacts between fellow-sufferers, i.e., people who had to cope with the same problems after a cancer diagnosis.

At this moment in The Netherlands, eight self-help groups for cancer patients are nationally organized. An important instrument for most of these organizations is the volunteer ex-patient who already has been through the illness and its consequences. This volunteer tries to support new cancer patients by means of personal (face-to-face) contact in which an exchange of experiences and feelings can take place (7,13). Of course, nonorganized contacts between fellow-sufferers also take place.

In this chapter we describe some aspects of the contact between cancer patients. From a social-psychological perspective we examine the process of social comparison as a means of elucidating the motives for seeking contact with a fellow-sufferer. These motives are closely related to problems experienced by cancer patients. The main problems cancer patients can experience are also described according to a theoretical model on coping with cancer. Insight into the main problems experienced by cancer patients is necessary in order to determine the possible effects of contact between fellow-sufferers.

Results of a study we carried out with 498 cancer patients provide further information on problems experienced by cancer patients and on contact with fellow-sufferers, and the method of this study is briefly described. A description of contact between fellow-sufferers is given, and the need for social comparison is presented against the background of the actual contact with fellow-sufferers. The first contact with a fellow-sufferer and a further account of the contact is presented, and the effects of contact with fellow-sufferers are described.

SOCIAL-PSYCHOLOGICAL PERSPECTIVE ON COPING WITH CANCER AND CONTACT WITH FELLOW-SUFFERERS

In a theoretical model we developed on coping with cancer, the following four main problems a cancer patient may confront are distinguished (5,6,12).

1. *Uncertainty*. Uncertainty can be defined as the experience of a lack of information in an area that is important for the patient. Uncertainty can refer to questions about the illness or treatment as well as to questions about where and how to get help for various problems.

2. *Negative feelings*. Negative feelings often occur in cancer patients. Fear, anxiety, and depression are mentioned most frequently in the literature. Other negative feelings include apathy, sorrow, feelings of shame, and loneliness.

3. *Loss of control*. This concept can be defined as the feeling of being unable to handle, manage, and influence events. Loss of control can be related to several events. A cancer patient may believe that he no longer has a hold on his own situation and that he cannot make plans for the longer term (e.g., as a result of admission to a hospital).

4. *Threats to self-esteem*. A patient whose self-esteem had previously been based on his own body, his achievements, and his relations with others may believe his self-esteem is threatened when cancer has been diagnosed or after treatment (e.g., mastectomy).

We assume that a patient wants to see a reduction in uncertainty and negative feelings, tries to get a (fresh) hold on his new situation, and wants to restore his self-esteem. A patient can use many means (coping strategies) to bring this about. One means is to seek contact with fellow-sufferers. Social comparison theory proposes that people first try to reduce their feeling of *uncertainty* by seeking as much objective information as possible ("hard" facts) (2), e.g., from experts such as the treating doctor or nurses. To the degree that objective information cannot be obtained in this way, a patient looks for it from other people, preferably people like himself. In the case of a cancer patient, these persons are fellow-sufferers who have to go through the same problems. In this way a patient can clarify his ideas about his illness and treatment and about possible solutions, despite the fact that he has no objective information available.

Social comparison theory also proposes that in the case of *fear* people need to seek out the company of comparable others, i.e., people in the same situation (8). Such contact can reduce fear through mutual support, trust, confirmation, and caring. It can also enable people to evaluate their feelings of fear. That is, by comparing themselves with people in the same situation, they can judge if their feelings are "normal" (1). Finally, social comparison proposes that people strive for favorable *self-esteem* (11). In a threatening situation (e.g., cancer) social comparison theory proposes that the person wants to compare himself to someone who is worse off (3). Results from a study in 78 women with breast cancer confirmed this proposition (9,10).

It can be concluded that by means of social comparison patients strive to: (a) reduce or solve uncertainty (evaluative function); (b) reduce or solve fear and other negative feelings (direct stress reduction); (c) reduce uncertainty over one's emotion (evaluative function); and (d) maintain, restore, or enhance self-esteem ("enhancement" function).

It is possible that the above-mentioned "drives" oppose each other. For example, contact with a fellow-sufferer can reduce uncertainty but at the same time evoke anxiety. Although one can benefit from comparing oneself with other people, it is also possible that social comparison delivers "costs." Such a "costs/benefits" analysis can, among other things, explain why one cancer patient may express a need for social comparison (and seeks and makes contact) with a fellow-sufferer, whereas another does not.

METHOD OF THE STUDY

In order to gain insight into the background factors, extent, and effectiveness of aftercare by fellow-sufferers, we carried out interviews with two types of cancer patient for whom there was nationally organized aftercare by fellow-sufferers in The Netherlands. Through the cooperation of medical specialists in 15 medical centers across The Netherlands, the National Organization for Breast Cancer Volunteers, and the Hodgkin's Contact Group, we were ultimately able to interview 216 patients with Hodgkin's disease (or non-Hodgkin's lymphoma)—hereafter referred to as Hodgkin's patients—and 282 breast cancer patients who had had a breast amputation. Their socioeconomic and demographic data are presented in Table 1.

The mean age of the Hodgkin's patients was 40 and for the breast cancer patients 56. Most of the patients in both samples had received the diagnosis of their illness from their physicians within the past 5 years and had undergone treatment (operation, radiation therapy, or chemotherapy) within the past 3 years.

The interviews were conducted in the patients' homes during February and March 1982. Forty female interviewers with prior interviewing experience were selected from a pool of applicants and were specially trained in interviewing cancer patients. Each interview lasted approximately 2 hr. Most of the questions in the interview were structured, requiring subjects to provide specific information and ratings about their problems experienced such as uncertainty, fear, anxiety, depression, loneliness, sleep disturbance, loss of control, and threat to self-esteem. Specific

TABLE 1. *Socioeconomic and demographic characteristics of Hodgkin's and breast cancer patients*

Characteristic	Hodgkin's		Breast cancer	
	%	No.	%	No.
Sex				
Male	57	123	—	
Female	43	93	100	282
Age (years)				
0–30	26	56	1	3
31–40	32	69	7	20
41–50	18	39	21	59
51–60	13	28	28	79
61+	11	24	43	121
Marital status				
Married/living together	81	175	69	195
Divorced	1	2	3	8
Single	16	35	11	31
Widowed	2	4	17	48
Family income level (Dutch guilders per month)				
0–1,500	14	28	30	76
1,500–2,000	26	53	27	68
2,000–2,800	30	61	23	58
2,800 or more	30	60	20	51
Total		202		253
Type of education				
Elementary school	17	29	28	54
Beginning vocational school	27	46	26	49
Intermediate vocational school	12	21	13	25
Advanced vocational school	11	19	10	19
High school	28	48	17	32
College/university	5	9	6	11
Total		172		190

information was also gathered about coping strategies and received information (e.g., from their medical specialist) and support (e.g., the openness to discuss the illness in the family). Finally, extensive questions were asked about social comparison and contact with fellow-sufferers.

NEED FOR SOCIAL COMPARISON AND ACTUAL CONTACT WITH FELLOW-SUFFERERS

The need for social comparison with fellow-patients was operationalized by the question: To what extent would you like to know more about how other people who are in the same circumstances as you react to their illness and treatment? Respondents could answer this question by means of four alternatives: "not at all," "a little," "somewhat," and "very much." Table 2 presents the distribution of scores for this question.

It can be seen that about one-fourth of the Hodgkin's patients and one-half of the patients with breast cancer had no need for social comparison with fellow-sufferers and that, respectively, three-fourths and one-half of the respondents experienced, to some degree, a need for social comparison with fellow-patients.

By "contact with fellow-sufferers" we meant a form of *personal contact* that people have with one or more patients or ex-patients with the same illness through the media, face-to-face or telephone conversations about problems or experiences, correspondence, and so on. Of the 216 Hodgkin's patients, 109 (51%) had at some time had contact with fellow-sufferers; the corresponding figure for the 282 breast cancer patients was 156 (55%). We also found that, at the time of the interview, respectively, 22.5% and 16.3% of the respondents expressed the need for actual contact with a fellow-sufferer.

A need for social comparison does not always lead to actual contact with fellow-sufferers. The most important reason for not having contact is the fact that one does not know a fellow-sufferer. About three-fourths (74%, $n = 136$) of the respondents who expressed a need for social comparison but did not have contact with a fellow patient stated that they had not had such contact because they did not know any fellow-sufferer. One of every five of all respondents (21%, $n = 494$) reported that they would like to know ("somewhat" or "very much") more about how and where to make contact with patients (or ex-patients) who have (had) the same illness. It is also possible that the need for social comparison with fellow-sufferers is supplied in another manner, e.g., by reading information on fellow-sufferers or via others. In this manner 43.7% ($n = 215$) of the Hodgkin's patients and 66.3% ($n = 276$) of the patients with breast cancer indicated that they knew one or more fellow-patients by name but had had no contact with them. Of these respondents, respectively, 81% ($n = 94$) and 68% ($n = 186$) indicated that they knew or heard something about the condition of the illness of the(se) fellow-sufferer(s) and of those, respectively, 53.3% ($n = 75$) and 46.4% ($n = 125$) indicated that such information was useful.

Finally, it appeared that current need for social comparison with fellow-sufferers

TABLE 2. *Need for social comparison with fellow-sufferers for Hodgkin's and breast cancer patients*

Need for more information about how others who are in the same circumstances react to their illness and treatment	Hodgkin's ($n = 215$) (%)	Breast cancer ($n = 281$) (%)
Not at all	27.4	49.5
A little	23.3	19.9
Somewhat	23.3	20.3
Very much	27.0	10.3
Total	100.0	100.0

was not related to such prior contacts. Similarly, there was no relation between the duration of the contact with fellow-sufferers and the expressed need for social comparison.

FIRST CONTACT WITH A FELLOW-SUFFERER

For most of the respondents the first contact with a fellow-sufferer took place during the stay in the hospital or during the period of the first treatment (Table 3). Table 3 shows that most first contacts with fellow-sufferers are made during the first year after the first treatment; after that relatively few first contacts are made. About half of the cancer patients who had had contact with fellow-sufferers indicated that the first contact took place on their own initiative. Only a few (5%, $n = 263$) indicated that the first contact took place accidentally.

In Table 4 the various ways in which the first contact with a fellow-sufferer took place are presented. As can be seen, an important channel for the first contact was the fellow-patient himself regardless of whether he was an official volunteer. About one of three first contacts took place via a fellow-sufferer. The second most frequent way in which the first contacts took place was via relatives and friends. It is striking that the first contact with a fellow-sufferer for Hodgkin's patients takes place relatively often through a booklet or paper, whereas for patients with breast cancer this type of contact occurs on an infrequent basis. Finally, it is also striking that only a few first contacts with fellow-patients take place through professional caregivers.

ACCOUNT OF THE CONTACT WITH FELLOW-SUFFERERS

Personal contact with fellow-sufferers can take place by telephone conversation; one of every three patients who had ever had contact with a fellow-sufferer reported that they had regular or frequent contact by telephone. The greater part, however, are face-to-face contacts. Table 5 reports the location and frequency of such contacts.

TABLE 3. *Moment at which the first personal contact with a fellow-sufferer took place*

Time	Hodgkin's ($n = 106$) (%)	Breast cancer ($n = 156$) (%)
Before the respondent became ill	2.8	18.6
During the stay in the hospital or during first treatment	52.9	55.8
Within 1 year after first treatment	26.4	17.3
At 1 to 3 years after first treatment	8.5	3.2
More than 4 years after first treatment	9.4	5.1
Total	100.0	100.0

TABLE 4. *The way the first personal contact with a fellow-sufferer took place*

Mechanism	Hodgkin's (n = 108) (%)	Breast cancer (n = 155) (%)
Via a fellow-sufferer who was not a volunteer	18.4	35.1
Via relatives or friends	14.0	27.7
By way of a booklet	15.9	1.9
By way of a paper	16.8	0.6
Via a fellow-sufferer who was a volunteer	10.2	7.1
Via a nurse in the hospital	3.7	8.4
Via a medical specialist	5.6	3.9
By way of a radio or television program	5.7	2.6
Via the family doctor	0.9	1.3
Via other channels (e.g., social worker)	8.8	11.4
Total	100.0	100.0

It can be seen that for three or four of every 10 patients the contact with a fellow-sufferer takes place regularly or often in the hospital. About one-fourth of the patients with breast cancer and one of 10 of the Hodgkin's patients indicated that contact with fellow-sufferers took place regularly or often at the respondent's or fellow-sufferer's home. Only a few patients had contact with fellow-sufferers through group meetings.

Of those who had had contact with one or more fellow-patients, about one-third had contact with only one fellow-sufferer, one-third with two or three, and one-third with four or more. On average, respondents who still had contact with a fellow-patient(s) at the time of the interview had had such contacts with five

TABLE 5. *Location and frequency of occurrence of face-to-face contacts between fellow-sufferers*

Location	Hodgkin's (n = 105) (%)			Breast cancer (n = 150) (%)		
	Regularly or often	Sporadically	Never	Regularly or often	Sporadically	Never
In the hospital	34.3	20.0	45.7	42.3	22.8	34.9
At the respondent's home	10.5	28.5	61.0	28.0	30.7	41.3
At the fellow-sufferer's home	11.4	21.9	66.7	26.0	27.3	46.7
In the waiting room	14.3	12.4	73.3	5.3	10.7	84.0
In a group meeting for talk and conversation	7.6	10.5	81.9	8.1	2.0	89.9
In regional or national meetings	12.4	23.8	63.8	2.7	1.3	96.0
In occasional places	2.0	14.3	83.7	—	0.7	99.3

fellow-patients over a period of 16 months and were making personal contact one or more times each month. The most important reason for ending contact with fellow-patients was the lack of felt need or the perceived resolution of problems. Another important reason was the death of the fellow-sufferer.

EFFECTS OF CONTACT WITH FELLOW-SUFFERERS

With respect to the significance and effectiveness of contact with fellow-sufferers, no definitive conclusions can be drawn at present. At 1.5 years after the initial interview the respondents were again interviewed. In a later report "objective" scores (measured with different self-report scales) of the second measurement will be compared with the scores of the first measurement and related to contact with fellow-sufferers. What we describe here is what the patients themselves saw as the necessity for and significance of contacts with fellow-sufferers. At the same time, we should point out that people are often predisposed to reach positive conclusions about activities in which they choose to participate. It is nevertheless interesting to describe the significance patients themselves place on their contact with fellow-sufferers.

About half of both patient samples who had had contact with fellow-sufferers experienced that contact as meaningful or very meaningful for themselves. Two-thirds of the Hodgkin's patients and three-fourths of the breast cancer patients were satisfied or very satisfied with the contacts with volunteers or contact persons, and the same percentage said that they were satisfied or very satisfied with contacts with fellow-sufferers who were not volunteers or contact persons. Only a very small number of patients expressed dissatisfaction with these contacts. In these cases negative experiences in the contact with fellow-sufferers included recurrence of the disease, deterioration in health status, or death of the fellow-patient with whom they had had contact.

With respect to the significance of contact with fellow-sufferers for basic problems, the following effects were mentioned. In regard to *uncertainty*, 34% of the Hodgkin's and 17% of the breast cancer patients said that they had come to know more about the disease and its treatment through contact with fellow-sufferers.

With respect to *negative feelings,* 43% of Hodgkin's and 47% of breast cancer patients said that they came to feel better through the contacts they had with fellow-sufferers. About one-third came to feel less or somewhat less anxious through such contacts.

About half of the patients said that they had more *control* of their situation through contact with fellow-sufferers. One-fourth of the Hodgkin's and 38% of the breast cancer patients said that they had profited from the contact by the solution of practical problems. Approximately half of the patients saw their *self-confidence* confirmed or somewhat confirmed through the contact with fellow-sufferers.

Another positive benefit cancer patients ascribed to contact with fellow-sufferers is that it made them conscious that others have the same problems, and that they were not the only one with feelings of fear and uncertainty. Furthermore, contact with fellow-sufferers was particularly important for them in order to:

1. Have a better perspective on their own situation
2. Feel that they are understood by others
3. Be able to talk about their concerns and problems
4. Learn to see their own problems in the "proper" light
5. Obtain advice and good counsel
6. Help others with the same problems

SUMMARY

About half of the Hodgkin's patients and one-third of the breast cancer patients in this study were found to be in need of "somewhat" or "very much" information about how others who are in the same circumstances react to their illness and treatment. Just over half of the patients had at some time had contact with fellow-sufferers. The initial personal contacts with a fellow-sufferer take place during the stay in the hospital or during the first treatment period, and most of these contacts are made during the first year after the first treatment, frequently on the patient's own initiative. Most of these contacts are face-to-face. It was also found that there is still a relatively large group of patients who experience important barriers to getting in contact with a fellow-sufferer. Most important among these barriers is the fact that one does not know any fellow-sufferers.

Patients ascribe different positive effects to their contacts with fellow-sufferers, and few negative reactions are reported. The most important positive effects that were mentioned are the confirmation of self-confidence, the gain of control, and the reduction of negative feelings. Contacts with fellow-sufferers make patients more conscious that others have the same problems and that they are not the only ones with feelings of fear and uncertainty.

ACKNOWLEDGMENT

This study was supported by The Netherlands Cancer Foundation (Stichting Koningin Wilhelmina Fonds).

REFERENCES

1. Cottrell, N. B., and Epley, S. W. (1977): Affiliation, social comparison, and social mediated stress reduction. In: *Social Comparison Processes,* edited by J. M. Suls and R. L. Miller. Wiley, New York.
2. Festinger, L. (1954): A theory of social comparison processes. *Hum. Relations,* 7:117–140.
3. Hakmiller, K. L. (1966): Threat as a determinant of downward comparison. *J. Exp. Soc. Psychol.,* (Suppl. 1):32–39.

4. Holland, J. C., and Rowland, J. H. (1981): Psychiatric, psychosocial and behavioral interventions in the treatment of cancer: An historical review. In: *Perspectives on Behavioral Medicine,* edited by S. M. Weiss, J. A. Heid, and B. H. Fox. Academic Press, New York.
5. Molleman, E., and Pruyn, J. (1981): Verwerken van kanker [Coping with cancer]. Project Poliklinische Zorg Oncologie Patiënten. Studiecentrum voor Sociale Oncologie, Rotterdam.
6. Pruyn, J. F. A. (1983): Coping with stress in cancer patients. *Patient Educ. Counseling,* 5:57–62.
7. Pruyn, J. F. A., van den Borne, H. W., and van Poppel, J. (1983): De vrijwilligster in de nazorg voor borstkankerpatiënten (The volunteer in the after-care for breast cancer patients). *I. K. R. Bull.,* 1:17, 40.
8. Schachter, S. (1959): *The Psychology of Affiliation.* Stanford University Press, Stanford.
9. Taylor, S. E. (1982): Social cognition and health. *Personality Soc. Psychol. Bull.,* 8:549–562.
10. Taylor, S. E. (1983): Adjustment to threatening events—a theory of cognitive adaptation. *Am. Psychologist,* 38:1161–1173.
11. Thornton, D. A., and Arrowood, A. J. (1966): Self evaluation, self enhancement and locus of social comparison. *J. Exp. Soc. Psychol.,* 1:40–48.
12. Van den Borne, H. W., and Pruyn, J. F. A. (1983): *Achtergronden en betekenis van lotgenotencontact bij kankerpatiënten.* IVA, Tilburg.
13. Van den Borne, H. W., Pruyn, J. F. A., and Wegman, M. (1981): Zorg om nazorg van kankerpatiënten. Psycho-sociale nazorg door (ex-)patiënten en hun samenwerking met professionele instellingen [Care for after-care in cancer patients]. *Maandbl. Geest. Volksgezondh.,* 12:1060–1072.

The Quality of Life of Cancer Patients,
edited by N. K. Aaronson and J. Beckmann,
Raven Press, New York © 1987.

Quackery in the Quest of Quality

REFLECTIONS ON THE IMPACT OF UNPROVEN METHODS IN THE TREATMENT OF CANCER

Simon Schraub and *Jan Bernheim

*Centre Hospitalier Regional de Besançon, 25030 Besançon, France; and * Edith Cavell Institute, 1180 Brussels, Belgium*

EXTENT OF THE USE OF UNPROVEN CANCER TREATMENT METHODS

The past several years have seen an upsurge of public and professional awareness of diverse modes of detection and treatment of cancer that have as a common denominator the disapproval of the classical biomedical community because of their unproven nature. In the United States, it was mainly the laetrile controversy that propelled the phenomenon to the foreground and thus created a problem for the biomedical community, the government, and the public (2,3,6,11,16).

Several studies have attempted to quantify the extent of the phenomenon. In the United States, 75% of cancer patients are aware of unproven treatment methods, and 10% make use of them (6). Another survey among pediatric patients of the M. D. Anderson Hospital showed that 39% of children had received some type of unproven treatment (13). A Swiss survey by Hauser (12), covering 153 hospitalized patients in two medical oncology departments in Zurich, indicated that 26% of patients were aware of the existence of such treatments; 9% had considered them; and 23% had taken them along with classical treatment. In Lausanne, Jallut et al. (14) have noted that 40% of cancer patients have used some type of unproven method or treatment at some point in their illness. In France, it has proven difficult to obtain comparable data, notably because of patients' reluctance to answer questions by "orthodox" medical personnel (24); however, as many as 40% of patients appeared interested in unorthodox treatment modalities (9). In Belgium, among 110 patients attending a medical oncologist's clinic at the J. Bordet Institute, Brussels, 15% mentioned spontaneously that they were following some alternative treatment; another 11% admitted so on questioning; and another 9% asked the physician's opinion about such treatments. This total of 35% more or less actively interested patients is probably an underestimate of reality (5). These figures under-

275

score the vast extent of the problem and should be viewed as underestimates, since no data are available on perhaps the most important category of patients, namely those who do not survive unproven treatment to undergo subsequent classical treatment.

This state of affairs presents several research problems. The extent of the phenomenon no longer warrants the "benign neglect" attitude that has thus far been prevalent in scientific medical circles. Since unproven treatments are widespread, they are a public health problem. To put the most commonly utilized unorthodox treatment to a scientific test therefore becomes a necessity. It would not be wise to test all unproven methods because this would not be cost-effective and might even encourage the development of more such tests or treatments.

So far, only laetrile and high-dose vitamin C have been so studied (6,15,19,20,29) and proven useless, with some cyanide toxicity noted with the former (21). Another study, performed in Denmark, tested miscellaneous herbs used in the treatment of leukemia. These results were also negative. A phase 2 trial on mistletoe is currently being conducted in Denmark. At the initiative of the Swiss League Against Cancer and in liaison with the American Cancer Society, a working party has been created to document unproven cancer treatment methods. Insofar as such studies effectively demystify widespread ineffective treatments and turn the public's attention to proven treatments, they are cost-effective in terms of saved person-years and therefore constitute good public health policy. It is necessary to have more data on who develops and prescribes these treatments and who uses or requests such methods and why.

One aspect of the problem certainly concerns quality of life. Although it is suspected that the popularity of unproven diagnostic and treatment methods rests in part on the public's perception that conventional scientific methods are detrimental, to an unacceptable level, to quality of life, we must ask, conversely, how the unproven methods affect the quality of life of those cancer patients who do employ them.

UNPROVEN METHODS AND THEIR PROMOTORS

A list of some of the most frequently used unproven cancer treatments in Europe is given in Table 1; however, it is impossible to give details on all of them. Some (28) have been documented by the Swiss League Against Cancer, others by Schraub (24); still others have been documented by the American Cancer Society (1,2).

For example, one of the unproven methods, Iscador, or mistletoe, is employed throughout the world. The use of extracts of mistletoe is proposed by people linked to the *anthroposophy* philosophy, which considers the world to be composed of four forces that characterize, respectively, minerals, plants, animals, and man. The imbalance of these forces, determined by such factors as diet, psychological stress, and toxic substances, causes cancer. In the 1920s, R. Steiner, creator of

TABLE 1. *Classification of the principal unproven methods used in Europe*

Anticancer therapy based on a special medical approach
    Antroposophic medicine and Viscum album (Iscador)
    Homeopathy
    Chinese medicine and acupuncture
    Homotoxics theory (Reckeweg)
    Water–earth–things theory (Kappler)
Diet
    Anticancer diet (Breuss)
    Protein diet (Windstosser)
    Selective diet (Hay)
    Macrobiotic diet
    Lactic acid theory and isopathy (Kuhl)
    Moerman therapy
    Oil–protein diet (Budwing)
    Vegetarian anticancer without salt (Gerson)
Medicinal treatment
    Actinine, Bamfoline, Beres drop, bromelaïn, carcinogen virus, Carzodelan forte, furfural,
        honey jelly, oral Gelum R.D., germanium, ginseng, yeast, Laetrile (vitamin B17),
        Neytumorine, Petrasch's anthozim, oil, Polyerga, Polydine, red carrot juice,
        Resistocell, Revitorgan, Tumorestone, Wober-Mugos, vitamin C
Enhancement of host immune defenses and analogs
    Niehans therapy ("fresh cell treatment")
    Serocytology (Thomas)
    Thymus extract
    Curative serums (Bonifazio, Bal'a)
    Integral therapy and immunotherapy of Issels
    Biological treatment (Zabel)
Treatment based on the stimulation of aerobic glycolysis in the cancer cells
    Alternative medicine by run training
    Oxygen therapy (Van Aaken)
    Substitution of ferment by betacyanes (Seeger)
    Ozone therapy (Wehrli)
    Physiatrons (Dr. Solomidès)
Miscellaneous
    Bioelectronic (Vincent)
    Earth radiation and cancer
    Massage of reflexogen zone of the foot
    Microwave therapy (Samuels)
    Protozairs and carcinoma (Weber)
    Cure by mind
    Simonton treatment
    Irridology

the anthroposophy philosophy, proposed that the use of mistletoe could correct the imbalance. Diagnosis, location, and follow-up of cancer are made possible by a test called *sensitive crystallization,* which requires a drop of dried blood on a paper. The blood is then mixed with a solution of copper and dried again. The shape of the subsequent crystals gives the diagnosis of the cancer and its location. Different forms of mistletoe exist, according to the trees on which they grow. They are mixed with different metals and prescribed to patients, sometimes in combination with a special ambiance, diet, artistic activity, etc. The mistletoe extracts are known as Iscador or Viscum album. Scientific evidence on the efficacy of this drug is weak. Some authors (25) have described an inhibition in the growth of murine tumors that was not noted by others (5). Many clinical publications come from the Lukas Klinik in Arlesheim (Switzerland), which has specialized in Iscador treatment. They are not published in review-type medical journals (17) and are questionable from a methodological point of view. Some consist of randomized studies and have been published by Austrian medical teams but are also questionable because of the statistical methodology used (22).

Iscador was not allowed in the United States after an FDA examination. Nevertheless, it is widely prescribed all over the world. In 1978, two million ampules were sold in countries where Iscador is prescribed, and approximately 30,000 patients are treated with this substance each year (26).

Therapy by means of unproven drugs or special beams or waves produced by some type of machine must be differentiated from diet and psychological therapies. (It should be noted although the latter two categories can lead to disaster, they cannot be legally considered to be drug therapies.) In addition to these treatment methods, a great number of simple tests are being offered that profess to diagnose cancer or to indicate a "susceptibility to cancer." All these treatments are characterized by an unquantitative, imprecise, or mystical chemical or physical basis; hazy methodology; and publication only in, usually, self-serving, nonreview-type publications.

The initiators or promotors of these unproven methods usually fall into the following categories: quacks or embezzlers; more or less biomedically trained individuals and their followers; bona fide biologists and physicians who, frustrated by the complexity and slow progress of biomedical science, pursue a reasonable partial truth to its extreme and build it into a panacea. Many of the latter are not primarily after financial gain; rather, they appear to be sincere (4,24) and to have idealistic motives. Their own inclination to individualistic omnipotence, compounded by the derisive attitudes of classical scientists, tends to make many of them behave as paranoid "true believers."

Prescribing physicians may have similar motives, or, while remaining skeptical, consider nonproven methods to be a lesser evil compared with difficult and often unsuccessful classical methods, some of which, admittedly, are equally unproven [e.g., the chemotherapy of advanced non-small-cell lung cancer has never been proven to be of benefit to this particular patient group (23)]. In some European countries where young physicians have a difficult time making ends meet, unproven popular methods are undoubtedly not only a shortcut to helping patients but to making a living as well.

CLINICAL USE OF UNPROVEN CANCER TREATMENT METHODS

Unproven methods may be used in four different ways. First, the treatments or tests are given before or instead of proven procedures. This is probably not the most frequent situation, but it certainly poses the gravest public health hazard.

Second, the unproven methods are used alongside classical treatment "to be on the safe side" or to lessen its side effects. Often, both classical and alternative therapists will be, right or wrong, presumed to be intolerant of each other and will be kept in the dark by the patient. A number of clinical responses may thus be incorrectly claimed. It is less likely but altogether conceivable that actual biological antagonism may be responsible for some "combined" treatment failures. This situation seems to be common in France, where unproven treatments are proposed as adjuvant. The promotors of unproven methods may thus be able to ply their trade without exposing themselves to legal prosecution. It must be remembered that the "art of healing" is the legally enforced monopoly of medical doctors in most European countries.

The third circumstance is the application of these treatments to patients who are beyond effective classical treatment. In these cases, there may be understandable humanitarian motivations and even benefit, if only psychological. Finally, unproven methods are applied in cancerphobic patients in a preventive setting, sometimes after unproven tests have declared them to be at risk or suffering from cancer. This procedure of course leads to fictitious therapeutic successes.

WHY PATIENTS RESORT TO UNPROVEN METHODS

The factors leading patients and their relatives to unproven treatments are numerous. The aura of salvation surrounding these treatments is an apparent antidote to the aura of inevitable lethality that still surrounds cancer. The fact that about half of cancer cases are actually cured lags behind in public opinion, more so in Europe than in the United States. By and large, many more cases of fatal outcome of cancer are known to the public than are cures. Especially in the case of celebrities, cure is rarely "news"; rather, it is a "nonevent." Also, in one's immediate surroundings, one is much more likely to hear about a cancer fatality than a cure, if only because (mainly in Europe) a cancer diagnosis is often not clearly communicated to patients in order to protect them from unnecessary anxiety.

Cancer is still, as was tuberculosis in the nineteenth century, a metaphor for vicious, undeservedly pervasive, and inexorably fatal evil (27). It is also, largely unjustifiably, branded a disease of technological society. Classical treatment is usually highly aggressive and technological. Another significant factor is that some chemotherapies and radiotherapy carry a risk of secondary carcinogenesis and are known to decrease host defenses. In contrast with this grim picture, many alternative therapies have a "healthy" ring: They act by boosting "natural" host defenses; they do not treat the epiphenomenon (the cancer) but the whole person; they consist of natural products; they are devoid of side effects; they work only if the patient has the "faith" (11); they "purify" the intestine or the bodily fluids that are poisoned (this latter notion is in keeping with the feelings of many patients who regard cancer as a punishment for sins or a consequence of impurity). Thus, the modern desire to "go back to nature," vague popularizations of environmentalism, and archetypical irrationalizations all conjoin to make "soft" and "natural" treatment attractive.

The fact that resorting to unproven methods is usually more voluntary than entrusting oneself to a classical oncologist is in itself an incentive. In a great number of cases, it is not the patients but the relatives who take the initiative to seek alternative treatment. They wish to be helpful, and their anticipatory guilt leads them to leave nothing untried. Also, many unproven treatment methods allow the patient to play a much more active role than is the case with most classical treatments and indeed no longer to be "the one who undergoes" as in the etymological sense of the word "patient."

This is especially true for dietary and psychological treatment methods, which are in many respects automedication. Some of the cancer diets that are propagated are in fact in their general principles quite reasonable (fewer calories, less animal fat, more fiber) in the prevention of cancer. Others aiming at "starving the cancer" are clearly dangerous. All require the constant faith of the patient or his or her relatives. This feeling of personal responsibility may well contribute to some patients' quality of life.

Another interesting technique is "visualization," complementing classical treatments, as proposed by the Simontons (1). It aims at exploring the psychological factors that increase or inhibit the growth of the tumor and postulates that carcinogenesis must have been initiated or facilitated by a nefarious psychological context. The patient learns both to relax and to mobilize his mental energy in a visualized fight against cancer. He is also encouraged to reorganize his "wrong," psychoaffective life. Some of these activities may promote the patient's well being in terms of psychotherapeutic support (18). It should be noted, however, that this technique is not without risk. A patient of one of the authors, a young woman with advanced breast cancer, refused further chemotherapy and came back from a Simonton course in the United States convinced that her relationship with her husband and parents had been "completely wrong." She went on to create dramatic changes in her affective environment and appeared to be rather lonely at the end of her life. The notion that one can bring cancer on oneself by living incorrectly can create unnecessary guilt if the benefits of change cannot be proven.

IMPACT OF UNPROVEN TREATMENT METHODS ON PATIENT QUALITY OF LIFE

The necessary precondition for any quality of life is some quantity of life. Insofar as unproven therapeutic methods shorten survival, they offer less potential for quality. The oft-proclaimed notion that less stress may in itself lengthen survival is unsubstantiated in humans, if not in animals. The therapeutic value of treatments that do not stress patients must therefore not be sought in anything else than in quality of life. But also on this plane unproven treatments are unproven.

It cannot be denied, however, that we see patients who very ostensibly claim to have better quality of life under unproven treatment than under classical treatment. Some display serenity and confidence, others even the ecstasy that one sees associated with religious and mystic experience. It can be argued that in the present era of increasing secularization, unproven treatments can be a refuge for those disappointed by an imperfect world.

ONCOLOGIST-PATIENT RELATIONSHIP AND UNPROVEN TREATMENTS

Some oncologists claim that none of their patients resort to unproven treatment, ostensibly because they believe that they meet all their patients' needs. This suggests that they do not even see the tip of the iceberg. Insofar as some of these treatments may interfere with classical treatment, there should be no communication gap between physician and patient. Chances are that an attitude of openness to any subject matter, attentiveness to various patient needs, and unfailing support are the most effective ways to be informed of the patient's desire to seek help elsewhere and the reasons for doing so. Should the patient raise the subject of alternative treatment, it must be discussed rationally and factually rather than rejected out of hand. The arguments against the use of unproven treatment, as opposed to proven albeit imperfect treatment, are formidable. When the patient wants to use unproven treatment along with classical treatment, a case-for-case discussion is in order. When he or she wants to use it after failure of all available standard treatment, we should bear in mind that experimental treatment or continued palliative care is then a rational option. If the patient's interest in unproven treatment is based on emotional needs, he or she should then be encouraged to invest in more traditional outlets: the cultivation of human bonds and spirituality.

CONCLUSION

There is no proliferation of unproven treatments for such widespread conditions as heart failure, diabetes, or fracture. Standard treatment is effective and permits good quality of survival. Therefore, the message from the epidemic of unproven cancer treatments is loud and clear: Through classical but innovative research we must improve the rate of cure, the effectiveness of palliation, and patient quality of life.

REFERENCES

1. American Cancer Society (1981): Unproven methods of cancer management.
2. American Cancer Society (1983): Unproven methods of cancer management: Iscador. *CA-A Cancer Journal of Clinicians*, 33:186–188.
3. American Society of Clinical Oncology (1983): Ineffective cancer therapy: A guide for the layperson. *J. Clin. Oncol.*, 1:154–163.

4. Baum, M. (1983): Quack cancer cures or scientific remedies? *Clin. Oncol.*, 9:275–280.
5. Berger, M., and Schmaehl, D. (1983): Studies on the tumor-inhibiting efficacy of Iscador in experimental animal tumors. *J. Cancer Res. Clin. Oncol.*, 105:262–265.
6. Cassileth, B. R. (1982): After Laetrile what? *N. Engl. J. Med.*, 306:1582–1584.
7. Creagan, E. T., Moertel, C. G., O'Fallon, J. R., Schutt, A. L., O'Connell, M. J., Rubin, J., and Frytak, S. (1979): Failure of high dose vitamin C (ascorbic acid) therapy to benefit patients with advanced cancer. *N. Engl. J. Med.*, 301:687–690.
8. Davidson, C. S. (1984): Are we physicians helpless? *N. Engl. J. Med.*, 310 (17).
9. *Est Republicain.* (1984): Deux personnes sur trois prennent des médicaments sans voir le médecin. July 19.
10. Ewerbeck, H. (1982): Procédés paramédicaux et éthique médicale. *Med. Hyg.*, 40;3698–3701.
11. Greenberg, D. M. (1980): The case against laetrile, the fraudulent cancer remedy. *Cancer*, 45:799.
12. Hauser, S. P. (1981): Krebspatient und paramedizin. Kontakte, Theorien, Behandlungsweisen. Dissertation, Zurich.
13. Holland, J. C. (1981): Patients who seek unproven cancer remedies: A psychological perspective. *Clin. Bull.*, 11:102–105.
14. Jallut, O., Guex, P., and Barrelet, L. (1984): Les méthodes non prouvées en oncologie. *Schweiz. Med. Wochenschr.*, 114:1214–1220.
15. Laster, W. R., and Schabel, F. M. (1975): Experimental studies of the antitumor activity of amygdalin MF (NSC-15780) alone and in combination with beta-glucosidase (NSC-128056). *Cancer Chemother. Rep.*, 59:951–965.
16. Lerner, I. J. (1984): The whys of cancer quackery. *Cancer*, 53:815–819.
17. Leroi, R., Boeck, D., Franz, H., Hajto, T., Khwaja, T. A., Lanzrein, C. H., Linder, M., Ribereau, G., and Rentea, R. (1984): Neue experimentelle Resultate der Iscadorforschung. *Krebsgeschehen* 16:11–18.
18. Mack, R. M. (1984): Lessons from living with cancer. *N. Engl. J. Med.*, 311(25):1640–1644.
19. Moertel, C. J., Fleming, T. R., Rubin, J., et al. (1982): A clinical trial of amygdalin (laetrile) in the treatment of human cancer. *N. Engl. J. Med.*, 306:201–206.
20. Moertel, C. G., Fleming, T. R., Creagan, E. T., Rubin, J., O'Connel, M. J., and Ames, M. (1985): High dose vitamin C versus placebo in the treatment of patients with advanced cancer who have had no prior chemotherapy: A randomized double-blind comparison. *N. Engl. J. Med.*, 312:137–141.
21. Sadoff, L., Fuchs, K., and Hollander, K. (1978): Rapid death associated with laetrile ingestion. *J.A.M.A.*, 239:1532.
22. Salzer, G., and Havelec, L. (1983): Adjuvante Iscador-Behandlung nach operiertem Magenkarzinom. Ergebnisse einer randomisierten Studie. *Krebsgeschehen*, 15:106–110.
23. Simes, R. J. (19xx): Risk benefit relationship in cancer clinical trial: The ECOG experience in non-small-cell lung carcinoma.
24. Schraub, S. (1983): Les traitements parallèles du cancer. *Concours Med.*, 105(26):2979–3000.
25. Selawry, O. S., Vester, F., Mai, W., and Schwartz, M. R. (1976): Zur Kenntnis der Inhaltsstoffe von Viscum album, II. Tumorhemmende Inhaltsstoffe, Hoppe-Seyler's. *Z. Physiol. Chem.* 324:262–281.
26. Society for Cancer Research. (1980): Iscador. A summary review. Society for Cancer Research, Arlesheim, Switzerland.
27. Sontag, S. (1978): *Illness as a Metaphor.* Farrar, Strauss and Giraoux, New York.
28. Swiss League Against Cancer. (1985): Files of unproven methods in Cancer (Anthroposophy, Carzodelan Forte, Furfurol, Iscador, Polyerga Neu, Total cancer cure according to Breuss, Trypanosa, Wobe-Mugos). Swiss League Against Cancer, Bern.
29. Wodinsky, I., and Swinlarsky, J. (1975): Antitumor activity of amygdalin MF (NSC-15780) as a single agent and beta-glucosidase (NSC-128056) on a spectrum of transplantable rodent tumors. *Cancer Chemother. Rep.*, 59:939–950.

The Quality of Life of Cancer Patients,
edited by N. K. Aaronson and J. Beckmann,
Raven Press, New York © 1987.

Differences in Perception of Disease and Treatment Between Cancer Patients and Their Physicians

Jan L. Bernheim, *Ghislain Ledure, *Michel Souris, and
**Darius Razavi

*Edith Cavell Institute, 1180 Brussels, Belgium; * Department of Psychosomatic Medicine, University Hospital St. Pierre, 1000 Brussels, Belgium; ** and Institut Jules Bordet; University of Brussels, 1000 Brussels, Belgium*

Cancer and most of its treatments are anxiogenic for both patient and physician (4,13). The disease as well as the patient may cause the doctor to adopt unavoidable projective attitudes. In oncology, such differences in perception between physicians and their young patients have been demonstrated by Pfefferbaum and Levenson (11), who used questionnaire data. Derogatis et al. (2) have shown that physicians tend to underestimate the incidence and intensity of depression in their patients. Investigating the opinion of patients and nurses on the needs of patients to be informed, Lauer (5) found important differences. These aspects of perceptual differences have also been studied in the child (8,11,14). Obviously such differences between patient and caregiver have an influence on the quality of emotional support offered the patient and on the latter's compliance with his treatment (3).

What does the informer know? What does he want to communicate (content)? What does he really communicate and how (mode and form)? What does the recipient of information know? What does he ask for? What does he hear? What does he remember? What does he integrate? Such are several of the possible variables. Thus an item of information communicated (e.g., the nature of the disease) may, by using a particular language (e.g., technical), not be understood. Deliberately withheld information, such as prognosis, may be perceived at an infraverbal level. Individuals clearly vary in their perception, metabolization, and integration of information from various sources. Moreover, the disease itself may modulate the patient's receptivity.

Differences in perception also occur in relation to the transfer of information to the patient. The patient information problem cannot be reduced to the ethical question of truth-telling (or not), if only because the information is provided by a healthy person, who is likely to perceive the disease differently than the suffering patient. The communication of information and its reception are concepts that interact and are influenced by many variables.

283

A number of studies and observations highlight large individual variabilities in the reactions of patients to cancer. Their mode of coping behavior depends on their basic personality, which determines their defense reactions facing the disease (6,9). Cognitive, emotional, and behavioral processes are brought in motion by the psychic trauma of cancer. These processes can be assumed to serve the purpose of maximally preserving psychic and physical integrity. Thus on the cognitive and affective level, the process leads to minimization, denial of the disease and its consequences, or seeking of information in order to reduce uncertainties. The most frequently observed states are anxiety and minor depression. Some patients have a behavioral reaction, actively participating with the physician in fighting the disease. Others withdraw, unable to integrate the threat. In others, one sees an absence of obvious reactive behavior, apparently reflecting an acceptance of the disease and treatments. Obviously these reactions are dissociated here only for schematization purposes but are in reality closely interwoven into a complex psychic process.

The health care provider also undergoes a series of psychological reactions that may be quite variable (12). On the cognitive level, minimization and denial may, in fact, be shared by the physician and his patient. At the other extreme, one may observe dramatizations that are not always shared by the patient. On the emotional level, physicians' anxiety and depression have not been thoroughly studied. Defensive behavior and the capacity to sublimate in research are frequent and relatively successful evasions. On the behavioral level, aggressivity, flight, and certain stereotyped behavior are often observed.

STUDY SUBJECTS AND METHODS

The present study is an extension of a preliminary study already reported (7). Forty-three consecutive patients with miscellaneous malignancies who had undergone aggressive treatment were the subjects of the study. All patients were being followed by a medical oncologist (J.B.) and were or had been under standard or experimental protocol treatment in a university-affiliated cancer center (Table 1). These patients had been referred to this particular physician's clinic only on the basis of availability of appointments or the fact that they spoke only Dutch. (The latter can no longer be regarded in psychosociological terms as clearly distinct from French-speaking Belgians.)

The only "unorthodox" feature was that they had been regularly interrogated on their Anamnestic Comparative Self-Assessment (ACSA) score by the physician. Briefly, ACSA is the numerical expression of subjective well-being on a scale defined by the memory of the best and the worst episodes in the patient's life experience. Sequential scores generate a curve that allows calculation of the average subjective well-being during the various phases of disease and treatment. The pilot study and validation of technique have been reported extensively elsewhere (1).

TABLE 1. *Characteristics of patients[a] who received aggressive cancer treatment*

Parameter	No. of patients
Type of therapy	
Surgery	18
Radiotherapy	19
Chemotherapy	39
Diseases	
Hodgkin's lymphoma	9
Non-Hodgkin's lymphoma	4
Mammary carcinoma	
Adjuvant Tt	8
Metastatic	8
Chronic myeloid leukemia, multiple myeloma	2
Bronchial carcinoma	2
Acute leukemia	2
Head and neck carcinoma	2
Miscellaneous solid tumors (1 each of colonic, chorionic, ovarian, testicular, hepatocellular carcinoma, osteosarcoma)	6
Total	43

[a] Median age 47 years, range 16–72. Sex ratio, M/F: 14/29.

The physician's general attitude toward the problem of the patients' information is, as is often the case in Belgium, one of intuitive compromise between a theoretical desire to abide by the patient's right to information and a concern to be protective and encouraging. The physician stated that he tried above all to respect the patient's autonomy by letting the patient set the level of information. He tried to give an impression of availability and made all information negotiable.

The investigation was performed by two psychiatrists (G.L. and M.S.). The patients, referred by the physician, were seen by one of them in semidirective interviews. At the onset of the interview it was made clear to the patient that the psychiatrist was uninformed about him or his disease. The stated objective of the interview was to let the patient express his feelings about the disease, the treatment, and the ACSA to a sympathetic but independent observer who was not involved in the treatment.

The patient was invited to talk about the nature of his disease, the nature of the information about the disease that he had received, and his opinion about the truthfulness and completeness of this received information. He was then asked to express himself on the degree of aggressiveness of the procedures he was subjected to during the pretreatment period of diagnostic workup of the disease and during treatment. Patients spontaneously referred to the influence of the disease on their relational life and commented on their relations with the physician. They were encouraged to talk about their fears, hopes, and doubts concerning the disease and treatment.

Later, the psychiatrists interviewed the physician on his assessment of the various disease-related variables the patient had commented on. Thus the perception of both patient and physician on the same variables could be compared.

RESULTS

Patient's Knowledge on the Nature of the Disease

In five instances no clear statement of diagnosis was made by the patient (Table 2). Respecting his defenses, the investigators did not inquire more precisely. In these cases the psychiatrist's impression of the patient's knowledge was noted. For example, a 50-year-old man had been hypochondriacal and cancerophobic ever since he had undergone sternotomy for a benign goiter 5 years earlier. His general practitioner referred him to the hospital for yet another checkup. A diagnosis of bronchial carcinoma was made, described to the patient as "a growth," and was treated with radiotherapy. Since that time, the patient's attitude to his health problem had changed dramatically: He asked no questions of the oncologist, told the psychiatrist he had no idea what was wrong with him, and stated that he was given no information by the oncologist.

Seventy-four percent of patients correctly stated the cancerous nature of their disease. Those with a good prognosis (defined as a disease that more often than not is curable or minimally decreases the normal life expectancy) seemed slightly more accurately informed (81%) than those with a poor prognosis (70%).

Information on Diagnosis and Prognosis

According to the physician, 79% of the patients had been informed that they had a malignancy (Table 3). Seventy percent of the patients said they had been so informed. Eight of the 22 patients who had cancer with a poor prognosis (Table 2) had been told so after they had insisted on being completely informed. Each of these eight patients who had been told the diagnosis of a malignancy with a poor prognosis acknowledged having been so informed. Seven of the eight told the psychiatrist that the confirmation of their fears had been followed by feelings of hopelessness. Although genuinely wishing to be informed, they had hoped that the information would leave them hope of recovery. The fact that the communication of the diagnosis had been accompanied by prospects of effective palliation had not removed their feeling of hopelessness. It is noteworthy that information regarding fatality was not denied by the eight patients who had demanded it, whereas more benign information was more or less denied by six patients. Information of fatality appears irreversible, but more benign information can be modified.

At the other extreme, there were four patients who had not asked to be informed and to whom the oncologist had not volunteered information. One may ask the

TABLE 2. *Knowledge of nature of disease and prognosis*

Actual prognosis	Cancer		Dangerous disease, cancer not mentioned	Mild disease, not dangerous	Does not know	Total patients	
	Poor prognosis	Good prognosis				No.	%
Poor	11	4	3	—	4	22	51
Good	1	16	2	1	1	21	49
Total patients	12	20	5	1	5	43	—
Percent	28	46	12	2	12	—	100

Prognosis according to patient

TABLE 3. *Information on diagnosis and prognosis*

Prognosis given to patient according to physician	Expressed by patient to have been obtained from the physician					Total patients	
	Cancer		Dangerous disease, cancer not mentioned	Mild disease, not dangerous	No information		
	Poor prognosis	Good prognosis				No.	%
Poor prognosis	8	—	—	—	—	8	19
Good prognosis	—	21	—	2	3	26	60
Dangerous disease, cancer not mentioned	1	—	3	—	1	5	12
Mild disease, not dangerous	—	—	—	—	—	—	—
No information	—	—	—	—	4	4	9
Total patients	9	21	3	2	8	43	—
Percent	21	49	7	4	19	—	100

question why the oncologist preferred to refrain from volunteering any information to these particular patients whereas in other cases they were more informative. Whatever impression motivated him, these patients tacitly seem to have approved of his attitude, because to the psychiatrists they expressed no suspicions regarding the nature of their disease nor a wish to have been informed.

Of the 26 patients who were informed that they had a form of cancer with a good prognosis, five did not register the information as such. Three of these patients had Hodgkin's disease and knew the name of the disease but insisted that it was not a malignancy. Another patient said she could never seem to remember the name of her disease and had to look it up in her notebook. This patient had asked no further questions despite having undergone in the course of several years total node radiotherapy, a laparotomy, and chemotherapy. Another patient with breast cancer stated with some rancor that all she was told was that she had had "a tumor," which was a meaningless term to her. She had not asked for more precise information. We think these cases of deformation of the information are illustrative of certain patients' tendency to use negation and repression.

One of the patients who was told he had a serious liver condition without mention of malignancy knew he had hepatoma. His alcoholic wife had hit him with the information during a quarrel. During an interview at her request on the condition of her husband, she had impressed the physician as deeply caring and worried about the fate of the family, so that he had communicated to her the diagnosis and prognosis. This case highlights the danger of informing the family while keeping the patient in the dark.

The fact that eight patients stated not to have been informed, while Table 2 shows only five patients to be ignorant of their diagnosis may at first seem contradictory. The three remaining patients told the psychiatrist they might have cancer but doubted it. We take this to express a necessity to "have a way out." They denied having received information from the oncologist, though he insists that he duly informed two of the three patients. The third patient indeed was not informed. She suffered from preterminal colonic carcinoma. She had asked for no information and commented to the psychiatrist: "One should not ask such thing to a doctor. He wouldn't say the truth, and it is better like this anyway."

Opinion of the Patient on the Way He Was Informed of the Diagnosis and Prognosis

When interviewed by the psychiatrist about how they had been informed, 56% of the patients expressed the opinion that they had been completely, accurately, and truthfully informed (Table 4). The physician said that, in fact, only 30% of the patients were so informed by him. He qualified his information to 53% of the patients as "edulcorated" (i.e., incomplete in that after providing initial general information with neutral and rather positive overtones he had sensed that the patient

TABLE 4. *Truthfulness of information*

In the opinion of the physician	In the opinion of the patient				
	No or deceptive information	Edulcorated	True	Total patients	
				No.	%
No or deceptive information	7	—	—	7	17
Edulcorated	3	8	12	23	53
True	1	—	12	13	30
Total patients	11	8	24	43	—
Percent	25	19	56	—	100

could not tolerate more information. This impression was derived from the fact that the patient asked no further questions or had eagerly appeared to organize himself on the basis of the provided information, e.g., by saying that he would have been devastated had the news been any worse. The 12 patients who had received edulcorated information and believed it to be complete gave the psychiatrist an impression of optimistic hopefulness and appeared satisfied with their information status. At least two of the patients of this category maintained this attitude until the day of death.

When the oncologist had been fully informative or had completely withheld information, the patients concurred, with one exception. Six of the seven patients who had not been informed had cancer with a poor prognosis. Apparently, a tacit agreement existed between these patients and their physician to let these matters remain undiscussed.

The only patient (with Hodgkin's disease) who stated that he had not been informed whereas the physician was positive that the diagnosis was communicated had, in the judgment of the psychiatrist, a paranoid personality. The interview with the psychiatrist provided an opportunity to vent his aggressivity toward the oncologist. His disease put him in an unbearable situation of dependence on the doctor.

Attitude Toward Disease

It can be assumed that nearly all patients with cancer have some measure of anxiety. Only anxiety that was manifested verbally and behaviorally was taken into account by the physician and psychiatrists to categorize patients as anxious or not. Patients classified as "interested, not anxious" generally manifested a rational and composed behavior. "Indifferent" patients gave an impression of more or less benign neglect (or denial) toward their disease.

Whereas 65% of the patients manifested anxiety in the psychiatric interviews, the oncologists had noted anxiety for only 48% (Table 5). This finding might

TABLE 5. *Manifested attitude toward disease*

Attitude according to physician	Attitude according to psychiatrist			Total patients	
	Anxious	Interested, not anxious	Indifferent	No.	%
Anxious	19	1	1	21	48
Interested, not anxious	9	8	—	17	40
Indifferent	—	2	3	5	12
Total patients	28	11	4	43	
Percent	65	26	9	—	100

mean that the oncologist is less receptive to the signals of anxiety. An alternative explanation for the discrepancy is that some patients make a point to appear brave and unflinching, concealing their anxiety from their treating physician. Several patients told the psychiatrist that they did not want to burden their physician with minor complaints or worries in order not to discourage him.

However, in two cases the oncologist had perceived anxiety in patients who did not manifest it to the psychiatrist. One was a hypochondriacal patient with advanced lung cancer and the other a business man with metastatic testicular carcinoma, who, outside the strictly therapeutic relationship with the oncologist, made major efforts of suppression to maintain "business as usual."

Tolerance Toward Diagnostic Procedures

The anamnestic appreciation of the patient on the degree of aggressivity of diagnostic procedures was compared with the oncologist's opinion on these procedures. In general, the oncologist considered such invasive procedures as surgical biopsy, angiography, and diagnostic laparotomy as "aggressive," and categorized as "mild" such procedures as endoscopy, blood and bone marrow collection, radiography, ultrasound, and nuclear medical investigations.

In 70% of the cases, the patient and the oncologist agreed. In some cases of lymphoma, diagnostic procedures were not considered aggressive by the patient because he did not think of the surgery as diagnostic but, rather, therapeutic. On the other hand, the summation of a large number of procedures deemed "mild" by the physician, sometimes including bone marrow aspirations, was perceived as aggressive by as many as seven (17%) of the patients (Table 6).

Tolerance Toward Treatment Modalities

The categories "minor" and "major," in the opinion of the oncologist, were compared with "well tolerated" and "poorly tolerated" in the anamnestic apprecia-

TABLE 6. *Tolerability of diagnostic procedures*

Tolerability according to physician	Tolerability according to patient			
			Total patients	
	Aggressive	Mild	No.	%
Aggressive	5	6	11	27
Mild	7	23	30	73
Total patients	12	29	41	—
Percent	29	71	—	100

tion of the patient when questioned in these terms by the psychiatrist. The physician considered as minor the following examples of treatments: skin and lymph node surgery, splenectomy, single site or low dose radiotherapy, and chemotherapy by single drugs or that are not usually associated with subjective side effects. Mastectomy, ablative visceral surgery, multiple site, and/or high dose radiotherapy and polychemotherapy were considered major. Using these categories it appears that, overall, many patients express good tolerance for major surgical and chemotherapeutic treatments.

For radiotherapy there was good agreement between the physician's and the patient's point of view (79%), whereas for chemotherapy (70%) and surgery (55%) the ratings were less consistent (Table 7). For surgery, this discrepancy was due primarily to the good tolerance of seven of 15 mastectomies. One-third of aggressive chemotherapies were well tolerated and only one-fifth of mild chemotherapies were poorly tolerated. Overall, more treatments were described as well tolerated than the oncologist had expected.

DISCUSSION AND CONCLUSIONS

The special feature of the method we used resides in the interviewing of both the patients and the physician by an independent psychiatrist, which allowed comparison of the perceptions of the two parties. The semidirective interview technique, though not standardized, allowed classification of the attitudes and answers of patients into defined categories. The patients and the oncologist often had discordant views on the nature of the disease and the aggressivity of treatment.

These results emphasize the frailty of a physician's impressions of what his patient is experiencing and the vulnerability of their relationship to misunderstanding. The patients displayed a clear tendency to deny or to edulcorate the information they had been given on the nature of the disease and its prognosis. This phenomenon occurred only when the information provided had not included the notion of imminent fatality. In the latter case, such information appeared irreversible. It was the psychia-

TABLE 7. *Tolerability of treatment modalities*

Degree of aggressivity according to physician	Degree of aggressivity according to patient			
	Well tolerated	Poorly tolerated	Total patients	
			No.	%
Surgery				
Minor	6	3	9	31
Aggressive or mutilating	10	10	20	69
Mastectomy	7	8	15	—
Total patients	16	13	29	—
Percent	55	45	—	100
Radiotherapy				
Minor	14	2	16	55
Major	4	9	13	45
Total patients	18	11	29	—
Percent	62	38	—	100
Chemotherapy				
Mild	7	2	9	22.5
Aggressive	10	21	31	77.5
Total patients	17	23	40	—
Percent	42.5	57.5	—	100

trists' impression that the knowledge of impending doom had contributed to these patients' feelings of hopelessness. The question, for which patients such information is indeed an independent variable in their quality of survival, can be answered only by more detailed studies. Until better data have been obtained on the effects of truth telling and edulcorating, we think it is wise to maintain truth telling, assuming that it is gradual and negotiable. On a request for information, one should inform the patient of the potential risks of precise information and at first offer him the truth, nothing but the truth—but not necessarily the whole truth.

In particular, the oncologist author feels strengthened by these data in having adopted the following attitude to the frequent question: "Doctor, is it cancer?" The patient in another situation would probably not even consider asking a physician if he is suffering from an infectious disease. It is not really a meaningful question, as everybody knows infectious diseases span a spectrum from perfectly trivial to extremely severe. Similarly, cancer is not really an informative term, as it includes diseases that do not require treatment such as uncomplicated chronic lymphocytic leukemia and, at the other extreme, rapidly lethal conditions. After interactive exchanges, the information thus usually boils down to some intermediate situation that lends itself to efficient treatment and leaves the patient and the physician with rational hope for the best possible outcome.

In this study, although the physician tended to overdramatize the overall impact of surgical and chemotherapeutic treatments, he may have been less perceptive than the psychiatrists to the signs of emotional distress his patients displayed. On the other hand, several patients proved to have a major interest in displaying a courageous and optimistic attitude around their physician in order "to keep up his spirits," as one said.

Thus both the patient and the physician seem to be aware of each other's vulnerability and act accordingly by leaving some things unsaid. These results are to some extent similar to those of Derogatis et al., who studied North American patients (2).

With a nonhomogeneous patient population, as used in this study, some potentially important variables could not be distinguished. For example, the type and stage of the disease may be relevant variables (15,16). Also, longitudinal rather than cross-sectional observations could shed more light on the dynamics of perceptions, concerns, and defensive reactions. To better study the transmission of information, one needs data on the content, mode, and form of communication, and on the psychological characteristics of the physician and the patient. In order to better understand what patients are really going through, correlations are needed between their type and degree of emotional distress and some characteristics of their behavior. Such refinements to our perception of needs and emotions of our patients would probably improve the quality of the support we offer them, their compliance to treatment, and their quality of life.

ACKNOWLEDGMENT

This research was supported in part by grant 2822225500 of the Belgian National Lottery via the Nationaal Fonds voor Wetenschappelijk Onderzoek, and by a grant from the Franqui-Foundation.

REFERENCES

1. Bernheim, J. L., and Buyse, M. (1983): The anamnestic comparative self-assessment for measuring the subjective quality of life of cancer patients. *J. Psychosoc. Oncol.*, 1:25–38.
2. Derogatis, L. R., Abeloff, N., and MacBeth, C. (1976): Cancer patients and their physician in the perception of psychological symptoms. *Psychosomatics*, 17:197–201.
3. Green, J. (1983): Compliance and cancer chemotherapy. *Br. Med. J.*, 287:778.
4. Hinton, J. (1973): Bearing cancer. *Br. J. Med. Psychol.*, 46:105–113.
5. Lauer, P. (1982): Learning needs of cancer patients—a comparison of nurse and patient perceptions. *Nurs. Res.*, 31:11–16.
6. Lazarus, R. (1982): Stress and coping as factors in health and illness. In: *Psychosocial Aspect of Cancer*, edited by J. Cohen et al. Raven Press, New York.
7. Ledure, G., Souris, M., and Bernheim, J. L. (1983): Le cancéreux devant sa maladie: Comparaison entre l'appréciation d'un médecin oncologue et d'un groupe de ses patients. *Psychol. Med.*, 15:1629–1630.
8. Levenson, P. (1982): Information preferences of cancer patients aged 11–20 years. *J. Adolesc. Health Care*, 3:9–13.
9. Lipowski, Z. (1971): L'individu face à la maladie physique. *Rev. Med. Psychosom.*, 13:235–249.
10. Mulhern, R., Christo, J., and Camitta, B. (1981): Patterns of communication among pediatric patients with leukemia, parents, and physicians; prognostic disagreements and misunderstandings. *J. Pediatr.*, 99:480–483.

11. Pfefferbaum, B., and Levenson, P. (1982): Adolescent cancer patient and physician responses to a questionnaire on patient concerns. *Am. J. Psychiatry,* 139:348–351.
12. Razavi, D., Berger, N., Frisch, S., and Souris, M. (1982): Les médecins spécialistes hospitaliers et le mourant: Une étude comparative. *Psychol. Med.,* 14:895–902.
13. Ringler, K. (1983): *Coping with Chemotherapy.* Umi Research Press, Ann Arbor, Michigan.
14. Slavin, L., O'Malley, J., Koocher, G., and Foster, D. (1982): Communication of the cancer diagnosis to pediatric patients: Impact on long-term adjustment. *Am. J. Psychiatry,* 139:179–183.
15. Spinetta, F. (1982): A guide to psychosocial field research in cancer. In: *Psychosocial Aspect of Cancer,* edited by J. Cohen et al. Raven Press, New York.
16. Weisman, A. D. (1979): A model for psychosocial phasing in cancer. *Gen. Hosp. Psychiatry,* 187–195.

Subject Index